The Origin of the World

The Origin of the World

Science and Fiction of the Vagina

Jelto Drenth

Translated by Arnold and Erica Pomerans

REAKTION BOOKS

Published by Reaktion Books Ltd
79 Farringdon Road
London EC1M 3JU, UK

www.reaktionbooks.co.uk

First published in English 2005
English translation copyright © Reaktion Books 2005

This publication has been made possible with financial support from the
Foundation for the Production and Translation of Dutch Literature.

First published in Dutch by Uitgeverij De Arbeiderspers as
De Oorsprong van de Wereld by Jelto Drenth
Copyright © 2001 Jelto Drenth

Printed and bound in Great Britain
by Cromwell Press, Trowbridge, Wiltshire

British Library Cataloguing in Publication Data

Drenth, Jelto
    The origin of the world : science and fiction of the vagina
    1.Vagina 2.Women – sexual behavior – History
    3.Sex customs in literature
    I.Title
    306.7'082'09

ISBN 1 86189 210 1

Contents

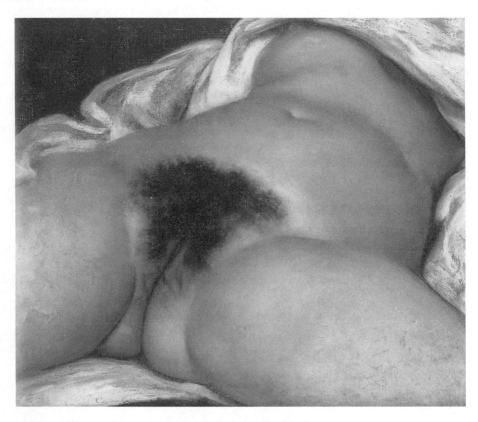

1 Gustave Courbet, *The Origin Of The World*, 1866, oil on canvas.

chapter one

On Femininity

What do you do when a publisher asks you if you are interested in writing a book about the female sex organs? The first problem, of course, is, do I have enough to say on the subject? And this leads directly to doubts about whether it is fitting for a male author to do the job. Wouldn't that be almost sacrilegious?

What motives can a man possibly have for 'getting to know everything there is to know about the female genitals?' And, not without significance: what motives are others likely to impute to him? Before you know what is happening, you have painted yourself into a raunchy corner. When I was fourteen or fifteen a precocious friend of mine – rather aptly called Willy – gave me a Christmas present, a paperback entitled *How to Stay the Night*, and although that book has long since gone astray, some of its instructions are still clearly imprinted on my mind. The intellectually puffed up dialogue went something like this: 'Of course, Eloïse' – the book had been translated from the French – 'you are right to assert that the sexual ecstasy of the female goes so much deeper, since her anatomy means that she has to open herself up so much more, with consequently far more fear to overcome but also so much more to gain, whereas the lust of the male, who hazards no more than his outer sexual organs, reflects a certain detachment, perhaps even hostility . . . '. And so on, with the author guaranteeing that well-chosen potential partners would fall like so many ripe apples into the lap of the amateur psychoanalyst spouting such psychobabble.

Western culture is replete with a wealth of images fostering the illusion that women are sexually dependent on the talents of men. Anyone reading the works of such once famous lovers as Casanova and Frank Harris is made somewhat queasy by their conceit and their casual assumption that the ladies they seduced would never have had such ecstatic experiences had they not had the good fortune of meeting the writer. Sleeping Beauty sleeps on, unable to rouse herself. For that she assuredly needs a prince.

That prince charges firmly for his educational mission. Life-long gratitude and unrestricted sexual access is the least of what he considers his due. It was not until recently that Dutch legislators introduced a change in the moral code by recognizing that rape may also take place in marriage (and constitutes a punishable offence). The old law was based on the premise that a married woman may not deny her husband sexual satisfaction, which was how the legislators once purposely put it. That too is deeply rooted in our culture. Children in some countries still sing a nursery rhyme whose subject, if we read between the lines, is premature ejaculation, the most common sexual problem that men struggle with. Rightly so. The man who cannot control his ejaculation fails in his duty towards women, thus forfeiting his conjugal rights. These rights are important, since cockiness and acquisitiveness play important roles in the encounter of the sexes. More vulnerable emotions hide beneath them. Deep down, men are convinced that female sexuality is far more exalted and transcendent than their own. Through female sexuality, man enters a paradise to which he would not gain admittance alone.

This opinion is far from new. In Ovid's *Metamorphoses* we are told how Hera, in a querulous mood about her husband Zeus' repeated acts of adultery, is put in her place by him – after all, women gain so much more pleasure from the act of love than men. When Hera makes bold to doubt this judgement, they seek the advice of Teiresias, who, following an unfortunate confrontation with two coupling snakes, had been a woman for seven years before being allowed to return to the sex in which he was born. Teiresias confirms Zeus's opinion. If sexual pleasure could be awarded ten marks, then a woman would receive three times three and the man just one. Hera is a bad loser and strikes Teiresias blind. Zeus makes it up to him by bestowing upon him the gift of unerring prophecy for which Teiresias is famed in mythology. It was Teiresias who revealed to Oedipus that he had murdered his father and bedded his mother.

In the Middle Ages, Gerard of Salo took a scientific interest in the question of how this greater sexual enjoyment of women could be explained. He gave four reasons: first, they receive the male seed; second, they release their own seed; third, they can sense the movement of the uterus during coitus; fourth, the friction of the male member causes them *pruritum et titilationem*. Small wonder that some women finish up in a never-ending circle of sexual pleasure.

And that is why the more intercourse women have they more of it they crave, inasmuch as choleric and saline vapours collect round the cervix, which explains why it is that the more intercourse women have the more prurient they become.[1]

When I began work on this book, I realized that this project was an excellent opportunity to pay close attention, for once, to the variability of human sexual behaviour. Sexologists often choose their speciality because of their interest in the wealth of the sexual field. The stories of the people who confide their problems to us never fail to lead to an enrichment of our knowledge about this particular area. It is remarkable that so many of our clients have difficulty in accepting the wide gamut of sexual experience. The crux of their problem often lies in the pursuit of some sort of sexual norm that fails to provide the satisfaction they seek. Most sexology clients want first and foremost to be normal.

While I was writing the book, a second theme emerged, namely the astonishing confusion caused by the fact that there are two sexes. History and anthropology in particular afford us glimpses of a universal desire to endow the differences between the sexes with meaning and to build bridges between them. In this, the genitals prove to be powerful sources of emotion. Hence it was inevitable that this book should have turned into a rich miscellany of bizarre facts.

chapter two

Searching for Words

Whenever I have my period (and that's only been three times), I have the feeling that in spite of all the pain, discomfort and mess, I'm carrying around a sweet secret. So even though it's a nuisance, in a certain way I'm always looking forward to the time when I'll feel that secret inside me once again.[1]

When people write or talk about female genitals and female sexuality, they generally stress that they are about to enter a sphere about which we know very little and one that is covered with a veil of secrecy. Shame and fear are rarely far away. The word 'pudenda', from the Latin for 'the shameful (parts)', reflects our feelings when we refer to these organs. In the Middle Ages, the phrase 'Women's Secret' was a generic term: every book on female health was referred to as a Woman's Secret, much as Baedeker is a collective term for travel books. In a 'Woman's Secret', the reader was likely to find various tips on health, and usually beauty hints as well.[2]

Sigmund Freud, too, was deeply conscious of the hopeless feeling that female sexuality always caused him. This was a territory he found hard to reconcile with his general views; he called it a dark continent. Classically educated readers will know that Pandora's box was a source of evil and disease. Is it pure chance that the word 'box' is a slang term for the vagina? This double meaning can also be found in Dutch, German and French (*doos, Büchse, boîte*).

Leonardo da Vinci took an intense interest in human anatomy, being one of the first to do so. He considered the sexual organs of men and women so repulsive that he believed mankind would long since have become extinct had not the rest of the body been so beautiful and the sexual urge so indomitable.[3] Leonardo made many studies of corpses, which may perhaps explain part of his revulsion. In this, he drew no sexual distinctions, and that redounds to his credit. Many artists have demonstrated that they found the male genitals well worth the trouble of detailed representation, but not the female organs. The knowledge women and girls themselves have of their genital organs is often equally slight. Here the Creator clearly went wrong, since without a mirror a woman cannot gain any real understanding of her parts (and even then she needs good eyes). Well over 20 years ago the New York psychotherapist Lucille Bloom asked 68 women, picked from the waiting room of a general practitioner, to draw their genitals (inside and out).[4] More than half 'forgot' the clitoris, and the younger subjects proved to be even more ignorant about it than the older.

A digression: *the clitoris*

> Above the nymphae lies the *clitoris*, being a round and slightly elongated body . . . It has two hollow bodies, a small apron string, various vessels, two erectile muscles, a foreskin and a small glans, whence its name of 'woman's rod'. This part, endowed with a tender feeling, is a woman's chief seat of pleasure during love-making, which has earned it the name of *oestrum Veneris*, or the Venus gadfly. The clitoris is generally quite small: it starts to appear in our daughters as they become nubile, and grows as they advance in age and gain a more or less amorous disposition. The least voluptuous stimulation causes it to swell, by means of the hollow bodies; and during the union of the sexes it attains a stiffness similar to that of the part distinguishing a man.[5]

The clitoris merits our special attention. In the Middle Ages it was rarely referred to in writing, simply because an organ whose sole purpose is the satisfaction of female lust was unmentionable by definition. Such lust was taboo. Since all things at the time were described by their function and purpose, Henri de Mondeville, in the early fourteenth century, postulated a more acceptable function for the clitoris.[6] He described it as the extremity of the urethra, and compared it with the uvula. What does the uvula do? At the time it was believed that it changed something in the air we breathe in and mediaeval physiologists also spoke of vaginal air currents, hence the repeated stories about fertilization by air.[7] If the clitoris played a part in reproduction, then the organ would no longer be taboo.

The comparison of the clitoris to the uvula has fascinating features. In this book we shall be dwelling in detail on the ritual removal of the clitoris (clitoridectomy) in childhood, and it is a striking fact that in a number of African countries the uvula, too, is often removed. The motive is preventative: the uvula is thought to pose a grave risk of suffocation during throat infections. In Ethiopia, the uvula of nearly all children is removed by traditional healers in the first months of life, which naturally leads to numerous medical complications.[8]

In 1997, the Argentinean writer Federico Andehazi published his novel *The Anatomist*, a book based in part on a historical figure: it describes the life of the Venetian anatomist Mateo Columbo, and how he discovered 'his America', the clitoris. That Colombo came up with a scientific description of the clitoris in 1559 and, what is more, far more realistically and reliably than any of his predecessors, is a historical fact. He even used to brag about it at great length, eliciting somewhat caustic comments from some of his younger contemporaries. In the novel, the reaction of the Inquisition to this faith-sapping discovery was the central theme of the whole drama. A hilarious parallel happened in real life: the author was awarded the foremost Argentinean literary prize for his book, but the woman whose name the prize bore refused to meet him. His prize money was sent to him by giro. Some secrets are firmly guarded even today.

In his own time, large sections of the population did not welcome Colombo's discovery. The sixteenth century witnessed witch hunts conducted with fanatical zeal and, according to the authors of the popular *Malleus Maleficarum* (Hammer of Witches), the witch's nipple was one of the main stigmata by which a witch could be identified.[9] Now, the nipple from which the devil fed his blood lust was found in the woman's secret parts. It seems more than likely that the clitoris was often taken for the witch's nipple. Thompson quotes an eye-witness account of an execution in 1593:

> After the execution was ended . . . and three persons were thoroughly
> dead, the jailer stripped off their clothes and, being naked, he found
> upon the woman Alice Samuel a little lump of flesh, in manner sticking
> out as if it had been a teat to the length of half an inch; which both he
> and his wife perceiving, at the first sight thereof meant not to disclose
> because it was adjoining to so secret a place which was not decent to
> be seen. Yet in the end, not willing to conceal so strange a matter, and
> decently covering that privy place a little above which it grew, they made
> open show thereof.

Did anyone in the audience really realize that the organ that so upset the jailer was a normal asset of every woman?

Pretty and ugly words

The mystery surrounding the female sex is also reflected in a dearth of appropriate words. In this book, I have tried to be sparing in the use of the word 'cunt', except where there is really no fitting alternative. 'Vagina' is very handy in conversations between doctor and patient (less so in lovers' talk), but the word is generally used as a synecdoche. The external part of the genitals is referred to as the 'vulva' in medical parlance. When women have complaints in this region, however, they do not generally use that word, though it is more common in English than, for instance, Dutch. Another way of referring to this region is as the 'labia', although further confusion arises from the fact that many women fail to distinguish the labia majora from the labia minora, referring to them jointly as 'my private parts'. Moreover, some women think their labia minora are their labia majora, certainly considering them the larger. For that reason, it has been suggested that the names be changed to inner and outer lips. Sex reformers often take exception to the use of the term 'pudenda', because they believe it reinforces a prevailing taboo and that female sexuality is, partly through this usage, condemned to permanent contempt. More flattering alternatives such as 'pleasure lips' have never taken hold, and few people will be sorry about that.

Traditionally, euphemisms have been common, for instance with parents anxious to teach their daughters the essentials of hygiene. 'Down there', is not very educational; with 'front bottom' and 'back bottom' some differentiation can at least be introduced. Not many parents make 'clitoris' part of their educational programme, with the result that daughters are sent into the sexual arena less well prepared than sons. Children certainly pass on scraps of information among themselves. The writer Lydia Rood tells us how, in her thinly walled home, she followed word for word as the girl next door showed Rood's daughter 'exactly where she had to fiddle about to get a nice feeling. I thought, good, I won't have to explain that to her myself.'[10] But the acoustics in most family homes are different, so that few parents have an excuse for not tackling this task themselves.

Nor do I really know how many women use special words, to themselves or to their lovers, for these particular regions. If your head itches, you say 'my head itches', but what does the woman think or say when she has an itch in her pubic hair? Isn't it taboo for many women to refer to it directly? Overcoming taboos leads to tension, and that tension may have a positive effect. For boys, scrawling dirty words on hoardings and lavatory doors is an erotic act. Crude, but effective. Adult males will sometimes use lewd words at intimate moments to increase and direct their sexual excitement. What do women do? I have done a little sounding out and have come to the conclusion that quite a lot of women use euphemistic expressions even in intimate relationships.

In D. H. Lawrence's *Lady Chatterley's Lover*, Mellors, the game-keeper, teaches Lady Chatterley the meaning of the word 'cunt', and what it stands for in his universe. Lady Chatterley acquires not only new feelings but also the words to express them. Lawrence wanted to use the book to send an unwelcome message to the world at large, and as well as a very small private edition, his book went through countless pirated print runs in the United States and in Europe. The British publishers, however, kept insisting on an expurgated version, which was why the author published his own edition in Paris in 1930. It was not until 1960 that Penguin produced an unexpurgated edition in England.

'Th'art good cunt, aren't ter? Best bit o' cunt left on earth. When ter likes! When th'art willin!'
'What is cunt?' she said.
'An' doesn't ter know? Cunt! It's thee down theer; an' what I get when I'm i'side thee, and what tha gets when I'm i'side thee; it's a' as it is, all on't.'
'All on't,' she teased. 'Cunt! It's like fuck then.'
'Nay nay! Fuck's only what you do. Animals fuck. But cunt's a lot more than that. It's thee, dost see: an' tha'rt a lot besides an animal, aren't ter? – even ter fuck? Cunt! Eh, that's the beauty o' thee, lass!'

That the salient terms have remained taboo is possibly due to their use as terms of abuse. The female genitals, no less than the male, are used to that end. To my mind, the female swearwords are somewhat coarser than the male. 'Don't be such a prick' is less abrasive than 'what a cunt you are'. In countries where clitoridectomy is a tradi-tional practice, the word for clitoris is part of the foulest oaths. Muslim fundamentalists in Egypt use 'mother of clitoris' as a swear-word for white tourists, and the worst insult you can fling at a man is 'son of an uncircumcised mother'.

Japan is an exception. Here parents enlighten their daughters about their *odaiji-no-tokoro*, their 'august important place'. Boys are told about their *odaiji-no-mono*, their 'august important thing'. For boys there is also a time-honoured synonym: the *ochinchin* ('honourable tinkle-tinkle'). In the 1980s Japanese feminists protested against this unequal treatment, and advocated the introduction of the term *wareme-chan* ('dear little slit'). Like so many emancipatory linguistic innovations, this term never became established.[11]

Naturally there are numerous synonyms for the female genitals, some of them highly individual. Clients sometimes tell me what terms they use in bed, and these are often first names (Joseph and Josephine is a pair I remember). In Paul Rodenko's adaptation of *The Thousand and One Nights*, a poetess challenges her lover 'to render with discretion and stylish grace what by its defenceless openness arouses your chivalrous desire to write verse' (in Dutch, the verb *dichten* has a double meaning – to write poetry as well as to fill, hence the pun). The lover comes back with such clichés as 'garden of pleasure', 'gateway of happiness' and 'hidden bower', but our critical poetess pours scorn on all of these. The short list of metaphors she herself prefers comprises 'the infant's cradle', 'the bird without feathers', 'the cat without whiskers', 'the rabbit without ears', 'the enchanted slipper', 'the cage without bars' and 'the wordless tongue'.

While Rodenko creeps into a woman's skin to come up with flowery expressions, Erica Jong gets a man to make her heroine, Fanny, recently initiated in every mortal sin, confront all the things with which her name is synonymous.[12] Lancelot, the bandit chief who would sooner mount a boy or a sheep than our hapless Fanny, knows his classics as well as the common vocabulary. Here a selection will have to suffice, for the list covers more than a page: 'the divine monosyllable', 'the best-worst part' (according to John Donne), 'the confessional', 'the third eye' (according to Chaucer), 'the marbled piece', 'box', 'bagpipe', 'fortress', 'fountain of love', 'sheath', 'bullfinch's nest', 'house at the bottom of the hill', 'the cream jug', 'the queen of hollows', 'the toothless mouth', 'the nameless nest'. 'Peach', 'rose', 'broad bean', 'fig' and 'passion flower' come from the herbal. Fanny listens in amazement. 'In me the poet is celebrated, even though the woman is insulted.'

At the beginning of the sixteenth century, there was a brief courtly tradition of exalting all the parts of the female anatomy in so-called *Blasons*.[13] From head to toe, in broad outline and minute detail, the praises of woman were sung, and not only her body parts, but also her voice, her mind, her virtue and her grace. The organ about which it all revolved was referred to as '. . .' (*con*) in the *Livre des blazons du corps féminin*, and was the only organ to be extolled in three blazons, including one on the '. . .' of a maiden. The last, written by Claude Chappuys, the king's librarian, contains the following verses:

... not yet ... , still a childish groove,
... my delight, my gentle garden,
Where no one has planted his tree or stock
... bonny ... with your vermilion mouth,
... my darling, my tiny dell
with your soft, shapely mounts
... adorned in high season
with a rich fleece of golden hair

All we do, utter or crave
all we wish, promise or aver
is to crown thee ... with honour
so that all may kneel and worship.

And I am content to tarry here,
close to you, ... to serve you
as the one who brings me the greatest comfort.[14]

Such paeans have been sung throughout the ages. Federico Fellini made a film about the life of Giacomo Casanova, and asked the poet Tonino Guerra, who had previously written the film script of *Amarcord* for a contribution. The poetic text unfortunately failed to get into the film, but Guerra had planned to put the following eulogy on 'the fig' into Casanova's mouth. The reader must bear in mind that Italians have always looked upon the fig as an exceptionally juicy fruit, juicier even than the plum. In northern Europe it made its debut in the dried form. Anyone looking at dried figs in their elongated cartons will be reminded of the scrotum of an old man rather than of an erotic female part.

The fig is a spider's web
a funnel of silk
the heart of all flowers
the fig is a door that takes you I know not where
a fortress for you to break down.

There are merry figs
figs that are utterly mad
figs wide and narrow,
figs for a couple of pence
figs voluble or stuttering
figs that yawn

or say nothing
even when you demolish them.
The fig is a white sugar mountain
a forest with prowling wolves,
it is a carriage drawn by fine horses;
the fig is a balloon of black air filled with fireflies;
an all-consuming oven.

When the time comes the fig is
The face of God,
his mouth.

It is from the fig that the world
has sprung, with the trees, the clouds, the sea
and the people, one by one,
and of all races.
From the fig, the fig, too, came forth.
Long live the fig!

Even more lyrical, and written from the feminine perspective, are the evocations in Monique Wittig's *Women Guerrillas*.[15] Here the heroic struggle of a primitive female horde to brave the threats of the other sex is described in a haunting poetic style.

Referring to the feminine parts, they say, for example, that they have forgotten the meaning of one of the ritual jokes. They mean the sentence, 'Towards nightfall, the bird Venus takes wing.' It is written that the lips of the vulva may be compared to the wings of a bird, which is why they are called the bird Venus. The vulva has been likened to all sorts of birds, for instance the dove, the starling, the weaverbird, the nightingale, the finch and the swallow. They say that they have dug up an old text in which the author compares the vulva to a swallow and adds that he knows no bird that can fly so well, and on such swift wings. However, towards nightfall the bird Venus takes wing; they say that they no longer know what that means.

I was curious to find out what terms lesbians use, and to that end I consulted a lesbian dictionary.[16] It seems to concentrate on a rather provocative use of language, and contains such terms as 'little pleasure', 'little box', 'bib', 'source of life', 'between-the-legs', 'woman's own', 'pussy', 'dusky down', 'juicy armpit', 'suction cup', 'joy lips', 'pleasure lips', 'Venus lips', 'mud flap', 'flood barrier', 'flower', 'daisy', 'little spot', 'stiff head', 'love button', 'tickle button', 'pearl', 'little mound', 'Shakespeare', 'Times Square', 'clit', 'clissy', 'joy groove', 'love groove', 'rosette' and 'little back door'.

This list seems to take us back to the 1960s, when feminist fervour caused women to coin their own words about female sexuality (if only to distance themselves from male-dominated sexual liberation ideology, which for women implied availability). It was also at this time that the term 'cunt power' emerged. We remember Germaine Greer, who argued so passionately in the Dutch underground journal *Suck* [17] in favour of 'regaining the power of cunt':

CUNT IS BEAUTIFUL
Suck it and see. If you're not so supple that you can suck your own fanny, put your finger gently in, withdraw and smell, and suck.

There. How odd it is that the most expensive gourmet foods taste like cunt. Or is it?

Squat over a mirror or lie on your back with your legs apart and the sun shining in, with a mirror. Learn it. Study its expressions. Keep it soft, warm, clean. Don't rub soap on it. Don't dredge it with talc. If you must douche it, do it with coolish water. Give it your own loving names, not the fictions of anatomy books, or the condescending diminutives that men use, like pussy, twat, box or the epithets of hate, like gash, slit, crack. What we need is a genuinely descriptive terminology of cunt.

WHY NOT SEND US A PHOTOGRAPH OF YOUR OWN CUNT, WITH YOUR NAME LABELED ON? If you can't get a photograph printed, send us the film, and your labels marked on a drawing and we'll do the rest. The results will be published.

If all else fails bring it to us and we'll kiss it for you.

In the end, Germaine Greer was the only one to have a close-up of her cunt printed in *Suck*, and not much later she left the editorial board, because the Amsterdam hippies thought the world of her message as long as they did not have to heed it.

It was inevitable that women should have gone their separate ways in order to come to know their own sexuality, no longer tainted with old stereotypes. In discussion groups, familiarity with one's own genitals was an important issue, and sometimes took the form of a group happening. The 'cunt film' of one of the 'consciousness-raising groups' has come down to us. Since the shared conquest of shame was so liberating, it had to be documented. The American sex therapist Betty Dodson went one step further in challenging the taboo on female sexuality when she encouraged members of her in-depth orgasm study groups to engage in collective masturbation. There is a video documentary, called *Selfloving*, about this group, and there are other instructive videos on the market, including one on finding your own G-spot.[18] A Dutch prostitute held several workshops at this time entitled 'In search of the whore within you'. In the United States, Annie Sprinkle caused a furore with shows in which she granted her audience deeper insight into their femininity with the help of a speculum and a pocket torch.

Much hard work was done to break down the old taboos, but whether or not large groups took the message on is difficult to judge. Sometimes the ban on calling a spade a spade evoked a special emotion, as in the poem by the Dutch poet and ship's surgeon J. Slauerhoff:

> Three butterflies flutter, side by side,
> In mid-ocean, forever banished from land,
> Three tender creatures on a raging sea.
> One might pass; if need be even two: lovers eloped –
> But three! What does destiny hold in its hand?
>
> Yet, I too am oft enthralled
> By three tender joys entwined,
> When normally no more than one
> Can pierce our grey existence?
> Then, far from the land in which I daily live,
> Her tiny mouth and two most gentle eyes
> Join in the smile so full of promise,
> And I founder and grow as wide as the sea,
> At first so small, and swelling to infinity
> Her love wafts over me until I leap up
> To own the other trinity, to make
> Her breasts heave, her body trembles
> From the spot I shall not name,
> Because it lies so deep, it is known only to me
> And I guard it as fiercely as the sea its secrets holds.[19]

chapter three

The Anatomy of the Female Genitals: The Facts

The internal organs . . . constitute a complicated system involving many different forms of storage and transport. The size of the elements varies from that of the spermatozoon (diameter of the head 3 micromillimeters), to that of a full-term foetus (3,500 cm³). Not only the size, but also the direction and speed of transit and the length of the stay, vary considerably. Thus the spermatozoa pass through the system with considerable speed, thanks to their own motility, but in view of the interval between ejaculation and fertilization (ca. seventy minutes), transport mechanisms in the system also come into play. The oöcyte (egg cell), by contrast, has a very low transit speed and remains in the Fallopian tube for several days before being transported to the uterus. Accumulation of blood and tissue in the cavum uteri (uterine cavity) over a longer period is undesirable, but the developing foetus must remain there for nine months and grow to a volume of approximately 3,500 cm³.[1]

These lines come from the first paragraph of an authoritative textbook on gynaecological diseases and reproduction. There may be some readers who will fear that by 'knowing too much' about such emotionally charged subjects as the secret parts of women some of the mystery of passion and love will be lost. It is for these readers that the above quotation from the anatomist B. Hillen is meant. However deeply he became immersed in the Women's Secret, his admiration did not grow any the less. The more we know, the greater our wonder.

We shall look at the different areas of the external female genitals with the help of an illustration from a classic and exceptionally well-drawn anatomical handbook, R. L. Dickinson's *Human Sex Anatomy*, published in 1949. The mons veneris and the labia majora are cutaneous regions characterized by a growth of tough, pigmented hair. Another characteristic is the somewhat dome-shaped curvature caused by a slightly thicker subcutaneous layer of fat. The labia minora can

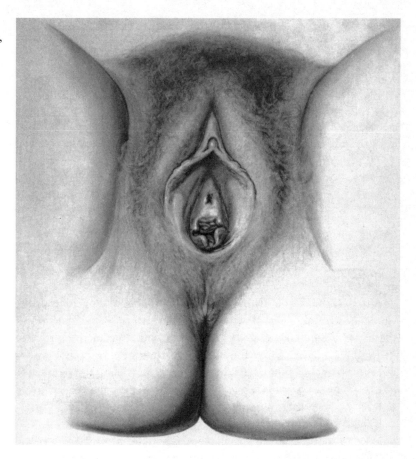

vary considerably in shape and size. In general, the margins are slightly
more pigmented than normal. Between the labia majora and the labia
minora lies a fold of skin whose depth varies markedly. The inner sides
of the inner lips form a transitional region. The skin at the outside
(keratinized, so with a dry surface) gradually makes way for mucous
membrane: smoother, moister, thinner and hence more vulnerable. It
may be compared to the mouth: going from the outside to the inside,
you can feel skin, the red covering of the lips, and the moist inner side
of the cheek. In medical literature the inner side of the labia minora is
referred to as the introitus; in older texts we sometimes find the term
'vestibule' or 'forecourt'.

   At the front, the labia minora merge into the prepuce of the clitoris.
The difference between it and the prepuce of the penis is that the glans
of the penis is fully enclosed in it while the glans of the clitoris is left
uncovered on the downward side. This area, however, curves down-
wards towards the opening of the vagina and between the labia. The

glans of the clitoris is in principle always hidden (unlike its representation in the drawing, which shows an introitus held open). Because in women, too, smegma (a whitish secretion) is formed between the glans and the prepuce, adult women should ensure that they uncover the clitoris when washing. In most women, you will find a thin fold in the mucous membrane underneath either side of the clitoris, which runs back into the labia minora (this fold resembles what is called the frenulum in men: the connection between the prepuce and the underside of the glans). The relationship between the various parts is so variable that when the labia move, the clitoris of some women moves too while in others it stays put.

If the labia minora are spread out, a small triangular area appears under the clitoris, in which the external urethral orifice can be observed. Beside that orifice two small openings can sometimes be seen, which are those of the excretory ducts of two glands. They are known as Skene's glands, named after the physician who first described them. Further back (at the bottom in our drawing), lies the opening of the vagina, surrounded by an irregularly shaped area: the remains of the hymen, popularly called the maidenhead. That name ought to be expunged, because it wrongly suggests that it is easy to tell virgins from non-virgins. On the basis of this simplistic assumption a number of extremely sexist rituals have been preserved; we shall be referring to them at some length in a later section of this book.

There are considerable variations in the appearance of the introitus (and hence not merely of the hymen). The effects of age, hormonal maturity, sexual activity and possible confinements all leave their mark. From the drawing, for instance, it can be inferred that this woman has borne a child. The hymenal ring is badly frayed at the rear on either side, a characteristic found in women who have had a child.

The internal organs are delineated above. The vagina lies behind the hymen. Its first section is enveloped by the solid muscular layers of the pelvic floor that enable a woman to constrict her vagina with some force. A few centimetres deeper, the vagina is surrounded by other pelvic organs, all of which have a more or less fixed place in the abdomen, yet share the space quite freely. As a result the vagina, which at rest is no more than a collapsed cavity, can expand quickly during sexual activity (when air is sucked in) and the uterus, too, can move slightly upwards, forwards or backwards, to the left or to the right.

The wall of the vagina is a mucous membrane with a number of folds or ridges (vaginal rugae). Deep inside, but generally not at the very top, the uterus opens into the anterior wall of the vagina. The uterus is

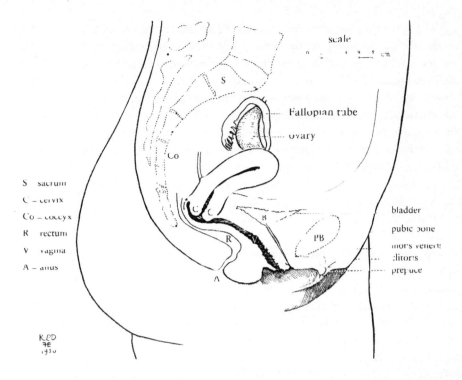

scale

Fallopian tube

ovary

S

Co

bladder

pubic bone

C C

B

R

PB

mons veneris

clitoris

prepuce

A

S   sacrum
C – cervix
Co – coccyx
R   rectum
V   vagina
A – anus

KED
7E
1930

3 Female pelvis
and contents.

a hollow muscle shaped like a somewhat flattened pear. The muscle fibres in the uterine wall are arranged in such a way that upon contraction (during menstruation and also of course during childbirth) the contents of the uterus are pushed out. The inner lining of the uterus is a mucous membrane with very special properties. The most significant task of the womb is reflected in the term uterus (derived from the Latin for the cavities of the earth from which the first creatures were said to have been born): in this mucous membrane a fertilized egg cell can nidate and grow until the moment that the child is able to live independently outside its mother. Menstruation is a reaction by this mucous membrane to changes in the hormone levels in the blood. These hormones are produced in the ovaries, where the cycle of changes is controlled by a biological clock in the brain, and the pituitary body, a gland at the base of the brain.

The outside of the uterus is lined with a serous coat derived from the peritoneum, as are all organs in the intestinal cavity. The peritoneum is smooth and moist, thus enabling all intestinal organs to move with respect to one another. That is not only essential for sex and reproduction, but also for the digestion of food. If adhesions occur after an operation or after appendicitis, the result is pain and functional impairment.

The two Fallopian tubes open into the upper side of the uterus, one on the left and the other on the right. Their shape is somewhat like a trumpet, which is what they are called in Latin (*tuba*). On either side of the opening lies an ovary, a small oval organ attached loosely to the abdominal wall by a stalk. Here every month an egg cell is brought to maturity during a woman's fertile years (provided she is not on the pill). At the moment of ovulation the egg cell is liberated and, fertilized or not, received by the Fallopian tube. The ovaries are also involved in the production of female sex hormones.

Embryology

At this point a detour into the field of embryology is necessary. This branch of science studies the development of embryos in the uterus, and, in particular, examines how the formation of organs is organized and controlled. It is in respect of the reproductive organs that the story becomes particularly fascinating, because male and female genital organs have a common origin. No matter how much the adult organs may differ, there are unexpected similarities between them. Doctors can take advantage of this fact: if they lack information about certain details in one sex, they can sometimes make use of what they know about the other sex. Sexologists know far more about men than they do about women – for instance how the erection is negatively affected by certain diseases or drugs. With some reservations, findings in the field of male sexuality can be used to predict how the female genital organs will react to certain factors.

Until the sixth week no sexual differences can be detected in the developing embryo, but thereafter the paths of the two sexes begin to diverge. Up to that point, the genital area seems most like that of the final state of affairs in the female: there is a genital opening and a swelling above it, roughly where the clitoris will eventually be found. Without hormone stimulation every embryo would develop into a body with female reproductive organs; however, when testosterone (the male sex hormone) comes into play, development in the male-genital direction ensues. Thus Eve did not spring from Adam's rib; every Adam was once an Eve. For quite a few woman theologians this is an important article of faith. In some diseases, female embryos too produce testosterone variants, and then develop along the path normally reserved for boys.

When testosterone does its work at the right moment, the swelling grows vigorously into an elongated organ, and the tissue surrounding the opening gives rise to a tubular structure towards the tip of the elongated organ. This is the urethra, which is surrounded by a separate spongy body (the corpus spongiosum) terminating in the glans. The slightly swollen sides of the genital opening become more substantial, growing together to form the scrotum. A small seam always remains visible along the middle line. The sex glands of both sexes are formed in the abdominal cavity, near the kidneys, but in the male foetus the testicles migrate through the groin into the scrotum. The canal facilitating that migration remains slightly patent, which is why hernias are so much more common in boys than they are in girls.

It is generally known that the testicles of boys descend quite a long way, and many people will have heard of some relative who has had to be treated for undescended testicles. Less well known is the fact that the ovaries, too, descend in the embryonic period, and that women too can have problems with undescended reproductive glands.[2] In such a case the ovary will be much too far from the uterus, the Fallopian tubes often incomplete and in any case not optimally patent. If both ovaries fail to descend, infertility results.

In sum, it is generally assumed that the following pairs of organs have a common descent:

ovary	testicle
labia majora	scrotum
clitoris	glans penis
labia minora	underside of penis, with urethra and surrounding layer of muscles

Here a caveat is needed: this analogy has been the subject of vigorous discussion for the past ten years, boosted by the American psychologist Josephine Lowndes Sevely.[3] She objects to such oversimplified comparisons and above all to the assumption that the clitoris is 'a small penis'. In her view, the clitoris, including its two crura, or 'roots', by which the organ is attached to the pelvis, is analogous to the two uppermost columns of erectile tissue of the penis (the corpora cavernosa). In other words, the tip of the clitoris is comparable to what remains of the penis when you remove the glans. She thus puts the question the other way round: where can we find the male clitoris? Her conclusion is that the male clitoris is situated directly beneath the rim of the glans penis, where the frenulum preputii (fold of the prepuce) is located. Men will know that this area has a special erotic sensitivity. Lowndes Sevely proposes that we call this area, in men and in women, 'Lowndes's crown'. In a footnote she points out that this would be the first anatomical term called after a female scientist. That is true enough; in the genital area, we have Bartholin's gland and Skene's gland; the oviduct is called the Fallopian tube, and a mature follicle is referred to as a Graafian follicle. Lowndes Sevely's aspiration is thus fully justified, but for the present it does not seem that it is being realized. The term 'Lowndes's crown' is nowhere mentioned outside her book.

Since the clitoris lacks an acorn-shaped glans, where is the region in women analogous to that? The glans clitoridis and the corpus spongiosum are the result of the growth of the small area underneath the clitoris, the small triangle with which the urethra ends in women, and the two small mucous glands. Lowndes Sevely calls this area the female glans, and postulates that it too is the seat of great sexual sensitivity.

The spotted hyena

Nature has provided one species of animal that is a striking illustration of embryological development: the spotted hyena (also known as the laughing hyena). Before birth, the females of this species are exposed to extremely large amounts of androgenous hormones, so much so that they are all born with external genital organs that are barely distinguishable from the male. A female spotted hyena thus has a penis that is nearly as large as that of the male, with a urethra that opens at the tip, where a fully developed glans can be seen. The labia majora are fused, forming what looks like a scrotum, albeit one without testicles. (Zoological textbooks usually speak of a clitoris in female spotted hyenas, but in the light of Lowndes Sevely's observations it would be more correct to call the organ a penis. An organ that has two erectile bodies on the upper side, and at the tip a fully developed corpus spongiosum with a urethra that runs up to the glans, looks quite unlike a clitoris. We will therefore not call it that.)

The penis of the female hyena thus has erections, and these have a social function.[4] On greeting each other, both males and females exhibit and sniff their respective penises, and an erection is an indispensable part of this ceremonial. It is thought that such behaviour wards off aggression, because these scavengers have strong jaws and might easily kill each other if there were no diversionary tactics during confrontations. In copulation, however, the female penis is flaccid, and the small muscles capable of pulling the phallus down are exceptionally well developed, as a result of which access to the urethral opening is kept relatively stable for copulation. This must be highly

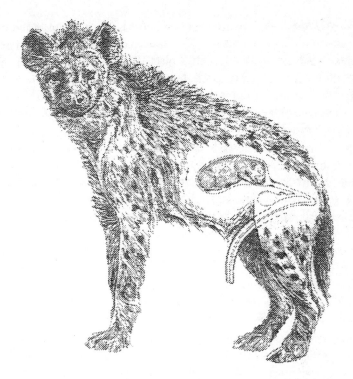

4 Spotted hyena, showing the genital organs during pregnancy.

effective since failure to conceive is relatively rare. However, the first parturition is admittedly attended by great difficulties, for the demands made on the urethra at that time are of course immense.[5] The illustration above shows that the birth canal of the female is not only twice as long as that of non-masculinized animals, but that a sharp bend has also to be negotiated during the expulsion of the foetus.[6] A special hormone called relaxin, produced in the placenta, renders connective tissue more elastic. Relaxin is present in large quantities in spotted hyenas during parturition.[7] (It is likely that relaxin plays a role in human beings as well. During childbirth a number of normally rigid joints in the pelvis become more flexible, the best known being the symphysis, a cartilaginous joint between the two pubic bones. In recent years considerable attention has been paid to the symphysis after childbirth, because women increasingly complain of after-pain in this region, where lasting instability may occur.)

In any case, when the spotted hyena gives birth, relaxin ensures that her urethra can dilate enough to allow the young to pass through, although large tears often result. Remarkably, this violent process is not apparently accompanied by exceptional pain, the female spotted hyena remaining reasonably calm. It is believed that relaxin may also have an analgesic effect on the central nervous system.

Objectively speaking, however, the first parturition is an almost impossible feat, and this is reflected in the result. Almost half of first-born cubs are stillborn or die soon after birth. Only during a second pregnancy do the young have a reasonable chance of survival.

Another painful detail is the fact that, due to the high testosterone level found in this species, the cubs are relatively heavier at birth than those of all other mammals. Pity the poor mother. At birth, the young already have a full set of teeth, including canines, and their behaviour shows signs of masculinity from the start. There is an average of two young per litter, and immediately after the birth of the second cub, the first subjects it to a furious attack.[8] A considerable percentage of second cubs is killed by the first-born or else the stronger monopolizes the mother's teats so effectively that the weaker starves to death. This is possible because the mother generally chooses an unused aardvark burrow for her 'birthing chamber', and the tunnels in it are so narrow that the mother herself is unable to get in. In order to suckle, the young must follow their mother out of their place of safety and it is easy for the stronger cub to block the exit and keep the weaker away.

Remarkably enough some twins reach adulthood all the same, but they are generally twins of a different sex. The female-female, female-male and male-male ratio ought statistically to be 1:2:1. If we include identical twins, there ought to be an even greater proportion of twins of the same sex. The conclusion is inescapable: if there are two sisters or two brothers, then one of the two is probably killed. If they are brother and sister, the chance that they will spare each other is greater. However, no twin comes away without a significant number of scars.

The spotted hyena is the only animal species that is so highly masculinized. (Animals can of course be affected by hormones from a polluted environment. In 1998, biologists discovered that female polar bears near Spitsbergen had suddenly developed small penises. In this case the assumed cause was exogenous. In the waters round Spitsbergen there is a great deal of PCB – polychlorinated byphenyl – originating in Russian factories and conveyed there by large rivers.) The question of why the hyena varies so greatly from the normal biological pattern has not been answered satisfactorily. Fratricide and sororicide also occur in some raptor species, but these species suffer from a shortage of food, so that the thinning out of the population is a functional necessity. That is not the case with spotted hyenas. 'Survival of the fittest' is an accepted principle of evolution, but why is its application to this species so extreme? Might the female hyena have tempted her partner with a fruit even more forbidden than the apple?[9]

Weak spots in the anatomy

The abdomen is a peculiar part of our anatomy. It is an enclosed area in which a number of vulnerable organs can do their work in safety, but it is also a part of our motor machinery, muscular power being tapped from this part of our body. The abdominal wall provides the necessary stability. It is a kind of football of muscles (cut into by the bony pelvis underneath) in which the pressure can vary enormously. If we watch a weight lifter, we can imagine why he supports his abdominal muscles with a leather belt. But there are also more trivial bodily acts that are accompanied by an abrupt increase in abdominal pressure. Cases in point are coughing, sneezing and emptying the bowels. For men this is a riskier process than for women because, thanks to the displacement of the sex glands through the groin, they have a natural tendency to develop inguinal hernias.

In women, too, the sex organs constitute a weak point, inasmuch as their abdominal cavity is in open connection with the outside world via the vagina, the uterus and the Fallopian tubes. Women have more abdominal infections than men. During menstruation, the cramps of the uterus are admittedly directed towards the cervix, but in most women a little blood and expelled tissue also enters the abdominal cavity through the Fallopian tubes.[10] This process is called retrograde menstruation. In general the white blood cells in the abdominal cavity can cope with a small amount of menstrual blood, but there are women in whom small collections of tissue form colonies on the peritoneum. The medical term for this is endometriosis. It occurs when there is plainly more material to be cleared up than the white blood cells can deal with, so that it is necessary for small blood vessels to grow into the colonies. The result may be an abdomen full of red spots, causing severe stomach pains in rhythm with the menstrual cycle. Endometriosis also means a high chance of problems with fertility.

Air in the abdominal cavity is another unwanted phenomenon. In patients with abdominal symptoms, an X-ray is always taken while the patient is standing up, without contrast; in this way air may be easily seen. Gases rise and in the abdomen they become visible as a thin crescent under the diaphragm and over the liver. Air in this area generally means pain radiating towards the shoulder. When a laparoscopy (an inspection of the abdominal cavity through an optical instrument) is performed on a woman, gas is deliberately introduced into the abdominal cavity, opening it up for easier inspection. The last action before withdrawing the instrument is to allow the gas to escape.

This is not always entirely successful; quite a few women complain of shoulder pain for a few days following a laparoscopy or sterilization.

Air in the abdominal cavity is easily distinguished from gas in the intestines (where gases are normally present), and in general gives considerable cause for alarm. The gas has usually originated in the intestines, thus indicating a perforation. In addition, there are gas-producing bacteria, and these are most unwelcome visitors. But air can also be introduced during orogenital sex, which can present surgeons with some extremely puzzling cases.[11] There are clearly some men who, at moments of great excitement, blow so hard into the vagina of their sexual partner that the various lines of resistance are overcome. To my knowledge this is the only example of a very unusual sexual predilection being brought to light by attentive surgeons.

Anatomy and age

This survey of the anatomy of the female reproductive organs would not be complete if it ignored changes occurring with age. When a child is born, it can sometimes be seen that the maternal hormones in the uterus have had a powerful effect. Some children, boys as well as girls, are born with swollen nipples, and sometimes a few drops of 'witches' milk' can be expressed from them. The genital organs of a girl can also make an unexpectedly robust impression. However, the effect of the maternal hormones is of short duration; for the next ten years or so there is no further growth in the genital area. All the parts are present (apart from the pubic hair), and primary school pupils can already derive a great deal of sexual pleasure from these organs, even while their reproductive functions are still in a sort of hormonal half-sleep. The onset of puberty, triggered off by changes in the biological clock, impinges on all organs.

To start with, the soft unpigmented hair with which the whole body is covered (at least in Caucasians) is suddenly joined by hair of a different sort in the armpits and in the genital area. These hairs harbour a special type of sebaceous gland in their follicles; moreover, in the anogenital region particular types of sweat glands are found whose structure somewhat resembles the mammary gland.[12] As a result, sweat from the pubic hair area has a distinctive smell from that time on. As the subcutaneous fat cells round the mons veneris and labia majora develop, the entire area becomes more curved and more elastic. The labia minora have little subcutaneous fat, but they grow because the skin does. The margins become slightly pigmented, from light to sometimes quite dark. The changes in the clitoris and prepuce are limited, but some growth can be detected in them as well. In the region between the labia, the mucous glands in the vestibule of the mucous membrane undergo some development, covering the area permanently with a thin, moist layer. Its function may be sexual, but the layer might equally well provide protection from the potential damage of the acid vaginal secretions to which this area is exposed from puberty.

This is because the vaginal wall, too, undergoes extensive development. The lining, which was smooth, becomes increasingly wrinkled (rugose) and more active in the production of fluid. Its length also increases. The vaginal contents gradually become more acid. The ideal pH value is 4.0; that measure provides protection against bacterial infections. The wall of the vagina is equal to so high a degree of acidity, but the area outside the hymen can to some extent be irritated by it. Spermatozoa, too, are vulnerable to acid: at pH 4.0 they are killed at once. If semen itself was not basic alkaline, and hence able to neutralize the acidity temporarily, reproduction would never take place. Here we are faced with clearly conflicting interests, since for a few hours following the ejaculation of sperm into the vagina a woman is exceptionally susceptible to vaginal infections.

The uterus also grows. The muscle layer becomes thicker, but the greatest change occurs in the inner lining. The reproductive function of the organ becomes more obvious: every month the thickness of the mucous membrane increases appreciably. Should a fertilized egg cell arrive, it can be captured for nidation (implantation). If that does not happen, the biological clock is reset. Hormone stimulation ceases, the entire layer is expelled and the uterus is encouraged to go into spasms, the better to get rid of the now redundant cell material. A specific type of mucous gland develops in the cervix and is at its most productive during ovulation, forming a mucus in which the spermatozoa can move to optimum effect. This cycle, too, has been handsomely depicted by Dickinson (see illus. 5).

The ovaries, finally, start their most active years. They have two functions. They transmit signals from the pituitary gland to the uterus by means of hormones, and they prepare one egg cell every month for fertilization. The egg cells have been present since well before birth, and quite a few of them die afterwards, but during the fertile years one egg cell will in principle react every month to the hormone cycle by growing and forming a surrounding follicle (secretory sac). The wall of the follicle starts to protrude from the ovary; some women feel the stretching of the wall as ovulation pain. After ovulation, the remainder

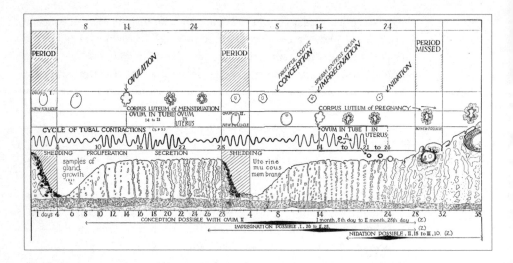

5 Ovulation, menstruation and nidation (implantation).

of the follicle produces the hormone progesterone. If the egg cell does not survive (that is, does not become fertilized or implanted), the ovary stops making progesterone and all that remains of the follicle is a minute scar.

The onset of physical maturity can vary by a few years. In the twentieth century there was clear evidence that the menarche (the first menstrual period) was appearing at an ever earlier age. Too early or too late can both – each in its own way – prove very trying and upsetting for young girls. A girl who already has pubic hair at the age of eight, when there is still perhaps mixed showering at school, can be badly affected, as can a sixteen-year-old who still has no breasts. In any case, this phase is naturally a memorable period in the life of a twelve-year-old girl; Anne Frank has given it a description with which we can easily sympathize. It is no small matter to discover that you are capable of bearing children.

The changes associated with the menopause are also universal. Its effects are largely due to the cessation of the production of female sex hormones, which means that a number of the pubertal developments mentioned above run in the opposite direction. Pubic hair does not generally diminish during this period; the continuous growth of pubic hair is controlled by the male hormone (which is produced in women to a lesser extent than in men, but nevertheless has some effect). Quite a number of women in fact start growing unwelcome hair at this time (for instance on the upper lip), which is explained by the assumption that the influence of the testosterone is no longer compensated by the oestrogen. The fat cells under the mons veneris and the labia majora reduce in volume, while the skin grows somewhat slacker. Nothing much is changed in the labia minora and the vestibule, but the mucous membrane of the vagina reverts to its pre-pubertal stage. The vagina becomes slightly shorter and the vaginal rugae disappear. If a doctor wants to give a graphic description to a patient of the changes during this phase of life, he might describe the wall of the vagina as being like velvet during the fertile years, and thereafter as like lining silk. At rest, the vagina is less moist; during optimum excitation an adequate amount of lubrication can still be produced, but if, on the basis of old routines, a quick response is expected, it will be found that the mucous membrane is more vulnerable. The acidity is lower, and hence the protective mechanism that wards off infection functions somewhat less well. The uterus becomes smaller and the mucous membrane of the inner wall shrinks to the pre-pubertal level. Last but not least, the ovaries no longer contain egg cells, and their hormone production becomes insignificant. The pituitary gland continues trying for some time to prompt the ovaries to greater activity, with the result that the control hormones of the pituitary reach improbably high levels.

Anatomy again: the personal experience

We expect biologists and anatomists to study their subject as objectively as possible – that is, unemotionally – but doctors know that their patients do not want to be treated as objects. Physicians are expected to be acquainted with the human body and the illnesses threatening it, but a doctor must also be able to share his knowledge with his patient in such a way that the latter grows wiser and more capable of looking after his or her own health. Nowadays many demands are made of the communicative skills of medical men, and fortunately attention is now paid to this matter during the various phases of medical training. That used not to be the case.

During my own medical studies (from 1963 to 1972) I was poorly prepared for my communicative duties. Communication was, of course, particularly difficult when taboo subjects were involved, and for most young medical students gynaecological examinations proved to be a source of acute embarrassment. We did not know what attitude to adopt and realized that the woman patient, too, felt far from at ease. Moreover, if we found something wrong with her, we often lacked the words to explain it to her in a way she could understand. Added to this was the fact that most women used to know very little about the biology of their reproductive organs. At the time, more so even than now, there were good reasons for doctors to enlighten their patients, certainly when it came to matters related to sex. But that was not something that students were taught.

Not long afterwards all that changed, the feminist movement playing an important role in this transformation. People spoke more openly about the emotional aspects of gynaecological examinations, a contact which many women found decidedly embarrassing, humiliating and alienating. Medical interest in abortions, too, was criticized; women, it was argued, had to be 'master of their own belly'. Stoked-up fury led to the publication of 'black books' and to other protests; in some gynaecological departments the call for change fell on fertile soil. Teaching supervisors saw to it that all housemen would be trained not only to undertake gynaecological examinations with skill, but to be aware at the same time of the emotional impact of such physical confrontations. In one hospital there was a group of women volunteers whose personal involvement made them experimental subjects and instructors combined. 'Information' became a key concept. A situation in which patients were no more than experimental subjects and were not told until later what was going to be done to them on the basis of the results was no longer in keeping with the times. It was replaced by a professional code that made high demands on communication skills – in principle even during the examination. A symbol of this development was the hand mirror placed beside the examination couch. The patient could watch the procedure if she wanted to. After all, for most women it would be a unique opportunity to look at their own cervix.

Since then, medical students have been encouraged to test their anatomical knowledge on their own body. An optional project introduced in the initial period includes a detailed written instruction for self-investigation. In sexological practice, discoveries in one's own body often leave the strongest impression. That is why, in this book on the female genital organs, woman readers are shown how to have such an experience. We shall accordingly treat the subject 'anatomy' as a manual for self-examination. If you, dear reader, happen to be a woman and are ready to take up this suggestion, the route to be followed is outlined below.

If you stand before a mirror and look at your abdomen, you will see the shape of your pubic hair. The pattern of growth in women is usually triangular; some women have a small strip of pubic hair leading towards the navel. During pregnancy, this strip sometimes darkens. Diamond-shaped pubic hair may indicate too high a level of male sex hormones in the blood. Perhaps your clitoris is visible, and perhaps the labia minora protrude a little between the labia majora. If you place your hand on the mons veneris, you can feel the pubic bone under the resilient layer of fatty tissue.

Now go and lie down, on a bed or slumped in an easy chair. With a hand mirror you will be able to see which parts of you are covered with pubic hair, something that varies considerably in women. On examining the labia you will probably notice that the edges of the labia minora are darker than the surrounding area, and often wrinkled in a particular way. Further back, the anus appears, and you will be able to see that in women, too, a small seam is visible in the midline between vagina and anus. (After childbirth it is likely that scars will be found in this region as well; cuts and ruptures are always found towards the rear.) Perhaps the clitoris has already appeared in your mirror, though generally the labia minora have first to be spread open.

If you hold the labia majora open, the labia minora and the clitoris are more easily observed. You will see that a small groove runs, on either side, between the labia majora and the labia minora (the sulcus interlabiales), and you may well spot some sebum (fatty secretion). At the bottom of the sulcus, the mucous membrane may be of a striking dark red colour, and this is because the colour of the blood shows through the very thin top layer. If you use two fingers not only to spread but also to pull the labia minora upwards, the clitoris with its prepuce and folds of mucosa below will become fully visible. This is the region Josephine Lowndes Sevely calls the crown. Direct the mirror a little further down, and if you manage to spread the labia minora more widely (for which you really need three hands) then a small triangular area – comparable to the glans penis in males – comes into view. It is generally quite obvious where the outlet of the urethra is located; the two pin-head-sized holes of the Skene's glands on either side of the urethra are probably too small to detect. On spreading the labia minora you will notice that the area between them is unpigmented again, and hence pink. In white women, the difference is not all that great, but the darker the skin the more striking the difference in colour. If you look another few centimetres further back you will find the opening of the vagina. In virgins, a circular fold (the hymen) may be seen. If you have had sexual intercourse, then this area will often look rather untidy, with a number of loose shreds round the opening. If you have had children, then often nothing of the hymen may be left towards the rear (and there may be scars from cuts and tears). Among the remains of the hymen, the opening of the vagina may be undetectable, but pressure (as during defecation) ensures that the opening comes into view.

Up to now you have been given a visual picture of your genitals. The exploration can be repeated by touch. You can feel the structure of the skin and mucous membrane with the tip of a finger, and with judicious manipulation it is possible to determine how the sensitivity in this area varies. Self-exploration enables you to focus attention on what the fingertip itself feels, and what feelings it produces in the region it touches.

When we speak about variation in sensitivity we are not just bandying words but are referring to hard facts. The skin has a number of different types of tactile corpuscle, and these are not evenly distributed in the region round the vagina.[13] The first type is attached to the root of a hair. You may know that cats partly feel their way through sensations in their whiskers. In the area covered with pubic hair, you can feel something even before the skin is touched. There are two other types of corpuscle that register touch (named after Meissner and Merkel), located near the mons veneris and the labia majora, and less densely distributed over the labia minora and the clitoris. The clitoris, for its part, has no touch sense, but the function of its Pacinian corpuscles is to register pressure. The labia minora contain relatively few corpuscles, although some of every type. The region near the hymen has the greatest concentration of the most primitive tactile organs: bare nerve endings capable of registering pain. Pain is the only tactile quality in this region! There are yet another two types of corpuscle (named after Ruffini and Dogiel-Krause), which probably register temperature fluctuations and which are believed to contribute a special sexual quality to this area's sensitivity. They are evenly distributed over the entire vulval area. Deeper inside the vaginal wall there are hardly any tactile receptors. This does not mean that a woman cannot feel anything when the inside of her vagina is touched. She feels that touch with the muscles surrounding the vagina, for muscles boast a sensory perception of their own. A muscle can feel how short or how long it is; in the muscles of our limbs this ability underlies our postural sense, enabling us to stand in equilibrium.

If you continue your tactile exploration with the mons veneris and labia majora, then the pubic hair is the seat of the first sensation. You can vary the pressure and friction of your hand. The resilience of the small layer of fatty tissue under the skin can be felt, and the pubic bone underneath. If it is a hot day, you will notice that this region perspires freely, and if you then smell your hand you will detect a specific odour. Armpits and crotch have the same type of sweat gland, but each has an odour of its own.

With your fingertip on the clitoris you can gauge the sensitivity of this small area. To touch the exposed glans you may need to use your other hand. Does touching the exposed glans feel nice, or not, and what about the prepuce? You should try to take note of that during a moment of sexual excitement as well. Does the sensitivity change, and is there any difference in the size or position of the clitoris? You can feel its shape under the prepuce. Next, run your fingertip over the edge of the labia minora, before returning to the midline. If you move your finger near the opening of the outlet of the urethra, can you feel anything there? How does the area round the (remains of the) hymen feel? If you do not yet move inside but continue a little further towards the back, you reach the place where the labia minora meet, and in most women that place forms a small recess. The mucous membrane is particularly tender in this area and quite a lot of vaginal complaints arise from this region. Further back you can feel a transverse band of muscle; it ensures firmness of the pelvic floor between the vagina and the anus. In medical textbooks this is called the fossa navicularis – the boatlike recess. If you again smell your probing fingertip, the smell will probably differ from that of the previous test. That is because this area has no sweat glands, but contains small mucous glands that keep it lubricated.

Now for the inside of the vagina. Past the hymenal region you will come to a number of muscular layers supporting the pelvic floor. If you are one of those women who find this a bit scary, your probing fingertip will probably meet stiff resistance, although the first circular muscle (sphincter) is in fact of modest calibre only. A little deeper in your fingertip will encounter two solid muscles to the right and the left, running from front to rear. These are the bulbocavernous muscles and they can play an active role in coitus. During the years of the sexual revolution much attention was paid to training programmes that aimed to increase the erotic capabilities of this muscular layer.

If your probing finger is moved back a little further as it goes deeper still, it will come upon the strongest muscle in the pelvic floor, namely the levator ani, the muscle that lifts the anus. Upon strong exertion, as when you have to resist a strong urge to defecate, you can feel the vagina becoming constricted from the rear to the front. Should you push your finger in as far as possible, you will have gone past all the muscles, and then the inside of your abdomen will feel wonderfully soft and giving. Your fingertip will easily be able to move five centimetres to the left or to the right, to the front and to the rear. In a women's therapy group at the Rutgers Foundation in Groningen, one woman who had never felt it before described the sensation as the feeling you have 'when you walk into a ballroom'.

We assume that you are in full control of your sphincters now, so that the other anatomical details can be explored freely. First, examine the wall of the vagina: if you are in your fertile years, the surface will feel velvety and rugose. After the menopause, this layer becomes much smoother and thinner. Normally, your finger will be against the front wall, but if you feel around, the wall will appear to have the same structure throughout. Press a little harder now against the front, and you come up against your pubic bone from inside. You can now feel, between thumb and forefinger, the breadth of the pubic bone, which can vary appreciably. In the midline a fleshy sausage-like structure runs across it: the urethra. Too much pressure in this region can cause an unpleasant sensation. Some women find that friction in this area during intercourse is unpleasant, and there are some who are left with an uncomfortable after-feeling, something resembling the irritation of a bladder infection. If you follow the urethra as far as possible and bend your finger, you will find yourself pressing against the bladder. If it is full, you will feel the urge to empty it there and then. Pull the finger back a little and continue pressing in the region behind the pubic bone. This is where the so-called G-spot is said to lie.

Every woman knows that the portio vaginalis uteri (that part of the cervix that extends into the vagina) can be found deep inside the vagina, but anyone trying to find her cervix for the first time by feel will not have an easy job. Women who are fitted with an intra-uterine device (IUD) are always advised to check during the first few months following the fitting that they can still feel the little strings protruding from the cervix after every menstruation. This often proves hard to do without further instruction because the cervix usually lies much further back than most women imagine. After the passage of the muscular layer, the vagina generally runs backwards in a kind of s-bend, which means that the cervix is located more at the level of the anus than that of the vaginal entrance. How can you tell for certain that you are touching the uterus? The surface of the cervix differs unmistakably from that of the walls of the vagina: it is not rugose but smooth, not soft but firm. To put it more graphically: if, in the depths of her vagina, a woman encounters something that feels like the tip of her nose, then she has come upon the cervix. Anyone expecting that the meeting of finger and uterus will also produce an internal sensation will be disappointed. The cervix has almost no tactile sense. Movement of the uterus can, however, be detected. With small pressure against the cervix it is possible to make the uterus wobble (especially by using two fingers in order to gain a better hold on the cervix), so you will have found out for yourself that this organ is able to move quite freely in the abdominal cavity. If you can take hold of it, you can easily move it a few centimetres to the right or the left.

Most women will have heard of a tilted uterus (the medical term is retroflected), and hence realize that the uterus does not apparently have one fixed position. It used to be thought that one position is right, another wrong, but this is now an outdated idea. In Europe, anteflexion (a slight forward curve) is the most common position, but in Asia retroflexion is more common. Older medical textbooks used to list a whole catalogue of symptoms allegedly caused by retroflex wombs, but of all these symptoms only a few minor complaints have survived. If a doctor discovers retroflexion during an internal examination, he can in principle try to manipulate the uterus and restore it to the most common position. This is often successful, but there is a good chance that the success will prove to be short-lived. As we have pointed out, however, this sort of treatment is no longer employed today because it serves no good purpose.

But back to the self-examination. The movement of the cervix can be felt – with the peritoneal nerves. That means that it is a very deep-down sort of feeling, an intestinal sensation so to speak. Some women find this extremely unpleasant, but others find it pleasurable during erotic excitement. The ovaries lie deep in the abdomen and generally somewhat towards the back, so that you cannot reach them yourself. During an internal examination by a physician, however, they can sometimes be reached, and the woman then feels this like a faint sickly pain. Perhaps the sensation is comparable to what a man feels when his testicles are gently squeezed.

That leaves us with the rear wall of the vagina. It is difficult to bend your finger enough to reach it. If you are really interested in feeling that area as well, your thumb is best suited for the purpose. Through the wall of the vagina you can then feel the area surrounding the rectum. Faeces may be present, in which case you will be surprised to find how clearly they can be felt. Bladder, vagina and rectum succeed one another seamlessly. If you go on feeling your way, you will be able to grip your coccyx between thumb and index finger. You might again smell your finger, and you will probably notice that the smell of the vaginal fluid differs from that found at the opening of the vagina.

For those who consider the anus a part of the genital area, another medical examination can be added, namely the recto-vaginal touch. Physicians use this when they want to probe as deeply as possible, in particular the area behind the cervix. This area is important because it is the lowest part of the abdominal cavity and if there is an infection in the abdomen then this area serves as a kind of drip-pan. Pain during a recto-vaginal examination is therefore an important signal that something is wrong in the abdomen. With the index finger in the vagina and the middle finger in the anus you can feel the solid transverse layer of muscles slide between your fingers, but then you will again be astonished to find how thin the double mucous membrane of the vaginal and intestinal walls feels to the touch. Endometriosis (see p. 29) often occurs in this region.

So much for the examination of your own body. You may find this section of the book too focused on the groin; erotic feeling is so much more than genital sensations. Nevertheless, I hope that this dwelling in detail on the variations in sensation will have given you some useful ideas. Some people cherish the conviction that sexuality is the side of life about which you should reflect least and which is all the better if you can throw yourself into it without reflection and with a partner you trust totally. But the chance of developing, knowing and cultivating your own sexuality is something that should not be ignored, and for that, information is necessary.

Sexologists meet many people whose sexual self-development has been far from automatic. In helping such people, it is often thought advisable to prescribe exercises, and in the therapeutic situation most people are more than ready to learn. In this process, they gain greater familiarity with the various sensations the body is capable of having, but also with awareness of these feelings. To take an example: it is confusing that from the hymenal region all perception is transmitted by the pain sense. A woman who is afraid of sexual penetration thus has her fears constantly reinforced. Every time she tries to get over her qualms, she finds that the pain sensations are too strong for her. Yet there are countless women who have learned without any problems that this over-sensitive feeling is readily overcome, for instance when they are eager to use tampons on a hot summer's day. Indeed, initial reluctance can give way to a pleasurable sensation if that is what you expect. What the body senses is 'elaborated' by consciousness into experience. In the best case, experiencing a physical erotic sensation influences another layer of feelings, the emotions. Making love can make you feel aroused, in love, emotional, ecstatic. Perhaps the physical sensation is not needed to reach these 'higher' emotions, but it is certainly a powerful aid. That is why developing the potential of the reproductive organs merits the effort of closer study.

chapter four

Physiology: On the (Sexual) Function of the Genital Organs

In 1966 William Masters, a gynaecologist, and Virginia Johnson, a psychologist, shocked American public opinion by the publication of their research into human sexual responses.[1] The shocking aspect of their method was that they had actually observed volunteers in the laboratory during all sorts of sexual activities. The image of a white-coated academic applying a variety of measuring devices to a sweating couple was hard to stomach for the average reader at that time. Funnily enough, not so many years later, Nancy Friday, investigating sexual fantasies in women, was told by a couple of respondents that this image had become part of the masturbation repertoire.[2] Masters and Johnson have enjoyed an unassailable reputation since that first publication, and their reputation was enhanced even further a few years later when they explained how they treated sexual problems with a brief therapeutic programme in which education and behavioural advice predominated. The effect of their research on professional sexology was immense. Up until that time sexology had been a medical speciality, but psychologists and social workers have seized the initiative in the field of the treatment of sexual problems from the medical profession every since. In the 1990s, however, the medical profession staged a comeback. Urologists developed various treatments for men with erection problems, and gynaecologists again took a more active interest in women complaining of painful sexual symptoms.

In their first book, *Human Sexual Response* (1966), Masters and Johnson summed up their observations in a chart, 'sexual response curve', depicting the course of responses of all their experimental subjects to sexual stimulation. They divided the curve into four phases: excitement (erections in men; lubrication and swelling of the vaginal introitus in women); plateau (a period during which sexual excitement is kept in check to increase the pleasure); orgasm and resolution (the decrease in physical and mental tension). In later years, Helen Kaplan advocated the inclusion of an earlier phase: that of desire.[3] By that she meant that physical arousal can be preceded by a mental process of anticipation, pleasurable expectation or preoccupation. The graph shown here is taken from a textbook of sexology.[4]

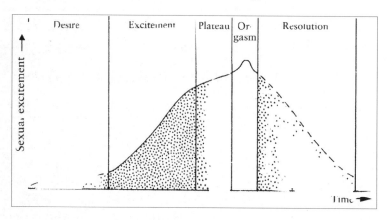

6 Graphic representation of sexual excitement during the various phases of sexual activity. The density of the dots is a 'measure' of interaction focus (dark) or a focus on personal mental and physical sensations (absence of dots).

The classical curve of Masters and Johnson is a useful device. People with sex problems often find the diagram helpful in conveying what they think is wrong with them. If the graph is drawn on a blackboard in a lecture theatre full of students, and the students are asked if they recognize themselves on it, most of them will nod thoughtfully. However, if the same group is asked to depict their own sexual feelings on a graph, quite different patterns usually appear. Master and Johnson were well aware of this fact, certainly in the case of women. For men, they present just one curve, because in men significant variations are only to be found in the time distribution, but for women they give us three curves, adding that these should only be considered as attempts to illustrate an endless number of variations. The curve shown in many later publications is always the male curve. This has given rise to the accusation that on the basis of the work of Masters and Johnson many attempts have been made to fit female sexuality into the male model.

Another objection that may be raised to the so-called sexual response cycle is that what are in essence totally different processes have been combined in a single figure. If desire, excitement and orgasm were each assigned a colour of their own, then more people might well recognize themselves on a tripartite graph. We shall now deal separately with each of these three aspects.

Sexual desire

The place of desire on the curve is illustrative of the idea underlying the use of this term. We assume that desire is a mental process preceding sexual behaviour and that it can be present even before excitement (and hence in the absence of physical arousal). Desire has an object; we desire something. Desire is undoubtedly connected with other mental processes reflecting one's mood. If one feels depressed, then sexual indifference is part of a whole complex of symptoms. As a rule, psycho-pharmaceuticals (drugs used in the treatment of emotional disorders) influence desire, generally acting as inhibitors. That is, almost always, an unwanted side effect; if a drug could stimulate desire (an aphrodisiac, that is) there would certainly be a market for it, but unfortunately there is more deception than efficacy in this field (and for that sort of deception you must go to a sex shop rather than to a pharmacy).

It must be remembered that a lack of desire does not imply an inability to produce the rest of the sexual response. If the initiative comes from another person, and that person is nice and erotically accomplished, then one can have all the sexual sensations even without being desirous oneself. Sexological literature contains an extremely instructive illustration of this point.[5] A married couple living in Scotland had a most satisfactory sex life. Their relationship had classical characteristics: the husband always took the initiative in their lovemaking, and the wife responded. Then the husband's initiative gradually began to flag. At first, no explanation could be found; the sexologist who treated them thought that their situation could be improved once the established role expectations were broken. No sooner said than done. The wife proved quite capable of taking the sexual initiative, and the husband responded well. Their relationship was once again harmonious. Some time later, however, it was discovered that the husband had an impairment of the pituitary gland. His prolactin output was out of control and an excessively high level in the blood was causing his lack of spontaneous impulses. After restoration of the normal hormone balance with drugs (the same kind of pills taken by women who do not want to breastfeed their newborn babies), the man's sexual initiative returned.

But things are even more complicated: in some people desire is part of lovemaking itself and not a preliminary phase. If we try to determine the part of desire in the entire sexual experience, then we do well to recognize that the linear model outlined above does not fit everybody, and that some people are better characterized by a more circular pattern. Feminists often object to the fact that sexology is based too much on the assumption that orgasm is the greatest good, in other words that the sexual experience is subject to some sort of natural direction. There are different positive experiences, which we shall temporarily classify as 'ecstasy'. 'Excitement' is not necessarily an appropriate term to define this peak emotion. There are certainly women (and men as well) who will tell you that their desire just keeps increasing. What we have here is undirected desire: a desire for desire.[6] Freud began his conceptualization of pleasure with a simple model: sexual tension is in principle unpleasurable (Unlust); the pleasure lies in its discharge (Lust). Lou Andreas-Salomé put Freud on a different path in one of her letters. 'Is it not then the great problem of sex that it not only strives to quench the thirst, but that it also consists in the yearning for the thirst itself, that the physical relief of tensions, of satiation, at the same time disappoints, because it diminishes the tension, the thirst. . .'[7]

When dealing with sexual desire, we have to say something about the role of the sex hormones. Hormones influence the operation of the brain, and many women experience this fact every month. In the first half of the menstrual cycle (that is, from menstruation to ovulation) oestrogens predominate and most women feel energetic, cheerful and extrovert. From ovulation to the next menstruation, the blood stream contains, apart from oestrogens, large quantities of progesterone, and this hormone has quite a different effect on the brain. It can make women grumpier, depressed, unsure, sometimes compulsive and less interested in contact with others. Since such pronounced mental effects are involved, it seems obvious that sexual feelings, too, will fluctuate. A great deal of research into this matter has been done. The founder of social sexology, Alfred Kinsey, concluded that quite a few women have their greatest spontaneous need for sexual stimulation when they are menstruating.[8] Later researchers have argued that it may well be during ovulation that a woman's need peaks, which would tally with a biological belief focused on reproduction. Some investigators have been able to demonstrate that sexual interest peaks around the time of ovulation, while others have found no evidence for this at all.[9]

With men, the situation is simpler. They have very few female hormones and the male hormone, testosterone, does not go through a cycle (at most, it has a diurnal cycle: it is highest in the morning). While a clear influence of testosterone on sexual feelings has been demonstrated, that influence should not be exaggerated. When a maturing boy produces practically no testosterone due to a congenital complaint (and hence remains undersized and grows no pubic or facial hair) he will develop no interest in sex. If, in somebody older, the testosterone blood levels drop sharply, the result is a loss of sexual initiative. The blood levels involved have to be exceptionally low because the range of the normal values is considerable.

In women, too, a certain amount of testosterone, much lower than in men, is present and probably also plays a functional role in arousing sexual desire. Women, however, vary much more in sensitivity than men.[10] Some women with extremely low testosterone blood levels do indeed complain about loss of spontaneous sexual desire, just as happened with the Scottish husband described above. Such extremely low levels will be found only in women who have been castrated (that is, have had their ovaries removed surgically) and who also use cytostatics in the treatment of hormone-dependent forms of cancer (for instance breast cancer). In that situation there can of course be quite other motives for placing sex low on the list of priorities.

Excitement

The term 'excitement' for this phase is rather misleading, for what is generally understood by excitement (think of girls mobbing the Spice Girls, their mothers cheering the Chippendales, or the general public during football matches) cannot always be equated with the emotional state of people during periods of great genital intensity. The term 'arousal' lacks this drawback – people can be highly aroused while remaining calm and serene. In the past, this serene form of arousal even used to be held up as a higher form of lovemaking, originating from India: the *carezza*. Couples engaging in this practice strove to attain optimal genital arousal and union, but not release. During contact between penis and vagina, the couple moved no more than was absolutely necessary to maintain the arousal of the genital organs; for the rest intimacy, symbolized by eye contact, was paid the greatest attention.

We cannot claim that the mental processes, the feelings, experienced during this phase are always distinct from those occurring during the phase we have called 'desire'. The accompanying physical sensations are quite specific, however, and we are not thinking only of the genital organs. The pulse and the blood pressure go up, and generally the breathing rate as well. In women, something always happens to their breasts. The nipples contract and become erect, while the areolas – the pigmented rings round the nipples – may grow larger. Fluid may accu-

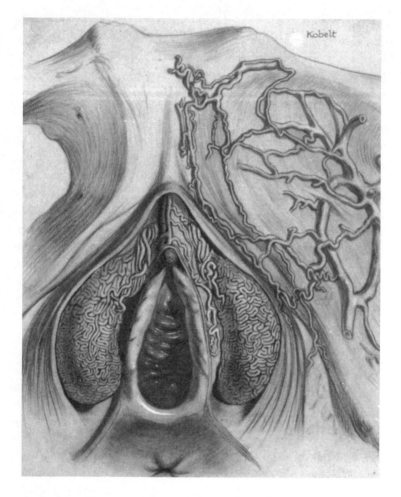

7 This drawing of the inner side of the labia minora shows the observations of the German anatomist Kobelt in 1844.

mulate in the breasts, increasing their volume by up 20 per cent. A specific skin reaction, called the 'sex flush' by Masters and Johnson, starts in the abdominal region and gradually creeps upwards to the breasts and neck. Arousal also leads to a near-automatic increase in muscular tension in many different muscle groups: in the abdomen and thorax, legs and groin, but also in the face and the feet. Some people deliberately use the muscular tension round the genitals to increase their sexual excitement.

Genital excitation is characterized by blood congestion. Round the vagina and uterus we find an extensive network of blood vessels, and the clitoris is a body of erectile tissue (comparable to the erectile tissue in the penis), which in the area between the vagina and the pubic bone is considerably larger than its external appearance leads one to suspect. The sole function of the clitoris is to swell up during sexual excitement;

during the phase shortly before orgasm that effect can be masked because the clitoris is pulled closer to the pubic bone (and perhaps also because, at this point, the prepuce swells considerably). The area between the labia swells up most of all, and here the pink colour becomes deeper. The labia minora are, as it were, pushed outwards and the opening to the vagina (the hymenal region) narrows a little. Masters and Johnson have called this region altered by sexual excitement the orgasmic plateau. Deeper inside the vagina, the blood congestion is even more visible. People lying in their own beds will rarely notice this, but in many laboratory investigations the colour of the vaginal wall is monitored as a measure of sexual arousal. Moreover, a high level of sexual excitement always entails the expansion of the vagina, which leads to a considerable quantity of air being sucked in; the uterus, too, is elevated. Masters and Johnson called this the 'tenting effect'. They were unable to show convincingly how it comes about, and in subsequent years it became a source of controversy among other investigators. Displacement is movement and movement generally implies muscular activity. The Egyptian gynaecologist Ahmed Shafik believes that the largest and strongest layer of muscles in the pelvic floor is responsible, and he has undertaken research to discover what stimuli produce a reflex response of the levator ani. A rapid inflation of a balloon in the vagina produces an appreciable contraction, but it lasts just a moment.[11] Roy Levin, a British investigator who has thoroughly examined the question of what really happens in the female genital organs, is not convinced that the prolonged and stable tenting effect can be caused by an ordinary skeletal muscle. He refers to an old and generally overlooked article by a Dutch anatomist, who stressed that a number of smooth muscle cells are present in the ligaments and connective tissue linking the pelvic floor and the genital organs.[12] Smooth muscles are found chiefly in our internal organs. Skeletal muscles govern our deliberate movements; they can be voluntarily controlled by the brain, while smooth muscles cannot. Smooth muscles are capable of remaining in a particular state of contraction for a considerable time. We owe our continence to that capacity of our smooth sphincter muscles; only when we have diarrhoea or an overfull bladder do we also make deliberate use of the ability to tense the skeletal sphincter muscles of our pelvic floor, but these are far less capable of supplying adequate counter pressure for long. Levin believes that the smooth muscles make a greater contribution to the tenting effect; Shafik argues that too few muscle cells are present to produce the effect.

Vaginal lubrication is the indirect result of blood congestion. All the tissues of the body obtain their nutrients and oxygen through the blood, but for that to happen the lymph (the almost colourless cell-free liquid) has to leave the capillaries, the delicate and thin-walled network of tiny blood vessels. It is the lymph that keeps an abrasion moist once the bleeding has stopped. The vaginal wall allows the lymph to pass through; the vaginal contents are thus diluted as the flow of blood increases; the vagina becomes lubricated and more slippery. In the vulval region small mucous glands add their secretion. The volume of fluid produced here is negligible, but it has more mucosity and thus probably helps to make the introitus feel smoother.

None of the bodily processes described here as contributing to sexual excitement have to be learned. The body knows how. Much as boys, even before puberty, occasionally wake up with an erection, so a girl's body will occasionally produce a spontaneous sexual response. True, women have to learn to register these reactions consciously and to interpret them correctly. At the beginning of my work in the Rutgers Foundation in the late 1970s, I examined quite a few young women who had consulted me about their vaginal discharges. They thought them abnormal and were worried that they might have a fungal infection or something similar. However, the examination showed nothing untoward. As doctors working in a sexual health clinic we were inclined to look on all genital symptoms as possible pointers to sexual dissatisfaction. I remember a girl who, when I asked if she might be in love, said 'Oh, I am, yes, terribly.' She herself had failed to see the connection between her feelings and her bodily reactions.

Orgasm

Orgasms do not come by themselves. If a man or a woman wants to have a satisfactory sex life, they must first find out how to master this phase of the sexual response cycle. They have to establish what makes the genital organs feel good. Some girls seem to begin this quest while still inside their mother's womb. The Italian gynaecologists Giorgio Giorgi and Marco Siccardi[13] made an ultrasound of a woman in her 32nd week of pregnancy and watched for 20 minutes while the foetus repeatedly touched her own clitoris with her right hand, accompanied by jerky movements of the pelvis and legs. Once her whole body had contracted, she relaxed. (The mother was an interested spectator, Giorgi and Siccardi pointed out, and rightly so, because there was little chance that she would have the opportunity to see her daughter masturbating later in life.)

In boys, the discovery of the orgasm is more of a matter of course. If an adolescent boy does not practise self-gratification, he is likely to have a nocturnal emission – a 'wet dream'. Often on waking up he notices more than just a wet patch in his pyjamas, and that generally makes him sit up and think. However, if they want to control their own orgasms, boys, too, have to pass through a learning phase. In girls, nocturnal orgasms also occur, but we assume that this is not a general rule. Moreover, if a woman does have a nocturnal orgasm she is often unaware of it. For that reason, when a woman asks for sexological help because she has never had an orgasm, we always ask her at some length about possible spontaneous responses, and it frequently happens that she then recalls certain experiences on waking up that might well have been orgasms. In women such events leave no unmistakable traces, but the failure to recognize a nocturnal orgasm is bound up with certain cultural assumptions. Everyone knows that boys have 'wet dreams'. Far less attention is paid to this matter in girls.

It has already been seen that desire, excitement and orgasm each has a dynamic of its own. The feelings of desire and excitement may not always be distinguishable, but everyone acquainted with orgasms will confirm that this response feels different. 'Release' is a description that many people would adopt. 'Surrender' and 'letting go' are also mentioned. Like excitement, this phase of the cycle has a mental as well as a physical component. In men, the physical component (the ejaculation of semen) is fairly unambiguous; in women the physiological aspect is less predominant and undoubtedly more variable as well. Some women are so involved in the mental aspects of their orgasms that they hardly notice the physical signs. Women will tell you far more often than men that they really are not all that bothered if they miss the occasional orgasm, and that this does not mean that some of their sexual encounters leave them with an unfinished feeling. Men will sometimes tell you that they measure the quality of an orgasm by the number of contractions they feel in their penis. No two orgasms are precisely the same, and many men use special techniques during masturbation to increase their orgasmic responses. If a man has an ejaculation that is truly 'superb', it usually means he has felt a large number of powerful contractions.

With women, I have come across this form of self-observation only once in lesbian sadomasochistic erotica (in other words in that sector of female sexual experience closest to the machismo side of the male experience). In *Jenny*, a story by Pat Califia, a Californian considered the figurehead of the lesbian S/M scene, Liz, a masochistic woman, is picked up in a disco by the most desirable woman there, the star of the

rock band Bitch. In the car sexual expectation is pumped up dramatically by verbal exchanges. Jessie has to drive, but Liz can do anything
she likes with herself provided she gives a running commentary to
Jessie. Finally, Liz is given permission to come:

> I needed more. I had waited so long that my orgasm was incredibly
> intense. My vagina clenched like a fist, then contracted and pulsed.
> I counted the contractions while I went on holding my vulva firmly,
> pressing against it.

Reflex physiology

Rhythmical contractions are the essential feature of the orgasm, and
once an orgasm 'breaks through', it can no longer be stopped.
Reflexes are direct bodily responses to a stimulus – that is, they do not
need the intervention of the brain. The classical example is the
knee-jerk reflex: a brief tap with a rubber mallet produces a sudden
kick. That response is involuntary; if you are relaxed you will find it
hard to suppress it. The tap upon the tendon below the kneecap (the
patellar tendon) is communicated to stretch receptors in the extensor
muscle at the front of the thigh, whereupon an electrical signal is
transmitted via a nerve to the spinal cord. Here just one signal jump
(synapse) across to another cell body, the neuron whose fibres run
back to the same muscle, suffices to produce a contraction. Another
example, involving a different sense, is the blinking reflex: a quick
movement towards the eye elicits a response by the eyelid. A visual
stimulus thus triggers a motor response. The whole cycle is completed
in milliseconds. Some reflexes are not transmitted by nerves but by
hormones. Lactation is a case in point. Stimulation of the mother's
nipple by a sucking infant stimulates the brain stem and releases oxytocin, a hormone that promotes the 'let-down' reflex during lactation.
This process takes a little longer than the last.

Reflexes are with us from birth (you might say that they are part
of our hardware). Functional psychologists refer to them as unconditioned reflexes. They do not have to be learned, though we might have
to learn how to use them to best advantage. Impatient parents often
turn on a tap if their toddler is taking too long to urinate. Anorectic
girls push their fingers down their throat, thus making abnormal use
of a normal reflex. If you feel that you are about to sneeze, you can
speed the process by staring at a bright light. Having an orgasm is
of the same order: the conscious manipulation of reflex possibilities.

What we have here is a complex reflex, quite a bit more complicated than the knee-jerk. When two people are having sexual intercourse, they are busy, among other things, with mutual manipulation of their reflexes. The same is true of parents who tickle their children.

Functional psychology deals not only with innate (unconditioned) reflexes, but also with conditioned reflexes. The classical example is Pavlov's dog. When a dog smells food, its stomach secretes gastric juice. With Pavlov's dog, passing a small tube through the wall of the stomach and the abdomen ensured the prompt observation of this phenomenon. If feeding is invariably preceded by the flashing of a red light, then turning on that light will lead to the immediate release of gastric juice. This experiment involves a simple reflex, and there are many other examples. Nursing mothers find that their breasts start to leak when they hear their infant cry, and this is no doubt a conditioned response. But more complex learned behaviour also involves conditioned elements. Just think of driving a car or playing the piano, and you will see that with some activities you can leave the job to your hands or feet almost without conscious control. Pianists speak of their 'muscular memory'.

This somewhat technical digression may help to explain the enormous variability of orgasmic responses, which applies to the stimulus as well as to the response side. On the stimulus side, the clitoris plays a leading part – the ability to respond to clitoral stimulation with an orgasm may almost be considered an unconditioned reflex. The Kinsey report on the human female pointed out that some girls start masturbating in infancy and experience what are undoubtedly genuine orgasms. Their conclusion was based on observations by the girls' mothers: their daughters stimulated themselves either by touching their clitoris manually or by rubbing it with a pillow or a teddy bear. The clitoris thus has a marked effect on what we may call the orgasm centre in the spinal cord, though it is by no means the sole orgasmic trigger. In 1976, Shere Hite made a comprehensive study of the sexual repertoire of American women. In the case of masturbation, direct clitoral massage (by hand, with a vibrator or with a warm stream from the shower head) was far more common than vaginal, that is penetrative, stimulation, but there was also a percentage of women who did not touch themselves at all. They were able to climax by the rhythmical contraction of muscles in the pelvic floor and in the thighs ('squeezing').

Eighteenth-century novelists were well aware of this fact. At the time, novels were thought to pose a grave threat to the impressionable sex. Bernard Mandeville played the devil's advocate when, in his *The Virgin Unmasked: Female Dialogues Betwixt an Elderly Maiden Lady and Her Niece,* he filled a whole novel with hypocritical warnings against novels.[14] Antonia, the niece, gives full rein to her imagination while reading plays and romances. Her bigoted aunt cannot admonish her enough, since she has caught Antonia behaving thus:

> . . . clapping your Legs alternatively over one another, squeezing your Thighs together with all the Strength you had, and in a quarter of an hour repeat the same.

In her short story 'No Joke', Kristien Hemmerechts has one of her characters use the same approach, following a confusing session with her gynaecologist.

> She shut her eyes and let it all happen again in the packed train. She tensed the muscles of her cunt, relaxed them, tensed them again, while concentrating on every detail of her consultation, letting his voice resound briefly in her head, tensing and relaxing, until something happened that could never have happened on the green imitation leather examination couch: she came. Startled, she opened her eyes and looked at her fellow passengers. No one was paying her the least attention. . . . She took her pocket mirror from her bag and wiped away some of the mascara that had started to run. There was not even a trace of a blush on her cheeks to betray her. The tremor she had briefly felt had been contained within. There was room enough inside her for small spasms without her frame having to take part. Should she do it again? Coming was healthy, or so they told you in all the books. And it kept you young.[15]

This method of tensing your body is similar to holding back your urine, and that is probably how some young girls hit upon the orgasm. One woman remembered that when she was about eight years old, she used to like going to bed early and would quickly drink a lot of water first. In bed, she would feel the pressure in her bladder building up and it became an exciting game for her to put off passing water for as long as possible. When the flow could no longer be stopped, she would squat beside her bed for a moment, next to a portrait of Paul McCartney pinned up at a strategic height. She would then whisper sweet nothings to him until the growing tension in her bladder and muscles would give rise to an orgasm. Then she had to make a dash for the lavatory.

Masturbatory squeezing is probably not all that uncommon. Quite a few parents have had to tell their small daughters not to do that sort of thing too openly. A young girl recalled that she would regularly sit in her playpen wriggling her body, and she had not the slightest doubt that the orgasms she attained as a result did not differ essentially from the adult variety. Her mother had told her gently that what she was doing was not wrong, but that she must not do it when others were watching. That had not been difficult. When she was at nursery school, a girl in her class did it quite openly, but clearly no one else knew what she was up to. Our young friend was shocked. What a dirty little girl, she thought, she doesn't even know you have to do that sort of thing in private.

Cycling and horse riding are another two 'natural' thigh-squeezing activities, which is why these two sports were considered unsuitable for young ladies in the nineteenth century. The invention of the treadle sewing machine, and particularly the type in which the legs had to move two pedals alternately, also gave rise to concern. This sort of movement was thought to pose a grave public health problem, since if sexual desire were aroused in an innocent young woman before marriage, a host of medical complications was bound to ensue. Stimulation of other skin areas, too, can bring some women to a climax. In the women's magazine *Viva*, one in six correspondents reported that they could be brought to orgasm by breast and nipple manipulation.[16] Another first-hand report came to me from a sixteen-year-old girl deeply in love with her young boyfriend, but prevented by her strict parents from being alone with him. Often her parents, her boyfriend and she would watch television together. Sometimes he managed to stroke her breasts surreptitiously under her loose-fitting sweater, and she would climax in perfect secrecy.

In her autobiographical *Don't Fall Off the Mountain*, Shirley MacLaine reports a conversation with a Parisian prostitute, whom she consulted prior to playing the part of Irma La Douce.[17]

> I asked her if she enjoyed physical love with her *mec*.
> 'Oh, yes,' she said, 'but not the way I used to.'
> 'What do you mean,' I asked.
> She seemed pleased to explain, as though she were answering a question she knew intrigued everybody. 'It's a question of your private place,' she said. 'My private place isn't here any more.' She patted herself and shrugged. She reached up behind her back, touching the place between her shoulder blades. 'When my *mec* caresses me here, that is all I need. But if a customer accidentally touches this place, I stop working immediately and give him his money back.'

Finally, there is Gina Ogden's remarkable study of the behaviour of fifty women who came to orgasm unusually easily. Thirty-two of them were able to climax without physical stimulation, purely by concentrating and using their imagination.[18] Masters and Johnson also mentioned this phenomenon. Their experimental subjects were mainly couples in a steady relationship with a positive attitude to sex. Among the women asked to satisfy their men manually, a few reported that they climaxed together with their partners without needing any other physical stimulation.

So far we have been dealing with the stimulus side of the orgasm reflex, but the response side too has an endless number of variations. The physical part, according to Masters and Johnson, is the series of rhythmical contractions of the sphincters in the pelvic floor, and that rhythm is identical in men and in women. Men are usually aware of what is happening when they climax: the spurting of sperm is automatically impressed on their consciousness. Women differ far more in the perception of their contractions. The intensity can vary considerably, involving a larger or smaller number of contractions, but is also reflected in the size of the region to which the reaction spreads. Thus there are women who can sometimes feel the contractions in the uterus, and if that feeling predominates, it is generally overwhelming. While the uterus produces no sexual response in some women, it is of paramount erotic importance in others. That fact used to be ignored by gynaecologists when dealing with illnesses and symptoms the treatment of which includes the essential, or at least advisable, removal of the uterus. Women find this a harrowing prospect, because it is felt more or less as losing their femininity. When women vented their concern about losing some of their sexual pleasure by a hysterectomy, gynaecologists used to be make light of it until recently; rightly in the case of some women but decidedly not with others.

Masters and Johnson did not content themselves with drawing just one curve when it came to depicting the sexual response of women, but they did start with the assumption that the physiological process is always the same. That view has been the subject of much debate since 1980, with particular attention to the G-spot, the female prostate and the female ejaculation.

The other orgasm: 'It's just another delicious, wet, beautiful thing that women can do'[19]

There have always been women (and their sexual partners) who did not recognize themselves in the Masters and Johnson model. For one thing, these two authors laid great emphasis on the primary importance of the clitoris. Women who enjoyed penetration and came easily as a result felt that they had been ignored. There were also women who came with an ejaculation and who were astonished at the quantity of fluid they felt running out of their vaginas during orgasm. Some years ago I had to reply to a letter from a very embarrassed young girl who told me that a pile of five towels was not enough to keep her mattress dry. Like all women who have this experience, she at first thought that she was leaking urine, but it did not smell like that. The older erotic literature often mentioned 'spurting' during orgasm, but in the twentieth century the phenomenon was thought to be no more than wishful thinking by male authors. In the Seventies a group of American sexologists tried to reconcile the various inconsistencies in the current physiological picture.[20]

For a start, some women with strong vaginal sensations were able to indicate fairly clearly where the most pleasurable spot in their vagina was located. This was at the front, a few centimetres in, the spot previously described in the older gynaecological literature by Gräfenberg. In their 1982 book, Kahn, Whipple and Perry decided to name the place the G-spot, in honour of the anatomist who first described it. It is found where the bladder passes into the urethra. In man, this area has developed into the prostate, which explains why the G-spot area is occasionally referred to as the 'female prostate'. During coitus, the spot is not effectively stimulated, but the necessary pressure and intensity can be attained with fingers (and in later years all vibrator makers have marketed devices curved in such a way that the G-spot can be reached by the woman herself). The spot swells and the woman may feel an urge to push down (like in defecation). At the point of orgasm, the G-spot has been found to produce a quantity of moisture, which in its composition indeed somewhat resembles the prostatic secretion of men. (Some men, especially homosexuals, also know of two ways of climaxing. Besides the usual stimulation of the penis, prostate massage through the anus can produce an orgasm, during which some men have quite different sensations.)

The story seemed at first to be quite straightforward, and in the early 1980s the search for the G-spot was considered a must for the sophisticated young woman (and her partner). Pelvic floor muscle training was part of it, for women who ejaculate are said to have greater muscle control. Josephine Lowndes Sevely has pointed out that women should try to acquire the habit, during high levels of excitement, of pushing rather than sucking in with their abdominal muscles.

Medical science, however, has always had difficulties with the G-spot and with female ejaculation.[21] It is not so easy to explain where the fluid is produced, especially if one is puzzled by the dramatic stories about large quantities. However, back in 1948 the pathologist John Huffman had given much attention to the structures surrounding the urethra.[22] There are tiny channels going to the urethra, and the number of them is variable. Moreover, some women have most prostatic channels near the bladder, others near the vulval end. So we can conclude that in man the prostate is a neat, well-defined, round structure surrounded by a capsula, and in women a certain amount of similar tissue is more dispersed and more variable.

The most graphic and convincing information about the G-spot comes from the part of the world in which the whole story began in the 1970s, the West Coast, and especially the Feminist Women's Health Centres there. Rebecca Chalker has collected the experiences of many women in *The Clitoral Truth*.[23] One woman reports that for a long time she used to think that the cold, wet places in the sheet after sex had been produced by the men she made love to, and it was only after she had her first experience with a woman that she realized how much she had overestimated the male share. Some of the stories mention large volumes of fluid and impressive fountains, but Chalker emphasizes that these are the exception rather than the rule. Quite a few women fail to notice this particular fluid because the quantity of vaginal lubrication is much larger. By way of comparison, it might be pointed out that, when yawning, you sometimes expel a very thin jet of saliva from the sublingual salivary gland. This happens to me quite often when I am reading the morning paper, as I can tell from the trace of tiny drops on the paper. The actual jet is something I have never seen.

Chalker believes that most women can learn to ejaculate, just as they can learn to have multiple orgasms. Anyone wanting to learn this form of sexual discharge can do no better than get visual instruction from a video.

I'd been working on my vaginal muscles for about a year before I saw a video of women discussing their personal experiences with ejaculation.
I first ejaculated after my lover and I watched a video about female

ejaculation together. Once we were sitting in chairs facing each other a few feet apart as we masturbated, and suddenly I began to ejaculate all over him for about 30 or 40 seconds. I don't ejaculate every time but I often do, and the amount varies quite a bit, and sometimes I do it without even having an orgasm . . .

Chalker includes a list of good videos. Incidentally, 'gushing' is a new hype in the porn market, but I assume the waterfalls these film makers present come from the world of special effects.

There is yet another physical characteristic of orgasms, namely dilation of the pupils. This is specific of orgasms; other high levels of excitement do not produce it. Because it is such a specific marker of an orgasm, Ogden used a pupillometer in her research (with women who climax without physical contact).

Satisfaction

Galen maintained that all animals are sad after coitus, except for women and cockerels.[24] Within the classical curve (which represents male rather than female responses) all tension disappears rapidly after orgasm. The blood pressure falls, the pulse and respiration level out, the spotting on the skin and the dark colour of the labia disappear, and the swelling of the labia, breasts and uterus subsides. There is one aspect specific to this phase: a little sweat can appear over large areas of the body that has nothing to do with exertion. Even when we reach orgasm in a relatively relaxed manner, this sweating may spontaneously appear.

An orgasm premotes a return to normality. If a woman has been aroused but has failed to have an orgasm, it may well happen that she has a bloated, sometimes obviously painful feeling in her abdomen afterwards. Among women who consult gynaecologists for apparently inexplicable abdominal pains, there are some whose sex life is characterized by anorgasmy and high-frequency intercourse (often imposed by their husbands, so that these women are sometimes scarcely aroused by sexual contact). But the model of growing tension, release and satisfaction is certainly not characteristic of all women. There are some who are rendered even more passionate by orgasms and who not only have several orgasms in succession, but also feel that every successive orgasm is more intense than the one before. Teiresias definitely had a point there.

chapter five

Virginity

Our world is full of dangers, but it is doubly dangerous for the young, who are unaware of the threats all round them, and, in their inno-cence, do not even suspect their existence. The instructive book of experience still lies closed before them. They believe that luck will never desert them, and are unaware that countless young brothers and sisters have become unfortunate victims of the temptation of their own foolish tendencies in the first spring of their lives. Thus, without even knowing it, they are in constant danger of losing their finest and best possession, their innate innocence and purity, and with it all claims to earthly happiness.[1]

The transformation of a girl into a woman begins with the develop-ment of breasts and the first period. Some girls are very happy about this, but for others their changed body means a summons to an adult world that they are far from ready to enter. If a girl needs a bra while she is still very young, she does not usually welcome it, nor the changed way in which boys and men let their eyes stray over her body. It confronts her with some hard facts – that various romantic possi-bilities await her and that it would be a good thing if she knew what to do about them. She will go on having new experiences for a number of years, either because of her own desires or because others provoke her into them. Life becomes a series of first times. In social sexology this is called the step-by-step sexual interaction career. The chart opposite illustrates the average age of boys and girls as they pass a number of milestones in their lives.[2]

The first coitus, the deflowering, is high in the hierarchy of important life events, but that does not necessarily mean that it is so special for every individual. Sometimes the first French kiss proves to be a far more memorable experience. The writer and actress Annemarie Oster

8 The growth
of experience
in teenage girls
and boys.

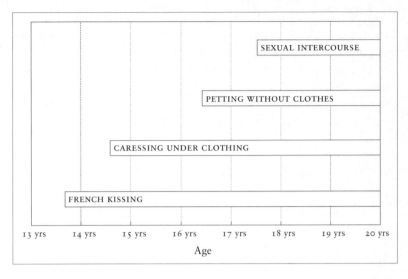

has described her first time, shared with the notorious actor and musician/songwriter Ramses Shaffy in the deserted Amsterdam Theatre after the New Year's Gala:[3]

> I was thirteen and had never been kissed. That kissing meant something soft and wet squirming into your mouth had never even occurred to me. At the time, you did not read about such things in ladies' magazines.

The memory was so precious to Annemarie Oster that a good forty years later she plucked up courage and asked Shaffy if he still remembered it as well. The reply, 'in his most intimate actor's intonation', was, 'Of course . . . Long time ago, wasn't it?'

By contrast, here is the story of a young woman's deflowering. She realized that it had been a rather flat event. 'Were you ready for it? Pretty much. Was it exciting? A bit. Did it hurt? Not really, because I was using tampons by then. How did you feel afterwards? Don't actually remember.' But her first French kiss was a colourful and vivid memory. She was playing in her room with a girlfriend, and two boys came and joined in the game. After a while, suggested some French kissing, and she still remembered replying, very pertly, 'I'll have to talk about it with my friend first.' They had sat for a while on the top step of the stairs weighing up the pros and cons, and then they went back inside and said that they would like to. The memory of the actual French kiss was less vivid. 'A bit yucky, I think.' A boy who was in love with a girl who he knew had more experience than he did, realized while they were petting that he could not possibly refuse her a French kiss. It made him feel sick, and after thinking up some excuse he ran back home to rinse out his mouth and brush his teeth.

French kissing is also sometimes associated with great fears. A woman friend reported that following her first experience of it, which she found repulsive, she had not dared to swallow her spit all the way home from the fairground for fear she might fall pregnant.

Christian ideals of chastity

The special impact of one's first sexual intercourse is of a different order from that of one's first French kiss. Deflowering touches on such cherished qualities as innocence, purity, goodness and unblemishedness. The Christian faith endows virginity with a religious aura. Mary's virginity is her chief attribute, and the Annunciation, the proclamation of her unique and sacred task, is one of the most important topics of religious art. Mary's virginity was so appealing that in the Middle Ages there was a growing belief that Mary herself was immaculately conceived. In the New Testament there is no mention of Mary's parents, but they are found in the Apocryphal Gospels.[4] Their names were Joachim and Anne, and their marriage remained childless for 20 years. At the time, childlessness was considered a disgrace, a punishment for a secret sin, so that when Joachim wanted to offer a sacrifice in the temple, the priest forbade him to do so. Anne poured out her heart to her servant Judith, who was also lacking in compassion. Next she sought solace in prayer, sitting under a laurel tree, in which she spotted a bird's nest. When that touched her emotions and caused her to give free rein to her sorrow, the angel Gabriel appeared and assured her that she would soon be bearing a child. Joachim, too, received a similar message. In the thirteenth century, the story was embellished further with their reunion by the Golden Gate in Jerusalem, Anne's conception thus being transformed from a physical into a spiritual event. The result was the dogma of the Immaculate Conception: during her conception and her birth, Mary was free of original sin.

There was a great need for miracles and idols in the Middle Ages. During the sixth century, Anne's body was taken to Byzantium and the cult of Anne was strongly fostered from that religious centre. Her greatest popularity came during the fifteenth to seventeenth centuries, and it is assumed that the flowering of bourgeois culture contributed to that popularity, since Anne, even more so than Mary, was the ideal homemaker, the venerable grandmother. She also, of course, had a model curriculum for the job as guardian of fertility.

For Christians, chastity and virginity are synonymous with excellence. When the need for monogamy and the immorality of premarital sex are stressed, it is nearly always for religious reasons. In the summer of 1994, 25,000 teenagers assembled on the lawn outside the Congress building in Washington to bear public witness to their commitment to enter marriage in the virgin state. 'True love waits,' was this counterculture's slogan. They planted 25,000 virginally white little cards in the green grass on which could be read: 'I believe that true love waits. I hereby promise God, myself, my family, all those I date, my future partner and my future children to remain sexually pure until the day I take my solemn marriage vows.' Ever since, a whole range of virginity rituals has swept America, most of them mass meetings, where hordes of parents solemnly place a virginity ring on their children's fingers. In support of this campaign, information on the use of condoms is suppressed as far as possible, and much is made of the fact that condoms can split. The United States is a minefield for AIDS educators.

In 1997, Congress passed the Welfare Reform Act, setting aside $50 million for programmes whose 'exclusive purpose is teaching the social, psychological, and health gains to be realized by abstaining from sexual activity'.[5] In judging the reliability of contraceptive methods, a distinction should always be drawn between *method failure* (the chance that the method may fail even when applied correctly) and *user failure* (the chance that the method is not used properly). American abstinence promoters usually refrain from referring to the chance of succumbing unprepared to temptation, and in any case do not feel responsible for the high percentage of unwanted teenage pregnancies. They behave like a condom manufacturer who insists that every condom failure must be blamed on the stupidity of the users.

In the United States family values are chiefly a Republican battle cry, but as early as 1994 Bill Clinton set aside a budget of $400,000 for 'Abstinence Only' sex education at high schools. Clinton is in good company: in Swaziland King Mswati III himself appealed to the unmarried women in his country to refrain from sex for five years and to adopt a sex-deprecating code of behaviour. To that end these women were asked to wear tassels of wool as a sign to men that they were to be left in peace. Despite the fact that, in his thirties, he is one of the last remaining absolute monarchs, his subjects can no longer be counted on to follow all his whims. Mswati himself failed to set a good example. Thus he was made to pay a fine to the father of his eleventh wife, who had charged him with abducting his daughter. Clinton, of course, is also not the most obvious advocate of chastity, though the Monica Lewinsky affair has thrown a fresh light on American public morals. The legal wrangle in which the president became entangled hinged on the question of whether he had perjured himself with his claim that he 'did not have sexual relations with that woman . . . Miss Lewinsky'. People may well snigger; can someone really claim that he has not had sex when he has had oral satisfaction several times? But in 1991 the Kinsey Institute presented a questionnaire to a group of 600 students,[6] with a series of questions of the type: 'Would you say you "had sex" with someone if the most intimate behavior you engaged in was . . . ?' There followed the familiar hierarchy of French kissing, breast-stroking, breast-kissing, touching of genitals, oro-genital contact, and anal and vaginal coitus. The results justified Clinton's claim: 60 per cent of America's hope for the future believed that you had not had sex if you went no further than fellatio or cunnilingus. Even if you had experienced anal sex, 20 per cent of the students believed that you had remained a virgin in the technical sense.

The authors did not publish this data until January 1999, in the *Journal of the American Medical Association*. The chief editor of *JAMA* was dismissed for publishing the report at that particular moment: The political implications of the timing were thought unbecoming to a scientific journal. The research was replicated in the UK in 2001.[7]

Virginity is an important subject of moral reflection for quite a few adolescents. Children's telephone advice services regularly have to answer the question: 'How long do you have to have been going steady with a boy before you can sleep together?' Counsellors believe that, ideally, every adolescent should be able, on the basis of sound information, to make up her or his own mind. The ideal outcome of the educational message is reached when the individual succeeds in living up to her or his own moral standard. If a girl has decided for herself that she will not go to bed with a boy before her eighteenth birthday, and then only if she has had a serious relationship with him for several weeks or months, then it is a valuable thing for her to act accordingly.

Israel Schwartz is a New York social sexologist who has made a special study of first-time coitus, and has compared the sexual behaviour, emotions and morals of American and Swedish students.[8] In both countries the average age at which girls lost their virginity was just under seventeen, the partner usually being some two years older. The Swedish women found this in keeping with their sexual code of conduct, for sixteen was the age that, typically, they considered an acceptable moment for this step. The American women in general had moral objections to losing their virginity at that age. Their ideal was on average closer to nineteen than to eighteen, so that they had let themselves go almost two years too early. Not surprisingly, therefore, they felt much greater regret, guilt and anxiety about their first time than the Swedish girls; they had also been more neglectful about contraception. In addition, the Americans had double standards: they believed that sixteen was acceptable for boys. The Swedish women, by contrast, felt they had the same sexual rights as men. The results of this investigation provided clear confirmation of the existence of a cultural stereotype: the morals of Americans are more restrictive, but barely influence their behaviour. The result: hypocrisy and a great deal of anxiety.

The construction of a moral framework of one's own – a conscience, including in sexual respects – is an important individual step in human development, regardless of whether parents and the social environment issue strict or tolerant guidelines. Some engaged couples still take it for granted that the bride will be a virgin on her wedding night, though their attitudes about what – until that night – is acceptable lovemaking may vary greatly. Sexologists are sometimes told by devout women that their engagement was far more erotically exciting than their marriage, since the couple had felt free to do adventurous things with each other because they stuck firmly to the basic rule of virginity before marriage. These stories are countered by couples who panicked at the least sign of passion.

In Josien Laurier's *A Heavenly Girl* (1993) 'the girl' grows up in fear of the Lord in a strictly orthodox Protestant home. Her only prospect of leading a different life lies in the gospel group Echo, in whose midst she becomes aware of an unexpected and precious talent. She is due to give her first solo performance on Christmas Eve. At about the same time she falls in love with Eddie the guitarist. Flouting her parents' orders, yet filled with near-sacred certainty, she decides to surrender her virginity to Eddie.

> A deflowering, she suddenly thought. The day after tomorrow it would
> be exactly four years since she had her first period. That had been at
> Christmas. A small Christmas present, she had thought at the time. This,
> this was the right moment to be deflowered. It must happen. What a
> strange thought. But it was the right thing. Absolutely the right thing. . . .
> She would tell him straight out, just the way she was feeling. 'Eddie, it
> was Christmas, exactly four years ago, that I had my first period.'
> Became a woman, she thought. 'And now I want you to take me.' If she
> puts it like that, he is bound to do it it. . . . In that way she will give him

something to believe in. Leave the dirty side behind. It all becomes more noble, more beautiful. Perhaps God will confirm it.

She fully realizes that she might fall pregnant, but accepts it. If things go wrong, she will know soon enough. Even while saying grace before meals her ecstatic thoughts persist. 'In the church. On the cold floor of the church. When everyone has gone, since Eddie has the key because his father is the pastor.'

Her contempt of her parents' narrow minds serves as counterpoint to these thoughts. But there never is a single moment of deliberate rebellion. Her decision is her personal reading of her piety. Although her parents probably have no inkling of what is going on in their daughter's mind, they decide that her concert with the gospel group must be called off. The girl does not defy them. The book ends in a suffocating minor key.

Proofs of virginity

Christianity is certainly not the religion most obsessed with virginity. In 2001, the Turkish minister of public health caused a feminist uproar when he decreed that all women wanting to take a course in health care had first to pass a virginity test.[9] One of his predecessors had started a controversy in 1992 because in his former post as director of a psychiatric hospital he had subjected all female staff to a monthly virginity test to protect them from possible sexual abuse. A paradoxical policy was obviously being pursued here. In Turkey, with its long secular tradition, feminists and traditionalists may have viewpoints that are exceedingly far apart, but a compromise solution is often found.

In Istanbul and Casablanca, too, teenage girls preserve their virginity by avoiding just one step in their reckless, trend-setting sex life, in which anal sex plays a prominent part. At the beginning of the 1980s, Soumaya Naamane-Guessous interviewed 80 young women in Casablanca, and the stories she heard confirmed the picture of an animated but highly ambivalent sex scene.[10] If you wanted to be 'with it', then you had to be prepared to go most of the way because the pressure from male admirers was unrelenting. Girls who preserved their virginity often gained little erotic satisfaction from their sexual escapades, since men usually paid little attention to the clitoris. Moreover, women often did not dare to let themselves go in their excitement lest they become too 'weak' to keep their vagina unharmed.

Modern Christianity differs from Islam in having no specific interest in proofs of virginity. The worst thing that can befall a strict Dutch Reformed bride is standing pregnant before the altar. In such a situation, she is not allowed to wear a white bridal dress, and in some Dutch Reformed churches bride and bridegroom are called to account before the whole congregation.

However important virginity may be in orthodox church circles, what happens during the wedding night is not considered the family's business. This was not always the case. In the Middle Ages, the lustful feelings that could accompany sexual contact between man and woman were viewed with suspicion.[11] Much weight was given to the story of Tobias and Sara when it was brought to the attention of the faithful, the better to drive home to them that pleasure is wrought with danger. It may not always be a mortal sin, but it is certainly a venial one. Sara had been married to seven men, all of whom had been killed on their wedding night by the devil. Lust is obviously the domain of the devil Asmodeus. Sara took Tobias, a kinsman, for her eighth husband because the laws of kinship demanded it, but Tobias's father had so little faith in the marriage that he had a grave dug on the wedding night. The archangel Raphael had, however, given Tobias the following piece of advice:

> The devil wields his power over couples that ignore God and surrender to their lust like horses and mules. Abstain thou therefore from touching her for three days while you pray together with her . . . , when the third night has passed, then take the virgin unto thee in the peace of the Lord, more out of a desire for children than out of lust.

No sooner said than done – Tobias survived the deflowering of his Sara and the three nights of abstinence became known as the Tobias nights. St Jerome, the church father who was so active in propagating the ideals of abstinence, had to adapt the original text in the Book of Tobit to some extent, but thanks to his version French bishops and priests were able to make some extra income: newly weds were expected to honour the Tobias nights; if they wanted a dispensation that could be arranged, but not cheaply.

Virginity is an excellent thing to have, but should we take every woman who claims she is a virgin at her word? In 1999, the touring Kneehigh Theatre Company, based in Cornwall, staged *The Itch*, an adaptation of *The Changeling*, a play by Thomas Middleton and William Rowley written in 1653.[12] In *The Itch*, Beatrice-Joanna is the capricious, spoilt child of a good family. She is used to getting her own way by manipulating others. Her father has found her a fiancé, but she herself has set her heart on another admirer. Her own choice knows what he wants to do: he proposes to challenge the official candidate to a duel. Beatrice-Joanna considers that too risky. Knowing that her father's servant, De Flores, cherishes a burning passion for her, she decides to persuade him to do away with the fiancé for an agreed sum, after which she will arrange his escape. De Flores has his own ideas. He wants not her money but her virginity in exchange for his bloody deed, and if any escaping is to be done, it will be by the two of them together. He has the dead body removed and they wait and see how things develop. De Flores turns out to be a persuasive suitor. Beatrice-Joanna succumbs to his argument that her complicity has made the two of them fellow-sinners. On top of that De Flores's passionate love for her makes a compelling case.

Meanwhile, following the disappearance of the fiancé, a marriage with her own candidate is agreed, but Beatrice-Joanna is afraid he might discover that she is no longer a virgin. She rummages through the dressing case of her future husband and comes upon a large quantity of magical potions. Luckily the little phials all state what they are intended for. One is a pregnancy test, and she realizes that she might be pregnant, but that is something she will not have to confess to for another few months. Next to that phial she discovers a virginity test, which is naturally more urgent. Luckily again the instructions are quite plain:

> Give the party you suspect the quantity of a full spoonful of the water
> in the glass M, which upon her that is a maid makes three several
> effects: 'twill make her incontinently gape, then fall into sudden sneez-
> ing, last into a violent laughing; else dull, heavy and lumpish.

Beatrice tests the reliability of the potion on her maid (following a series of searching questions about her virginity) and the three phenomena do indeed occur in the predicted sequence. If her fiancé were to ask her to drink the draught, Beatrice thus knows precisely what she will have to do. To make doubly certain, Beatrice changes places on the bridal night with her maid, whose purity has been established but who is prepared to make this sacrifice for a large reward. Later that night De Flores and Beatrice-Joanna share their bed again, with perverse enjoyment, but towards daybreak, they begin to fear that their deceit might be discovered. Fortunately, the maid then appears, admitting frankly that lust has made her forget the time. She continues to be a threat, of course, so De Flores sets fire to the house, killing the girl. But the murdered fiancé has a brother who sows doubt in the bridegroom's heart, and when he applies moral thumbscrews to his bride, she denies adultery but confesses to the murder. This does not please De Flores. He stabs his lover, and before he cuts his own throat he informs the bridegroom that he, De Flores, possessed the now dying Beatrice-Joanna on her wedding night. Curtain. Tremendous applause. Sixteenth-century theatregoers apparently could not have enough of such gory scenes.

The hymen

The virginity test in *The Itch* sounds less than convincing, but is there a better method? Among Muslims, as among Hindus, proof of the bride's virginity during the wedding celebration is still a moment of great emotional impact, such proof being entirely dependent upon the flow of blood from the maidenhead. Unfortunately there are girls who do not bleed at all the first time they make love. This is a scientific fact that those who adhere to these rituals wholly ignore. It is all very much like a manufacturer who sells a householder a burglar alarm that only works every now and then. The buyer can therefore never be absolutely certain who will be there when she comes home. Much the same happens with the hymen: it does not always do what (according to some people) it ought to do.

In the earliest medical literature you will even find long discussions on whether or not the hymen really exists. The gynaecologist M.M.J. Reyners has examined this subject thoroughly in a book on the circumcision of girls.[13] The following jingle is said to date back to Roman times:

> Est magnum crimen
> perrumpere virginis hymen.
> (It is a great sin to break a virgin's hymen.)

In the second century AD, Soranus of Ephesus, by contrast, denied the very existence of the hymen. Albertus Magnus wrote in the fourteenth century that

> there exist, in the cervix and at the entrance of the womb of virgins, membranes made of a tissue of veins and extremely loose ligaments which are, once seen, the proven signs of virginity, and which are destroyed by the act or even by inserting one's finger; whereupon the small quantity of blood in them flows out.

That sounds quite modern and correct. The word hymen was not in use in the fourteenth century, but a century later it made its debut in medical literature. Vesalius was the first to puzzle his head about what a non-intact maidenhead implied.[14] In 1537, he was present at the dissection of a noble girl who had died of a lung infection but had also suffered from 'hysteria'. Her hymen displayed a tear; Vesalius assumed that she had 'deflowered' herself with a finger, either for frivolous reasons or because she was aware that vaginal stimulation was a cure for hysteria. Vesalius himself was familiar with this treatment. He had written his doctoral thesis on a book by Rhazes in which the author described this midwifery practice.

In the seventeenth century an animated polemic re-emerged concerning the existence of the maidenhead. The most famous Dutch physician of the time, Reinier de Graaf of Delft, wrote about it in somewhat jocular tones:[15]

> In plumbing the secrets of nature, the search for the maidenhead has caused no small unease and difficulty, even to the most quick-witted analysts who have squabbled and fought most stubbornly over it. Some have asserted boldly that its discovery would run counter to the provisions of the law and the course of nature, others scream and shout themselves hoarse, asserting that it can be found in all dissected maidens, so that failure to find it must be due to negligence or ignorance. But not even they can agree on its independent existence, place and form.

De Graaf thus keeps his own options open, but a century later the matter was settled. 'De hymenis existentia nemo dubitat,' wrote the forensic anatomist Brendelius – no one doubts the existence of the hymen. Every girl is born with a hymen; its variation in shape and thickness can, however, be considerable. Even experienced physicians find it hard to judge whether or not a hymen is intact. To put it even more strongly, forensic paediatricians are aware that while tears often appear in the hymen of young girls after they have been raped, only a few weeks later the former condition is often restored. An authoritative opinion on whether or not a hymen is intact thus continues to be elusive, and if a hymen is intact no one can say if defloration will go hand in hand with loss of blood.

It is scarcely conceivable that these facts should be unknown in Islamic countries with their onerous virginity ceremonials, but the rituals can apparently not be done away with without cutting out the heart and soul of their culture. Defloration is not always a sexual act. In the Egyptian countryside, the bloody act is performed in many villages on the wedding day by a *daya*, the woman who also performs the circumcision of girls.[16] Like the *mohel* at a Jewish circumcision, the *daya* keeps one of her finger nails long and sharp for her work. The best *daya* is the one who assaults not only the hymen but also the wall of the vagina, for that releases more blood onto the white sheet that the father later parades. And this ritual can also bring about infections, as the physician Nawal al-Saadawi established on more than one occasion.

The bloodstained sheet is proof, not only of the bride's virginity, but in many cases also of the bridegroom's virility. In addition it reassures the bridegroom's parents that the bride was worth her price. M.M.J. Reyners used to practise medicine in Tunisia, where he saw many brides, accompanied by their mothers and mothers-in-law, in his consulting room, women who came to him for *el certifikka sbiyya*, a virginity certificate, before the signing of the marriage contract. And as we might expect, on one occasion he found that the prospective bride was pregnant, and that the family probably suspected it. That meant the girl might be killed in the consulting room, for a male relative in the waiting room was prepared to restore the family honour with a knife.

During the wedding night, the bridegroom is expected to deflower his bride, and all the guests want to see the bloodstained sheet, the colour of the blood being of great importance. The bride saves her sheet carefully and if it stays a bright pink, pale pink or scarlet, she will be proud of it all her life. 'My blood was a very beautiful pink, a shade that you hardly ever see . . . ' It is also believed to have magical powers:

> My sheet was very beautiful and they talked about it for a long time afterwards. The old women quarrelled among themselves over passing it across their eyes. Apparently it can protect you from blindness.

In the male sexual experience of many cultures, defloration is considered a source of extra excitement and satisfaction. In Shakespeare's *Pericles*, pirates abduct Pericles' daughter Marina, and revel in her virginity. The brothelkeeper in whose hands she then falls tells his servant how to sell her in the market:

> . . . take you the marks of her, the colour of her hair, complexion, height, age, with warrant of her virginity; and cry, 'He that will give most, shall have her first.' Such a maidenhead were no cheap thing, if men were as they have been.

We know from bawdy Victorian writings (for instance *Fanny Hill*) that very high fees were demanded for a virgin, fear of syphilis driving the price up considerably. According to Reay Tannahill, the London price for a virgin had risen to at least £100 at the beginning of the nineteenth century.[17] By about 1880, the going rate had dropped to £5, due not to a fall in demand but to the enormous rise in supply. This was because virginity could be easily restored.

Arthur Golden's *Memoirs of a Geisha* was published in 1997. It deals with the life of Sayuri, the Japanese protagonist, in the 1930s and 1940s. Golden presented the book as a biographical work, but it turned out to be fiction, though based on lengthy interviews with a former geisha. The author is a Sinologist and Japanologist and worked for many years in the Far East. As a girl, Sayuri is trained to become a geisha, which entails, among other things, wooing by a number of protectors. The training period is rounded off in her fifteenth year with the *mizuage*, the defloration, by the man who buys the right to it. Sayuri offers each candidate a small box of sweet rice cakes, which means that they have her agreement to make an offer. In her case, too, a doctor is summoned to the house to verify her virginity, and is asked by the madam if he can tell whether there will be much blood spilled during the defloration. He is unable to say, but the man who eventually deflowers Sayuri is also a doctor, and is in fact obsessed with blood. He even keeps a collection of tiny glass phials with small swabs, pieces of bandage or wadding soaked in samples of blood obtained by him from desirable women patients. Sayuri's blood, too, has ended up in his collection. Sayuri herself is completely ignorant of this aspect of her body. Her madam is a remorseless businesswoman who knows how to play off several candidates against one another, and the sum the doctor eventually pays her is not only the highest she has ever been paid for a *mizuage* but about three thousand times what clients usually paid in those days for an hour in the company of a geisha. After the *mizuage* the doctor loses interest. There follows a second round of bidding, in which a man can become the patron of, and hence acquire the sole right to sexual congress with, the geisha. For as long as this patron can afford her company, she will be his exclusively. The normal work of a geisha – keeping men company, as a rule in a teahouse – is a chaste affair. (Golden's book became a bestseller, but his source has let it be known that she feels he has given a false picture of her.[18] In particular, she denies having been deflowered for money. Golden for his part claims that he has everything on tape.)

Japan is a country with a fascinating sexual culture, difficult to fathom. In his book *Pink Samurai*, Nicholas Bornoff gives us a detailed survey of the astonishingly varied erotic nightlife of the Japanese. A famous place in Tokyo was the Lourdes, a *no-pan kisa* (nightclub without panties). The most exclusive room was below ground, and the ceiling was a one-way screen showing the room above, where the girls – without panties – brightly lit by the reflective floor, could be ogled at leisure. There is now a cheaper, more contemporary version of the geisha, aimed at tourists and very convenient for students wanting to earn a little money on the side. Nowadays there are also meeting houses in which women are entertained pleasantly but chastely by friendly young men, and are happy to pay enormous sums for the privilege. This is one result of the fact that, in Japan, wives are in total control of the family budget. One half of all married men complain about getting too little pocket money from their spouses. The Japanese also have a unique attitude to erotica: there is a rich supply of pornographic strip and animated cartoons called *manga,* some of which are explicitly meant for teenagers. Another curious fact is that the paragraph on incest in the *International Encyclopedia of Sexuality* mentions mother-son incest only. In Western sexological writing, this form of incest comes low on the list, because it is thought to be the rarest form of sexual abuse by blood relatives. It was nevertheless the subject of a number of Japanese soap operas in the mid-1980s, the mothers concerned being the classical suffocating mothers who kept an eagle eye on their son's academic attainments. In Japanese culture this is not so outlandish; top jobs are reserved for graduates from the top universities, and these have strict selection criteria. Some mothers have admitted that for this reason they decided to take charge of their sons' sexual relief, because otherwise the boys ran the risk of being distracted from their homework by girls.[19]

The obsession with female blood of Sayuri's deflowerer is perhaps not as rare as we think. Golden's description of the teahouse recalls the Chinese brothel. The Sinologist and diplomat Robert van Gulik, best known for his detective stories, set in a mysterious Japanese atmosphere, also wrote a scholarly study of sexual behaviour in China.[20] He mentions the 'six girdles' (*liu-tai*) used to soak up virginal blood and usually kept in special baskets. Van Gulik quotes a poem dedicated to the man who discovers on his wedding that his bride is no virgin:

> Tonight a splendid wedding feast was held,
> But when I prepared to explore the fragrant flower,
> I found that spring was already past.
> What use to inquire after much red or little red?

Nothing to be seen, nothing to be seen!
I return to you the piece of white silk.

Menstrual blood is also capable of arousing very strong emotions. When the sixteenth-century Chinese scholar Li Mao-yüan visited the hot springs near Loyang, where the famous courtesan Yang Kuei-fei had bathed many centuries before, his eye fell on a few red spots on a rock. He was told that these spots were thought to be the menstrual blood of Yang Kuei-fei, and when Li Mao-yüan heard that, his heart was touched. As he left in his sedan chair, a woman's hand appeared for a second through the curtain. That night he was visited in his hotel by a woman who told him she was the ghost of Yang Kuei-fei. That ghost stayed with him until his death.

A hankering after virginity can also be found in Western fiction. In *Sweet Movie*, a film directed by Duŝan Makavejev in 1974, Miss World 1984 is asked for her hand by the richest man in the world, Mr Kapital. Naturally he expects value for his money, and so the bride is taken to a gynaecologist. In a near-sacred atmosphere the woman is placed on the gynaecological couch and over her shoulder we can see the doctor taking his allotted place between her spread knees. His face is bathed in a golden light, and his expression gives the cinemagoer a hint of the delights reserved only for the doctor and for the bridegroom. The gynaecologist plays no further part in the story, but we know that his life will never be the same again. The spectator follows this Miss World and the blows she suffers in her life. The husband (it goes without saying) is so well-endowed that their wedding night ends in a way that is usual with dogs but not with men and women: they cannot break free. She finally manages to escape her marriage and enters the sexual liberation commune of the German Expressionist painter Otto Mühl (at this point the film turns into a kind of documentary) and ends her life by drowning in a vat of chocolate. Makavejev's futuristic fantasy contains a miscellany of virginity symbols borrowed from various cultures.

Let us return to the Muslim world. As an illustration of the deep gulf between male and female attitudes to the virginity ideal, Reyners quotes Sheikh Jalal Ad din al Sayuti (second half of the fifteenth century) on the heavenly pleasures awaiting the Chosen in Paradise:

Every one of the Chosen will marry seventy houris, in addition to the legitimate wives he had on earth. Whenever he has congress with a houri he will discover that she is a virgin. In addition, the Rod of the Chosen will never flag. His erection will be everlasting. Every congress will give rise to special pleasures, to sweet sensations so unheard of on earth that, were anyone to experience it here, he would at once lose consciousness.

It is assumed that the avid longing by Muslim fundamentalists for martyrdom is connected with the prospect of exceptional carnal rewards held out by their spiritual leaders. But would the houris enjoy having sexual intercourse time and again, while remaining innocent and undefiled?

We must not forget that Mary may also be considered a champion of virginity. Even after the conception of Jesus, her hymen remained intact; that in any case is what a legend in the Apocryphal Gospels tells us.[21] When the birth was imminent, Joseph went to look for a midwife. He even found two, but when he returned with them to the stable, Jesus was already lying in his crib, wrapped in swaddling clothes. Mary smiled, but Joseph said, 'Do not smile, but take care lest they depart again and you need medicine.' The first midwife was allowed to see Mary; her name was Zélomi. Her amazement was great when she learnt that this baby had been born to a maiden, one who continued to be a virgin. She reported the matter to her colleague Salome, who seems to have had a more pragmatic turn of mind. She proposed making a personal examination of the state of Mary's hymen. 'And Salome placed her finger in her lap and cried out loud and said, "I have tempted the living God and lo! my hand is burning."' An angel then appeared and advised her to touch the newborn infant with her injured hand, and behold, the sickness was cured. The story of the two famous midwives was neglected in later centuries, but during the Middle Ages, paintings and woodcuts of the crib often showed two women on the periphery, one of whom ostentatiously supports one of her arms with the other. In Robert Campin's painting *The Birth of Jesus* (overleaf), Zélomi holds a banner with the words 'ecce virgo peperit filium' (behold a maiden has given birth to a child), while Salome's banner reads 'credam quin probavero' (I do not believe until I have examined).

Sham virginity

In the West, doctors are sometimes asked by Muslim mothers together with their daughters to issue the traditional virginity certificate, but more often the daughters turn up unaccompanied. They know that they have lost their virginity, and want a repair job. Or they are better informed than girls in their home countries, and realize that they have no guarantee that they will bleed, even if they are virgins. In Morocco, there are many proven ways to increase the loss of blood. Soumaya

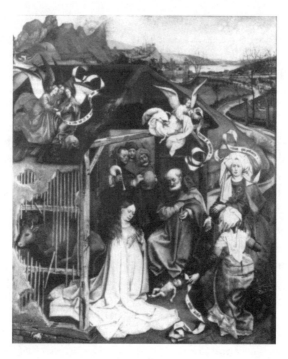

9 Robert
Campin, *The
Birth of Jesus*,
panel,
1420-25.

Naamane-Guessous quotes the fifteenth-century writer Suyuti, who listed nine of them. Ox bile in a ball of cotton wool imitates blood, but a suppository made of the plant silene is more effective. It irritates the vaginal wall so much that even the slightest touch will make it bleed. Men are not entirely ignorant of these tricks, of course, and Suyuti also mentions methods whereby a man can test his suspicions. Thus if a clove of garlic is pierced with a pin and then placed in the vagina, then in a virgin the smell of garlic will not be noticeable from outside.

Arnaldo de Villanova was an Italian monk who obviously enjoyed telling stories about his female compatriots.[22] At the time (about 1500), betrothals seemed to go on forever, and if the husband was engaged in commerce, long periods of separation were often unavoidable. Arnaldo describes at some length the mechanical means lonely women used to still their sexual appetite. He is not very keen on adultery, and welcomes the fact that the fear of unwanted pregnancies is bound to restrain many women. But even the bride who has been deflowered with a dildo must pretend that she is a virgin to her bridegroom. Neapolitan women would use leeches for that purpose, as we are told in the *Trotula*, the most influential compendium of women's medicine in mediaeval Europe. It first appeared in Salerno in the eleventh century and consists of a series of texts believed to have been contributed by one or more female physicians, including the perhaps mythical Trotula. In her 'De curis mulierum' (On the treatment of women), she writes:

> What is better is if the following is done one night before she is married: let her place leeches in the vagina (but take care that they do not go too far in) so that blood comes out and is converted into a little clot. And thus the man will be deceived by the effusion of blood.[23]

That method is also mentioned by Tannahill in her account of practices in nineteenth-century London brothels.[24] Some of these brothels employed a physician who signed certificates of virginity. Prostitutes used small bags of blood introduced beforehand; substances were squirted in that had a mordant effect on the wall of the vagina. There were surgical interventions as well. Tannahill also tells us that in Tokyo a 'rebirth of the hymen' ceremony was quite common during the 1920s, because 80 per cent of Japanese men wanted to have a virgin for their bride. To that end, plastic surgeons sewed a piece of sheep's intestine into the vagina shortly before the wedding day.

Good clinical practice for Dutch physicians implies discussing the various possibilities with girls who ask them to restore their virginity.[25] What has she thought of doing herself, and is her fiancé prepared to join in the deception? The latter is usually responsible for the fact that the girl's hymen is no longer intact. No doubt the deception often involves the use of chicken blood or a small cut in the finger. If the girl is on the pill, she will easily be able to produce her withdrawal bleeding on the wedding day. But some brides insist on a restorative operation, and sometimes the partner also insists on it, even though he knows that the girl is no longer a virgin.

According to gynaecologist W. M. Huisman, two methods can be used for the restoration of virginity. If the woman can visit the clinic shortly before her wedding day, the vaginal wall just inside the hymen can be stitched from left to right, so that upon entry of the penis the suture must tear the mucous membrane on one of the two sides. In a more drastic operation, the mucous membrane is folded in a double layer at the level of the hymen, turning into a kind of flap. With both methods there is, however, no guarantee that there will be bleeding. This type of intervention requires from most Western doctors a degree of detachment, because it means collaborating in the preservation of a culture in which women always come off worst and in which virginity in daughters (and chastity in wives) are undoubtedly the main pillars of family honour. Where these attributes are so revered, it seems obvious there will be gossip, and where there is doubt, women have to undergo the most humiliating practices to protect their honour:

The members of my family who live in the countryside said I was no longer a virgin because I lived in the town, where all the girls are wanton. My mother then called in two 'ârifates who spread my legs in the full light and in the presence of my grandmother. They testified that my maidenhead was intact . . . I was terrified that they might discover that I had already had superficial contact, but they never noticed that detail. All they were interested in was my maidenhead.[26]

By superficial contact, this girl probably referred to the method known as the 'brush stroke', by which the penis is moved, not in, but across the vagina. The girl was clearly convinced that an expert could tell that she had permitted 'brush strokes', and that makes her story all the more poignant. 'Ârifates are females employed by the ministry of the interior with special powers to issue sworn virginity certificates. It is assumed that their expertise also extends to judging the colour of the mucous membranes, and that the friction produced by a male organ, or contact with sperm, causes the mucous membranes to grow darker.

In KwaZulu-Natal a different standard is applied. Here there is a centuries-old virginity ritual that has recently been advocated most strongly as a means of preventing the spread of AIDS.[27] Every month there are ceremonies at which thousands of young girls wear their traditional virginity skirts. They undress and are examined by *amaquik-iza,* slightly older girls who, though they have boyfriends, have not yet had intercourse with them. These 'virginity inspectors' are government-trained and will receive a very official-looking certificate. This ritual might be described as a form of peer education, and the traditional message it proclaims is that, if you have contact with the opposite sex, the two of you may permit each other quite a few pleasures but penetration is strictly for after marriage.

Western doctors do not usually look all that closely at the female sex organs. Following cases of rape, they are sometimes asked to pronounce on the nature of the injuries as part of the legal proceedings. Pain during intercourse is the only reason for making a detailed examination of the opening of the vagina, and the doctor's diagnostic work always reconciles the patient's story with the visible signs of violent interference. Only in very young children does one sometimes have to let the picture speak for itself. Paediatricians know that they have to be extremely careful with their opinion in such matters.

The man who can initiate us into quite a few 'genital details' is Robert Latou Dickinson. This American gynaecologist studied his own patients as well as the bodies of the dead with great application and endless patience. The second edition of his magnum opus, *Human*

Sexual Anatomy, was published in 1949, when he was nearly 90 years old. In his view, the essential contribution of an anatomist lies in making anatomical drawings, and his book is a true delight to behold. He provides overwhelming proof that there is an enormous variation in shape, but his attempts to interpret that variation are not always wholly convincing.

His aim was to be just that. He patently began his work in the expectation that after lifelong study the observer must, like a kind of Sherlock Holmes, be able to tell someone's sexual curriculum vitae from their genital anatomy. By the end of his life, however, he realized that he had been chasing an illusion and he emphasized that every interpretation of the anatomical picture must be in part determined by what the woman herself has to say about her experiences. In his drawings, this information is always included. Dickinson postulated that an intact but yielding hymen was usually the result of masturbation or of manual erotic approaches by a sexual partner; coitus would as a rule cause a tear in the hymen, because he assumed that coitus usually involves greater violence. He also looked for other signs of self-gratification, and gained the impression that certain observable facts can be attributed to masturbation. Growth and increased corrugation of the labia minora are two invariable results; he described the labia minora of woman who are sexually active (by masturbation or intercourse with a partner) as cockscombs. In virgins, this phenomenon is generally due to friction during masturbation. At the time, laymen claimed that masturbation led to enlargement of the clitoris, but Dickinson was unable to confirm that view.

In the course of the twentieth century, the belief that the development of juvenile into adult labia had a mechanical cause was challenged by doctors who attributed a greater and autonomous role to sex hormones. These had just been discovered, and their precise function had still to be established. The question, simply put, was: are there young women who are not yet interested in sex (no masturbation, no intercourse) but who nevertheless have what looks like fully adult genitalia after puberty? And conversely, are there sexually experienced women whose genital development does not take them far beyond the infantile state? These are real questions, to which the answer has not yet been given, and probably never will be, since medical research financers are unlikely to release funds for that purpose.

Dickinson was a practical man with a passion for observation, but he does not come across as a methodical investigator. Clearly, he himself did not always know exactly what to do with his observations. The pleasure his book continues to provide is predominantly visual.

The illustration reproduced here on page 81, for instance, shows that men and women have identical types of corrugation in the sexually sensitive areas. A charming observation, no doubt, but one that does not get us very far.

Back to the Muslim girls, who await their wedding night in fear and trepidation. Confusion threatens them on all sides. If a girl has never had intercourse and yet fails to bleed on the first night, where does that leave her? Undoubtedly there are some girls who, in their ignorance, conclude that they cannot be virgins. They are thus pre-destined to feel shame and be ostracized through no fault of their own. From infancy, daughters are watched over anxiously and given all sorts of nonsensical advice to prevent damage to their maidenhead. During physical exercise, they must not spread their legs too wide; under no circumstances must they shin up poles or slide down the banister . . . Some mothers watch their daughters with bulldog tenac-ity. The slightest irregularity in the menstrual cycle can cause utter panic. The girl's naked body may be scrutinized in the bathhouse for a whole range of ominous changes. At home, some mothers listen secretly when their daughters sit down to pass water. 'When a virgin pees, you can hear a sharp sound (psss) but if she isn't a virgin any more she makes a heavy sound (pshpsh),' according to one of the girls interviewed by Naamane-Guessous.

Many Turkish and Moroccan girls can accept the fact that they will marry a man their parents have chosen, but abduction remains a constant threat for them. In July 1999, the Dutch television network VARA showed 'The Turkish Bride', which told the story of a sixteen-year-old girl abducted by the family of a boy who wanted her for his bride against the wishes of her parents. She was freed by the police, and the kidnappers (the prospective bridegroom and his uncle) received gaol sentences. Three years later, the girl nevertheless mar-ried her abductor. Although she maintained before the camera that she had married for love (and her memory seemed to have complete-ly deserted her when it came to her earlier joy at being freed by the police), the programme left a nasty aftertaste. It appeared that, after what had happened to her, the girl had had no other way of saving her honour.

Turkish doctors are not in an enviable position either. They are often consulted by women who tell them all sorts of tales ('I landed on a fence with my legs apart'), and then ask for a restorative operation. Such an operation is illegal as well as morally objectionable, for it means the (generally male) doctor is colluding with the woman to perpetrate an extreme deception on a man. Should this become known,

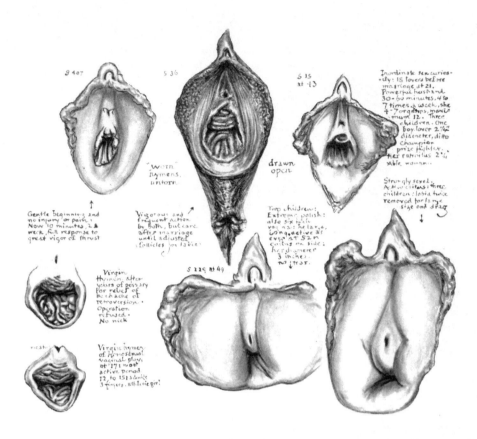

The handwritten annotations accompanying the illustration read:

♀ 4.07

5.36

"worn hymens, untorn."

Gentle beginning and no injury or pain: Now 10 minutes, 2 a week, full response to great vigor of thrust

Vigorous and frequent action by both, but care after marriage until adjusted (follicles on labia)

5.15 at 43

drawn open

Two children: Extreme polish: also six inch vagina: he large, congestive at every at 52 m coitus on side; her diameter 3 inches; no stress.

Inordinate sex curiosity: 18 lovers before marriage at 21. Powerful husband 30–60 minutes, 4 to 7 times a week, she 4–7 orgasms, maximum 12. Three children. One boy lover 2½" diameter, ditto champion prize fighter; her rami 2¼" sable woman.

Strongly sexed: Active clitoris: three children: labia twice removed for large size and drag

5.229 at 49

Virgin hymen, after years of pessary for relief of backache of retroversion. Operation refused. No nick

Virgin hymen of homosexual vaginal play, at 17, most active period 12 to 15: 3 days, 3 fingers; athletic girl!

10 Hymens stretched, nicked, worn and gone.

the doctor too will go in danger of his life. No wonder that the operation costs a fortune, five to twenty times as much as an abortion.[28]

W. M. Huisman tells an even more harrowing tale about a Moroccan girl raped by her uncle when she was thirteen.[29] She had returned to Morocco for the marriage of her sister, and when she took her sister into her confidence, she was urged never to tell their mother. It so happened that the sister had been raped by the same uncle, and when she had told her mother, the mother had laid the entire blame on the victim. Only a considerably older man could be found as a husband for the sister. Huisman's patient had got wind of her parents' plans to get her married off the next year, and she was terrified of disgracing her family because she was no longer a virgin (and might perhaps have to pay with her life because of it). She corresponded with Dr Huisman in deepest secrecy, to try to overcome her fear of visiting his surgery. Practically speaking, too, an appointment was not an easy option since all her comings and goings were kept under constant supervision. By the time she managed to make a visit to the clinic, a marriage had in fact been arranged for her. On a Friday afternoon, the

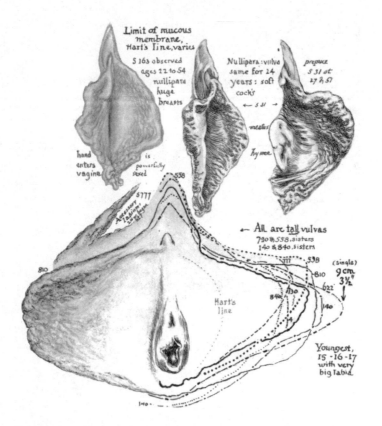

Limit of mucous
membrane,
Hart's line, varies

S 163 observed
ages 22 to 54
nullipara
huge
breasts

Nullipara : vulva
same for 14
years : soft
cock's

prepuce
S 31 at
27 & 57

← S 31 →

hand
enters
vagina

is
powerfully
sexed

meatus

hymen

558

S777

All are tall vulvas
730 & 558 .sisters
140 & 840 .sisters

Hart's
line

810

538

(single)
9 cm
3½"

810

622

730

140

840

Youngest,
15 - 16 -17
with very
big labia

140

11 Corrugated
minora in
fullest develop-
ment.

'quick method' (stitching up) was used on her. Next Saturday, she flew to Morocco, and months later a letter arrived from her through a girlfriend. 'You said that it might turn out to be painful. It was painful, not for me but for my husband. You also said it was not certain if I would bleed; I did bleed.'

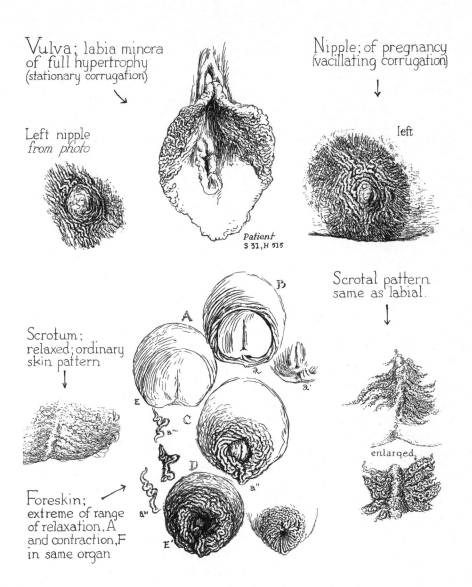

Vulva; labia minora
of full hypertrophy
(stationary corrugation)

Left nipple
from photo

Nipple; of pregnancy
(vacillating corrugation)

left

Patient
S 31, H 515

Scrotum;
relaxed; ordinary
skin pattern

Scrotal pattern
same as labial.

Foreskin;
extreme of range
of relaxation, A
and contraction, F
in same organ

enlarged

12 Various corrugations, but the pattern of the puckers is the same.

chapter six

The Power of Freudian Ideas

The Sleeping Beauty

She was too young for spinning silk,
this needled her; she lay as dead,
as was foretold in years gone by
when she imbibed her mother's milk.

But as befits a fairy tale,
enter Prince Willy, fair and wicked.
He reached the tower through the thicket,
and kissed her cheeks, so wan and pale.

Her parents, who were fast asleep,
must have heard her bedsprings creaking;
what they saw was beyond speaking.
They begged the Prince with anguish deep:

'Please don't quicken fresh young life, sir.
No more banging, just revive her!'[1]

Even without the double entendres of the poet Driek van Wissen (some
of which were unavoidably lost in translation), the tale of the Sleeping
Beauty is a poetical allusion to the destiny of a growing girl. The prince
on the white horse for whom she must wait remains a popular
metaphor. He comes from Mars, while she is destined to languish on
Venus.

Fairy tales and myths provide glimpses of our collective unconscious, but their certainties are in sharp conflict with the anatomical and
physiological facts. The previous chapters lead to just one conclusion:
ever since the Garden of Eden, men and women have had different

preferences in lovemaking, certainly when the woman places her own orgasm high on her list of priorities. Were we in a questionnaire to ask: 'Which do you find the *easiest* way to come to an orgasm?' we predict that, among male respondents, the sequence of preferences will be fairly uniform, with coitus indisputably in first place. The answer we might expect from women is much less certain. It might well be that no particular form of stimulation will score more than 30 per cent, though vaginal intercourse will certainly be defeated by oral and manual stimulation (by one's partner or oneself), and also perhaps by a vibrator. The conclusion: it is in the interest of men that in society's common perception of heterosexuality, coitus has become a synecdoche for sex, and it was only right and proper that the women's emancipation movement in the 1960s should have dwelled at such length on the question of what actually defines sex.

Here, feminism came up against a powerful bastion. The message that normal sex must necessarily lead to coitus and is thus essentially bound up with reproduction has been preached with great emphasis for centuries, for instance by the Christian church. In his encyclicals, the present Pope continues to stress that reproduction is the only righteous purpose of sexual intercourse. Forms of sex aimed solely at pleasure are sinful and delinquent and can be punished by death. That quite different views are possible had been known for a long time. The *Book of Conversations with Friends on the Intimate Relations Between Lovers in the Domain of the Science of Sexuality*, published in the twelfth century, was written by As-Samau'al ibn Yahya, a Jewish physician who had converted to Christianity.[2] The author admitted that some women obtain much greater pleasure from their clitoris than from coitus, which could only be explained by assuming that they had Sapphic tendencies. He drew a very flattering picture of this group: they were more intelligent and sophisticated than the average woman; they were erotically active and assertive, and they moved in elegant and culture-loving circles.

Psychology was quick to come up with its own interpretation of sexuality, and the new science, too, described all sexual acts that were not focused on penetration and reproduction as pathological or morbid. The word 'perversion' was introduced for these transgressions. In the late nineteenth century, when, following the extremely prudish Victorian period, there was a revival of positive interest in sex, the female orgasm became an important problem. Freud, the father of psychoanalysis, was well aware that many women failed to have an orgasm during coitus. It was his interpretation of that fact that has left its mark on women to this day. Freud did not merely point out that some women could be brought to orgasm by penile-vaginal contact while others could not, but added a value judgement in favour of the first group. His point of view is shared by many people and that is why we shall be examining clitoral and vaginal orgasms in some detail, together with a number of critical comments on Freud's approach.[3]

The clitoris–vagina dilemma is bound up with the psychological working-out of the difference between the sexes, and in Freud's psychology this process plays an important role in the development of the growing child. The discovery of the difference between the sexes is alarming for girls and boys alike: how is it possible that a girl should not have a willie, when every boy has one? This lack gives rise to penis envy in a girl; she wants that body part that you can hold in your hand when you stand up peeing. Daddy has got one, and her little brother as well. Mummy hasn't, but she has got breasts, and sometimes a baby in her belly. That is quite something; thus the daughter is at a disadvantage all along the line, so small wonder that she becomes acquainted with jealousy. Penis envy is born.

What happens next? The little girl turns against her mother. All her life, her mother has been the most powerful authority, so that if there is so great an injustice it is bound to be Mummy's fault. Her compensating desire becomes focused on her father, who has been a more absent figure throughout her life. He has a penis, and that is something she wants to keep close to. She may never have a willie, but a baby is something wonderful as well, and Daddy is certainly able to take care of that.

To complete the picture, let us now consider a boy during the same phase of life. When he realizes that there are human beings who have no penis, he gets a terrible fright. His logic (which is not yet very rational) tells him that that can only mean that he, too, could lose his willie. Why and how? It is bound to be a punishment for some terrible sin. Has he been a sinner then? Perhaps he has been too possessive about Mummy, and Daddy might be cross with him about that, because Mummy really belongs to Daddy. Might Daddy get cross enough to cut his son's willie off? Daddy still has his own willie while Mummy has not, so if anyone cuts off willies it's likely to be Daddy. Best to keep on his good side then, and to distance himself from Mummy. That is not easy, since all the good things in life so far have come from Mummy. He will have to force himself to withdraw from her, and his greatest aid in that is their sex difference. Thanks to his willie, he is quite different from Mummy, better in fact, and that is something he is pleased to recognize. He becomes an individual; he builds up strong boundaries around his ego. In the years to come he will be less able than his sister to empathize with other people. That makes him a bit like Daddy, so that is who he will identify himself with from now on.

But to return to the girl and her wrestling with sexuality. Freud was convinced that, by virtue of some primal knowledge, boys and girls had a picture of just one sex organ, the penis. If any information about female anatomy should come the girl's way, then that information would be about the vagina and not about the clitoris. That small organ, which she already possesses and which she may well have already played with on quite a few occasions because it gives her such lovely feelings, is never mentioned. What little knowledge filters through to her concerns the vagina, where later, with the help of a man and his penis, something very special will happen to her. Let's hope it is well worth waiting for; if she has had any experience of clitoral pleasure, she will henceforth suppress any inclination in that direction. Should she continue with (clitoral) masturbation, she must expect to be punished. It might even stop her from having babies! Woman's bisexuality calls for a clear choice (the word 'bisexuality' in psychoanalytical literature easily leads to confusion; it does not mean that women can love other women as well as men, but that they have the choice between a clitoral and a vaginal, a male and a female, sexuality).

According to Freud, it is only right and proper that women should suppress their clitoral sexuality. Clitoral lust is a childish form of sexuality, in which the little girl is actively fixated on herself, and hence in conflict with what she is expected to become. She has to overcome her aversion to boys, stop competing with them, and accept the fact that her pleasure will come from her surrender to a man and his penis. If she forgoes her clitoral satisfaction, her vaginal desire will grow automatically, and if a prince on a white horse should enter her life, she will see that *one* penis is enough to afford the highest pleasure to a man and woman alike. She will recognize her maturity once she is able to have orgasms during coitus. Her clitoris will have been superseded. She has grown into the kind of woman who, in Vienna in about 1900, satisfied all the demands of propriety – the type of woman who in Schnitzler's play *Reigen* (best known as *La Ronde* in the French film adaptation) may be seduced in six versions by any man who desires her.

His theory about infantile sexuality earned Freud great opprobrium in Viennese academic circles. In John Ford's film of Freud's life, the presentation of these ideas to a university audience was greeted with hisses and boos, and with demonstrative spitting on the floor. Yet their acceptance did not take very long. Ever since, such terms as 'castration anxiety', 'penis envy' and 'frigidity' have been part and parcel of the psychological terminology. There was a time when educated circles talked about 'clitorals' and 'vaginals' as blithely as we nowadays talk about extraverts and introverts.

By 'frigidity', orthodox Freudians still refer to the inability of women to achieve orgasm through coital stimulation. In everyday speech, the definition of 'frigidity' has been extended to lack of sexual desire, or downright aversion to physical contact. The word 'frigid' has become a term of abuse, a combination of all sorts of female attributes on which men are not very keen. Can Freud be blamed for that? In any case, his writings reflect the fact that he grew up in an age when a man could permit himself to make all sorts of contemptuous remarks about women with great assurance. In Freud's work we can recognize Nietzsche's dictum: 'Everything about woman is an enigma and everything about woman has one solution. It is called pregnancy.'[4]

What are we to make of a woman who cannot have an orgasm during coitus, but responds passionately to clitoral stimulation? For Freud the answer was obvious: she has failed to accept her femininity, sticks to an active sexual role and has not succeeded in overcoming her jealousy of the primacy of male sexuality. In short, she suffers from a masculinity complex. Marie Bonaparte had this to say on the subject in 1933:

> . . . women, it appears, may be divided into three main types, each of which responds, in its own way, to the traumatic shock that every girl experiences on first realizing the difference between the sexes. The first type soon succeed in substituting the desire for the penis for that of a child, and become true women: normal, vaginal, maternal. The next abandon all competition with men as feeling themselves too unequal, renounce all hope of obtaining an external love object and, socially and psychically, achieve a status among humans like that of the workers in the anthill or hive. Lastly, there are those who deny reality and never accept it; these cling desperately to the psychical and organic male elements innate in all women: the masculinity complex and the clitoris.[5]

This last group is of course the most interesting to psychoanalysts. Karl Abraham has called them hysterics of the vengeful type. In literature, the model is Brunhild, Wotan's favourite and most belligerent daughter:

> Nevertheless, in many clitoridals of long date, successful analytic treatment remains difficult . . . Such *partial frigidity*, though limited in *vaginal anaesthesia*, has often a poorer prognosis than that for *total*

frigidity; . . . doubtless owing to the essentially hysterical nature of their inhibitions.

This partial form of frigidity, in my opinion, is not only the most obdurate to treatment, but also the most frequent. The number of women so afflicted is far greater than men think, given the dissimulation women generally practice to hide their deficiencies in the erotic sphere. Also, the manner in which women endure this kind of frigidity varies greatly from one to another. Some resign themselves as to a command from on high and are content, for consolation, to remold *all* women in their own image. According to many clitoridals, those who boast of the pleasure experienced with the male must be braggarts or liars, or at least exceptions.

Other clitoridals compensate their inferiority in the sexual act, obvious though it is, by a kind of pride in their condition. They never surrender to a mutual passion and remain 'independent' and aloof from the man; this enables them, at need, to be self-sufficient, in particular through masturbation, which is always possible to such women. Some clitoridals, however, more honest with themselves, are well aware how much they suffer.

That, if you like, is plain speaking, and, as we shall see, Marie Bonaparte knows it all so well because she is largely writing about herself. It is remarkable that so many female disciples of the founder of psychoanalysis should have developed his ideas so consistently, often writing about them in such blunt and indigestible terms. Thus Helene Deutsch has made much of female masochism, alleged to be inherent in the abandonment of active sexual objectives.[6] In her view, childbirth is the peak of female erotic pleasure. Freud always surrounded himself with a coterie of women who absolutely agreed with him that the weaker sex was inferior by virtue of the lack of a penis. To them, the penis was all that counted. 'Anatomy is fate', Freud had decreed.

For many years, the most prominent female objector to that view was Karen Horney. She had an open mind about the social influence to which both men and women were subjected. At the time, women were generally modest and obedient. That had nothing to do with their lack of a penis, but was due to their inferior social status. Horney came across penis envy too, but she considered it a pathological phenomenon and not an inevitable phase in the life of all women. And if some women felt envious of the male sex organ, how about men's envy of the female power to bear children? Horney and her successors tried to establish whether it was really true that only after turning their backs on the clitoris did girls find out about their vagina. There are all sorts of indications that very young girls experience vaginal excitation, stimulated by vaginal masturbation. And if both these organs can give rise to pleasure, what reason is there for always considering them separately? 'And I do not see why . . . it should not be conceded that the clitoris legitimately belongs to and forms an integral part of the female genital apparatus.' Is she also trying to suggest that there is no reason to make so much fuss about women who resort to clitoral stimulation if they want an orgasm? She does not say that in so many words, but she implies that 'frigidity' is so common that psychoanalysts should stop considering the condition pathological, if only for methodological reasons.

Horney's remained a voice crying in the wilderness. We have some difficulty in understanding why this controversy was so violent, but then quite a few deeply rooted convictions held at the time have come to seem very strange to us. From 1910 to 1912, the Wednesday night meetings held in Freud's house revolved explicitly round the harmfulness of masturbation (in men), and the question of whether masturbation led to neurasthenia.[7] At the time, neurasthenia was considered a disorder of the nervous system, characterized as degeneration. In contrast, the neuroses were considered to be psychical exhaustion caused by stresses of an infantile origin. Masturbation could naturally lead to neurotic misery when it produced all sorts of negative feelings. Freud, however, maintained that, though masturbation sometimes helped to reduce tensions, it nevertheless caused nervous debility. In that respect, his views were still close to those of Tissot, the remorseless eighteenth-century opponent of masturbation, whose main work, *Onanism, a treatise on the diseases caused by masturbation,* was a worldwide bestseller in its day.[8] One of the dangers of masturbation, according to Tissot, was withering of the spinal cord, which is a diagnostic description familiar to neurasthenia. In the circle round Freud, Wilhelm Stekel was the only defender of the innocence of masturbation. His persistent attitude led to his exclusion in 1912 and to his resignation as editor-in-chief of the *Zentralblatt für Psychoanalyse.* Anyone championing the clitoris in those years was thought implicitly to be defending adult masturbation, or lesbian love, for at the time no one could imagine how clitoral love between a man and a woman could be possible. That, too, we read in Tissot. When he deals with clitoral self-abuse, like As-Samau'al ibn Yahya, it inevitably ends up with lesbianism.[9]

Outside the world of psychoanalysis, too, there was the firm conviction that the male makes an essential contribution to the female orgasm. Thus we can read in *Ideal Marriage*, the international bestseller published by the gynaecologist Theodore-H. van de Velde in 1923:

> . . . then we must, for a start, recall to mind that the orgasm, and everything connected with it, physically or mentally, can occur without ejaculation by the man. Thus a highly responsive woman may have more than one orgasm before her less sensitive spouse has reached his own climax.
>
> While that is an incontrovertible fact, it is no less certain that in normal intercourse the ejaculation of sperm is the most important factor in the orgiastic satisfaction of a woman.

This is a remarkable illustration of how observation can be overruled by archaic certainties. Van de Velde was a declared opponent of coitus interruptus, because it robbed women of their strongest orgasmic stimulus.

Freud's influence also had a lasting effect on the more fashionable advocates of psychoanalysis. Freud's most prodigal son was Wilhelm Reich. Reich's social involvement led him to Marxism at an early age. In later years he 'was dragged into the black ooze of occultism', with sectarianism, strange life-threatening experiments with radioactivity, insanity, and a lonely death in prison as a tragic outcome. Alexander Lowen continued along Reich's original lines and became the founder of bioenergetics, which continues to be a popular neo-Freudian form of therapy, involving work not only with words but also the use of body language.

Bioenergetics has always had a great appeal for women therapists. However, this movement too is dominated by men, and the women knew that they must never utter the c-word.[10] Lowen enjoined men to refrain from trying to control their orgasmic discharges, and to surrender unreservedly to their instinctive core. Women, provided they had surmounted their masculinity complex, would be dragged along willy-nilly by the tumultuous force of the male libido. At the same time, Lowen told women that multiple orgasms were a fable, and that women who thought they had them had in fact no more than superficial genital reactions (he must have been unaware of what Teiresias had told Zeus and Hera). In 1975, women for the first time held a separate meeting. It should be stressed that this took place well after Masters and Johnson had made the results of their physiological studies known all over the world, once again giving a prominent place to the role of the clitoris. In their anonymous replies to a questionnaire by Alice Kahn Ladas, women bioenergeticists (all of whom had undergone analytical therapy) dared at long last to admit that their clitoris continued to be an important seat of pleasurable stimulation, even during coitus. At the same time, they challenged Lowen's pronouncement on multiple orgasms. And there were countless respondents who refused to be fooled into believing that their multiple orgasms were of an inferior kind.

Shortly after the enquiry, Alice Kahn Ladas came into contact with two doctors, Beverley Whipple and John Perry, which rekindled her interest in vaginal sensitivity and culminated in a theory about the G-spot. A vaginal locus of non-clitoral orgasms had at last been discovered. It must have been a bitter pill for Freudians to learn that the penis was not at all suited to G-spot stimulation. Phallocracy was being assailed from all sides.

Even Helene Deutsch, perhaps Freud's staunchest woman disciple, had to concede at the end of her career that Freud's orgasm theory had a fundamental flaw.[11] Everyone had meanwhile come to appreciate the fact that a clitoral woman could rarely if ever be made to have vaginal orgasms by psychoanalytical treatment, even once all her conflicts and anxieties had been settled. Even more confusing was the fact that some women of the Brunhild type proved to be intensely vaginal. Something was clearly wrong. Freud had meanwhile died. Would Deutsch have dared to oppose him so vigorously had he still been alive?

Orgasm wars

Not everyone is as obsessed with the intricacies of the female orgasm as psychoanalysts are. Some women think that having an orgasm is very important; others are to some extent indifferent to them. However, if women have sex with their partners, then orgasms play a significant part in the relationship. In particular, if the partner is a man, the woman's orgasm can become an area of conflict. Some men look on their partner's orgasm as a reward for excellent behaviour, much as their teacher's good marks in their school exercise book used to be her seal of approval. If *she* fails to come over the threshold, then *he* can never be sure about his prowess as a lover. In couples, an orgasm can be experienced as a present to each other, but for some women it feels a little like ransom money.

Female bisexuality can be extremely confusing for a man. Thirty years ago, a friend confided his regrets about a brief relationship to me. His girlfriend had an insatiable longing for vaginal sensations. She liked best to straddle him, when his penis in her vagina afforded her an ecstatic, unconfined sense of euphoria, 'like a baby's at its mother's breast', as she put it. However, he had discovered that if he pulled her forward so that her clitoris was pressed against his pubic bone, she would be overcome by an animalistic spasm that ended in a noisy orgasm within a minute. Not just once either: he had counted ten orgasms in less than half an hour on one such occasion. He felt like a little boy with a new Dinky toy. She was angry, and broke off the relationship, because, she said, he begrudged her the best part of her lovemaking.

Man's own desires led to the invention of simulated orgasms. Anja Meulenbelt, a feminist leader in the Netherlands in the 1960s, always brought the sexual element up for discussion. In one of her consciousness-raising groups she asked those present if they had ever faked an orgasm, and a large majority raised their hands. Her aim, of course, was to make everyone resolve firmly never again to yield to macho pressure (as those who had raised their hands obviously intended to do), but among those women who did not raise their hand, there were quite a few who were thinking, how clever, and what an idiot I am not to have thought of doing it myself. The trick was nothing new. In 1848, Auguste Debay published his *Hygiène du mariage*, in which he advised women to fake orgasms 'because men love to share their own pleasure'.[12] In the 1950s, Eustace Chesser's *Love Without Fear* was one of the most popular sex-education texts. In it we can read:

> Both [partners] should play their parts. And here it should be noted that *simulation of orgasm* is within the power of any intelligent woman. Eve, who proves so adept in the practice of feminine arts which harmlessly deceive the male, can, once her eyes are opened to the need, simulate orgasm so well that it is almost impossible for the man to detect that genuine orgasm has not occurred![13]

In 1992, he was commended in *Cosmopolitan* magazine, the (woman) writer of the article finding it unfair to withhold a reward from men who tried so hard to please their partners. That article in *Cosmopolitan* was quoted at length in the article 'Faking it. The story of "Ohh!"' by an Australian research group in the faculty of women's studies at Sydney University.[14] They interviewed small groups of women and men about fake orgasms, and concluded that satisfying women was tough work for the men. Luckily, they had their hands free, for their own pleasure was attained automatically – the male libido saw to that. In return, the women made it their business to shield the men from doubts about their technique. It is obvious that women can do so convincingly, for they all faked orgasms on occasion although almost all the men interviewed were certain they had never been fobbed off with a fake.

You can look on the faked orgasm as a product brought onto the market because there is an overwhelming demand for it. Anyone who has seen a pornographic film will no doubt have noticed that the orgasms of the actresses look extremely stereotyped, and certainly most unconvincing to female viewers. Commercial TV stations have produced documentaries giving titillating background information on this subject, and when the porn actresses interviewed are asked if their orgasms were real or faked, their answers vary a great deal. In the film *Broken Mirrors* by Marleen Gorris, first shown in 1984, a novice in a brothel is taught by a seasoned prostitute how to fake highly convincing orgasms with minimum effort:

> Coming off! All of them want you to come off. As if we had nothing else to do. So don't just lie flat on your back panting like a short-winded performing poodle, because they won't fall for that. They may be stupid but not that stupid. You could try saying, 'Well, I've come twice already today,' a bit sulky, a bit anxious, lots of batting of the eyelashes, 'and I don't really know if I'll be able to manage it again.' Well, he'll be banging away, and at just the right moment you hold your breath a bit (*she shows her how*), not too much, not too little, and you cry out 'oh', perhaps, gently for a moment, and there you are, he feels like the top bonker of Baghdad and you're in line for thirty quid extra.

Men have learned by now that they are occasionally taken for a ride. In the film *When Harry Met Sally* (1989) there is an unforgettable scene in which Sally cuts her friend Harry down to size. Harry has been boasting a bit; he knows for sure that no woman can fob him off with a fake orgasm. In response Sally, in the crowded restaurant in which the scene is set, produces a spontaneous orgasm, impressive and extremely noisy. In the silence that follows, as she sips her glass of wine contentedly, an elderly lady at the next table says to the waiter, 'I'll have what she's having!'

In the course of civilization we have strayed a long way from the sexual response cycle in which sexual behaviour is considered to be an automatic biological process. When two people make love, the process becomes complex and cultural aspects come to the fore. Actual experience is coloured by expectations, and both partners take the assumed expectations of the other into account. But there is in the male-female relationship in particular the danger of believing that one can tell the other's wishes, because 'all women/men like that'. The stereotypical picture is embedded in our language. We speak of 'foreplay', 'intercourse', 'climax', and 'after play', as if the importance of the various elements of intimate contact were the same for all people and fixed for all time. The media contribute to the survival of this idea. Every sexual encounter in a film will confirm the view that there is a natural inclination for penetration, as well as the expectation that the woman is so carried away by the dynamic force of the man that the two automatically climax together. Filmgoers are wont to extol the love scene in *Don't Look Now* (1973), which is exciting as well as exceptionally aesthetic. Although the woman is mainly on top and seems to dictate the rhythm and intensity of the act, this scene too fits into the classical sex scenario.

Two investigations illustrate particularly well how the orgasm 'works' in a relationship. At the end of the 1980s, Willeke Bezemer researched the relationship between sexuality and power aspects in heterosexual contacts.[15] The problems she looked at were of two kinds: women who suffered pain during intercourse and men with erection difficulties (both of them secondary, that is problems that were not present at the beginning of the relationship). Women with unexplained abdominal symptoms and men with addictions were then included in the experiment. It was quite an undertaking to recruit participants in this research; in the female abdominal pain group the researcher had to accept that it would prove impossible to persuade partners to collaborate. The question that interests us here is female orgasm. About half of the women had regular orgasms but only a quarter of the men had a clear picture of their wife's pattern. Thus 44 per cent of the men assumed that their bedfellow always had an orgasm, although this was true in only 19 per cent of the cases. Even when the woman never had an orgasm, there were husbands who took it for granted that their wives always climaxed.

Bezemer's research had a limited scope, but Gerda de Bruijn collected written information from many more women. In 1985, she wrote the bestseller *Making Love with a Man: Can It Really Be Done?*, but she had already contributed an article in 1983 to the *Journal of Sex and Marital Therapy* called 'From masturbation to orgasm with a partner: how some women bridge the gap – and why others don't'. The first thing to emerge from her research was the effect of the woman's attitude when she fails to have an orgasm: it is because at that particular moment she feels no need to have one. If the woman is bent on having an orgasm, then most will see to it that their lover does something with her that is not too unlike what she herself would do if she were masturbating alone. That often means finger and tongue stimulation rather than penetration, but if penetration is appealing to her then the classical copulatory movement (in and out, up and down, piston-like) is not very effective. Women who do climax readily during penetration often move in a more or less circular way, which means that friction is applied to the labial and clitoral area. Ask random subjects for a definition of intercourse, and you will generally get a formulation in which 'the penis moves inside the vagina'. It is very unusual to define intercourse as a movement of the vagina round the penis, but for some couples that is a more appropriate description. In this method of lovemaking too, time is always an important factor. In general, every woman needs about five minutes with every form of stimulation, and many women evidently find it difficult to ask for that time. There is a certain pattern that De Bruijn herself was told about, but that is also found in the literature. What is well known to be most effective for the woman (that is, enabling her to climax most easily) is judged by both partners to be part of foreplay. This means that at about the time that her orgasm is close, the main course is served, and the chance is missed. Some women realize full well how this works, but do not dare to ask their lovers at the crucial moment to go on until she has had her satisfaction.

De Bruijn concluded that the pattern shown in films (the man moves, in and out, and the woman follows his movements) does not work for most women. There are, however, women for whom that is indeed the most pleasurable approach, and it is in this group that intimacy, feelings of love, surrender and of being engrossed by the other are felt to be essential. De Bruijn ended her article, rather philosophically, with the assumption that most relationships are simply not good enough, not respectful enough, nor equal enough to attain the classical ideal. That is due not only to the individual man or woman, but to our entire culture. In her opinion, neither psychology nor sexology have much reason to be proud of their contributions.

In Taiwan the clash of the sexes became a public spectacle in an unusual way during the early months of 2002, when a tabloid circulated a secretly-taken video of an adulterous affair involving the ex-lover of the mayor of Hsingchu. The suspicion was that the dumped mayor had had mini-cameras installed as an act of revenge. Men were unanimous in finding the first 20 minutes of the video tedious and boring, while women breathlessly enjoyed watching the foreplay they had always yearned for but never experienced. For weeks on end millions of Taiwanese had scarcely any other subject of conversation. Never before had the conflicts of interest between men and women been so clearly expressed.

I do not know if many men have read De Bruijn's book. Whenever I recommended it to my patients, I noticed that they had great difficulty with the message. For men in general the motto 'When sex is good, it's great; when sex is bad, it's still pretty good' holds. If good sex for women is so much more dependent on a good relationship, then mediocre sex becomes far more distressing. Conversely, if you doubt the vitality of your relationship, you can always reassure yourself by making a success of your sex life. Some men try to do a little bit better in bed, and if they succeed in 'giving' her an orgasm that can be interpreted as: 'In that case, it can't be so bad with us after all.' There are women who climax easily, but who are not really happy about that in a shaky relationship. They know that their orgasm is a reason for their partner not to take their complaints seriously. They feel somewhat betrayed by their orgiastic powers. Some women have had unwanted, forced orgasms during sexual abuse. In therapies aimed at coping with sexual abuse the betrayal by one's own body is often the most painful part of the process.

Marie Bonaparte

Let us return to the psychoanalysts. Karen Horney could not earn Freud's approval, despite the fact that he fully accepted that the inferiority of women also had social roots. Marie Bonaparte held a special place in his heart, despite her rather nonconformist research into the vaginal orgasm. Her interest in this subject had a tragic side, and her life story makes *Dallas* and *Dynasty* pale into insignificance.[16] It is all too interesting not to examine it in some detail.

Marie's great-grandfather was Napoleon Bonaparte's oldest brother. In the years following the French Revolution, he used his position as president of the Council of Five Hundred to make his brother a consul. Then, while foreign minister and ambassador to Madrid, he was able to amass a considerable fortune. An affair leading to a secret marriage earned him Napoleon's displeasure, but by then he could afford to live in Italy in grand style. Napoleon then offered him the Italian crown on condition he agreed that his wife and children would not inherit the royal title. That was a blow below the belt, but other noble titles could be acquired for money. Thus the Pope had inherited a barony from the Farnese family that he upgraded into a princedom, of Canino.

Of the prince's large family (ten children from two marriages), Marie's grandfather Pierre was unquestionably the wildest. By the age of thirteen he had been involved in a knife fight and when he was fifteen he was thrown into gaol for supporting an illegal liberal movement. Following military adventures in South America, where he caught a tropical disease, he returned to Italy, only to be sentenced to death for killing an officer in connection with a plot against the Pope. The sentence was commuted into lifelong exile. After further peregrinations, he ended up leading the life of a country gentleman in the Belgian Ardennes. Hunting and women were his main preoccupations.

In 1848, the time was ripe for a return to Paris, where it even seemed that a political career was in store for him. After the death of his first wife, he secretly married Nina, the daughter of a Corsican brass manufacturer. Their first child was a boy, whom they called Roland, the name chosen for him telling us something about the hopes his father had invested in him. After Pierre had again committed murder, this time at the age of 57 (the victim was a journalist who had acted as second to a man Pierre had challenged to a duel), he was again banished to Belgium. Nina moved to England because she could not bear seeing her children treated as bastards and hence prevented from bearing the name of Bonaparte and their princely titles. One year later, the succession was settled in their favour.

In Marie's eyes, Grandmother Nina was the true phallic woman, one who took complete charge of her son's life. She found the ideal marriage partner for him, Marie-Felix Blanc, the immensely rich daughter of a stock-exchange speculator who, after being sentenced for insider dealing, multiplied his fortune by running a number of casinos. The wedding day was a scandalous affair; the bride's parents and countless guests waited in vain for bride and groom, who, on the initiative of the bridegroom's mother, had staged a kind of elopement to Nina's country house. The observation of convention between the nobility and the nouveau-riches clearly lacked subtlety in those days. Marie-Felix saw little of her husband, and under pressure from her mother-in-law quickly agreed to make a will leaving all her possessions to him. Marie-Felix died within two years of her wedding from the effects of her first confinement. Nina congratulated her son on this remarkable stroke of luck. There were rumours that both grandmother and father had had a hand in Marie-Felix's untimely demise, something of which Marie, the daughter, was well aware.

She herself was looked after until her tenth birthday by a constantly changing stream of nursemaids, not least during the period when she was being treated for tuberculosis. From an early age, Marie filled innumerable exercise books with her writings. At a later age she published these childhood fantasies, including the interpretations she came up with during her analysis. Her early preoccupation with her mother's death and her grandfather's reputation led to a lifelong fascination with murderers. In 1921, she sat in the public gallery during the trial of Henri Landru, who was said to have married and murdered ten women, and in 1927, she produced a psychoanalytic study of a woman murderer who had baffled everybody with the apparent senselessness of her deed. Revulsion and admiration competed for precedence in Marie.

During the interwar years in France, incidentally, Marie was in good company. The surrealists glorified Violette Nozières, a Parisienne who had led a double life from an early age, being the ideal daughter by day and a man-eater at night. In 1933, she poisoned her father, which earned her the death sentence, though she was eventually reprieved. In 1978, Chabrol made a film about her, with Isabelle Huppert taking the leading part. Jacques Lacan, the figurehead of French psychoanalysis, was fascinated by the Papin sisters, who murdered their employer and her daughter in the most gruesome way, and who inspired Jean Genet's play Les Bonnes (The Maids). During the last years of Marie's life she became a vociferous opponent of the death penalty. When she was 77, she travelled to the United States to plead for the life of the murderer Caryl Chessman, and she was deeply disappointed when her efforts to save him proved unsuccessful.

All in all, Marie was an unhappy child, brought up in regal isolation and desperately longing for fatherly love. Her life was riddled with anxieties and feelings of inferiority. When she was only sixteen she was the victim of blackmail attempts by a secretary to whom she had written love letters. At the age of twenty-five she married a son of the Greek king who was also a prince of Denmark. Her husband was thirteen years her senior, and must have had a number of qualities compensating her for her father's neglect. Alas, he was involved with an older man, and although it is uncertain if the two had a homosexual relationship, the prince took little sexual interest in his wife. Marie, for her part, had a series of lovers, all of whom helped to introduce her to the worlds of science and art.

The princess's complexes were chiefly about her looks and her femininity. The crux of her perceived deficiency in this area was her inability to have orgasms in the 'normal' way. She had already had a number of plastic-surgery operations when she first met the Viennese gynaecologist Josef Halban, and together they developed a theory that radically challenged the prevailing psychoanalytical ideas. Her basic assumption was that no woman could ever expect a man to accept that his lover needed anything more than the usual up-and-down routine. On the other hand she was well aware that stimulation of the clitoris is the most powerful trigger for female orgasms. It could not be denied that something was wrong with the anatomical relations of the sexual parts.

In 1924, Marie Bonaparte, under the pseudonym A. E. Narjani, published the results of a study among two hundred Parisian and Viennese women in the journal Bruxelles-Médical. She had measured the distance from the glans of the clitoris to the opening of the urethra

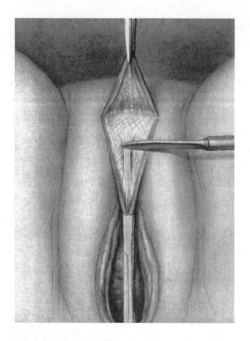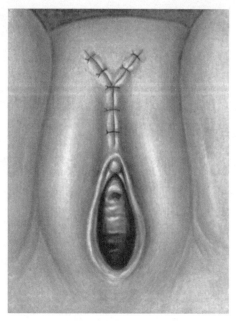

and found that this distance ranged from 1.25 to 3.5 cm. She divided the women into three groups: in the case of *paraclitoridie* the distance was smaller than 2.5cm, and she referred to distances greater than 2.5cm as *téléclitoridie*. She referred to a distance of precisely 2.5cm (10 per cent of her group) as *mesoclitoridie*. In one group of 43 women she had questioned about their sex life, all the women who had had orgasms by masturbation and not by coitus fell into the *téléclitoridian* category. There was a clear correlation of the distance between clitoris and urethra with body height, and Bonaparte suggested the possibility that the 'cold' reputation of Scandinavian women might well have a genetic cause. Anatomy is indeed destiny, but Halban believed that he could do something about it by surgery. In 1932, he published an account of *Klitorikathesis* in his *Gynäkologische Operationslehre*, from which the two drawings above are taken.

By cutting through the ligament by which the clitoris is attached to the pubic bone, the clitoris can be bent back, and the skin around it stitched tighter. Remarkably enough precisely the same skin incision is performed on men during operations, so hotly debated in the 1990s, to increase the length of the penis. In that case too the ligament is loosened. Halban tells us that, with two patients, he also shortened part of the labia minora, and that the mucous membrane between the clitoris and the outlet of the urethra can also be trimmed back in order to fix the position of the glans of the clitoris close to the opening of

13, 14
Relocation of the clitoris.
Left: Cutting the suspensory ligament of the clitoris. *Right*: The incision sutures. Position of clitoris after the operation.

the vagina. By the time he published his book, Halban had performed this operation five times, and he was careful not to commit himself as to its success.

It was not until 1949 that Bonaparte reported five such cases; we may take it that she was referring to the same women as Halban had treated. She had no follow-ups in two of the cases, and of two others she reported that they had more pleasurable sensations during coitus after the operation, but no vaginal orgasms. The fifth bitterly regretted her decision to have the operation and tried to get over her disappointment in a brief analysis. This woman had had the operation because she could only attain orgasm when straddling her partner during coitus, and that was not good enough for her. Bonaparte's psychoanalytical conclusion was that this woman's masculinity complex was exceptionally strong; in other words, she would only have been satisfied had the surgeon provided her with a penis.

The tragedy of the princess was that she herself had the operation, not just once, but three times, and without success. It was an embarrassment for the psychoanalytical community that every insider knew about this and also that she had these operations while she was being treated by Freud himself. The idea behind the operation must have been a repugnant form of primitivism for every psychoanalyst. While Freud did his utmost to rid her of her fixations and to get her to drop her active clitoral fixation, the patient herself was busy allowing an organ that she was expected to refrain from using to play the main role by means of a detour. And all that with a predictably poor result. Three times she denied Freud. During these years, Freud provided her with literature on clitoridectomy,[17] which we may consider a desperate and perhaps slightly sadistic effort to drive it home to her that even 'primitive' people realize that women must subdue their clitoris to attain full womanhood. In subsequent years the princess made a study of women who had had clitoridectomies. In one of her studies she does not conceal the surgical sin of her youth and humbly admits that her ideas were so many errors, and 'para-analytical' at that.

When precisely the cock crowed for her we do not know, or if she ever apologized to Freud for her betrayal. Her correspondence with Freud has only partly been published, and Marie's published letters were written during his last years, during which the princess made special efforts to get the old, ailing Jewish scholar safely out of fascist Austria and to London. Freud always held her in high regard. It was to her that he dared confess in a letter that he still did not know the answer to the pressing question 'Was will das Weib?' – what does woman want?

Since that time we have learnt a great deal more about Freud's life. And among other things we now know that he was not entirely opposed to fashionable but irrational treatments, for he himself underwent one of the rejuvenation cures that were popular at the time, namely Steinach's method, the subcutaneous division of the vas deferens. The idea behind this procedure is that sperm production on one side then stops, whereupon testosterone production increases.[18] The justification for this intervention seems to be just as dubious as that for clitoral displacement. It would be interesting to find out if Freud and Halban ever met and if they discussed the patients they had in common. Let us imagine an encounter in the foyer of the Burgtheater, during the première of one of the scandalous comedies of modern manners by Arthur Schnitzler. It would have been an awkward dialogue. Would Freud have dared to accuse his colleague openly of callously exploiting the problems of an unhappy woman? And what would Halban have replied?

Nor do we know if Halban proceeded with his clitoris-displacement operations. He reported five of these in 1932, and in 1949, as we saw, Bonaparte wrote about five women about whose operations she had been told. It may well be that both of them realized after these five operations that their theory was wrong. That would have testified to remarkably perceptive self-criticism on their part. Did Halban have any successors? At a World Sexology Congress in the 1980s an American researcher was conspicuously accompanied by his very beautiful, very taciturn wife. People whispered in the corridors that she had had an orgasm-enhancing operation. That had almost certainly not been Halban's work, but in 1983 the gynaecologist J. C. Burt and the psychiatrist A. R. Schramm published their experiences with an operation they called postero-lateral redirection extension vulvo-vaginoplasty. Their main criteria for performing the operation were recurrent bladder infections after coitus and deep sexual pain. The purpose of their surgical intervention was to change the angle of the vagina in the pelvis minor so that the thrusting penis would not rub so fiercely against the bladder floor. To that end, Burt stitched the labia minora together at the rear and tucked in part of the vaginal wall on either side. The result was, among other things, that the penis automatically came into closer contact with the clitoris, and there was a smaller chance of the glans penis coming up against the cervix. A negative consequence was that coitus from behind ('a tergo', as Freud called it) is almost impossible. To intensify the sexual impact even further, Burt combined the vaginal intervention with circumcision: he partly removed the prepuce of the clitoris.

Burt and Schramm spoke enthusiastically about the results: coital pain disappeared, there were no more bladder infections, and far less effort was needed to achieve an orgasm. Before the operation, three quarters of the women who had it admitted occasionally lying to their husbands about their orgasms; after the operation that proportion had shrunk to one half. The authors were true Freudians in the way they posed their questions: they asked which type of orgasm women would be prepared to give up, if they were forced to make a choice. The great majority of the satisfied patients (80 per cent) said they would give up clitoral orgasms. The psychiatrist Schramm had the impression that psychotherapy could not have made the same favourable impact on the feminine psyche and marital intimacy. Yet Burt's operation did not cause a great stir in sexology, and Burt himself was denounced in the press because he apparently performed his beneficial work on occasion without asking for the patient's consent.[19]

chapter seven

On Reproduction

At the beginning of this century, some anthropologists entertained the
public with claims that there were people, in Australia, for instance, or
in the Trobriand Islands, who did not know how children were made.
The role of the woman could not, of course, fail to be noticed, but that
of the man was said to be uncertain. Pregnancy was the result of a
woman having smoked a special fish on a fire, or having had a dream,
or having caught a bullfrog.[1]

Hans Ree, chess player and columnist, did not join in with the sniggering at primitive people. He admitted freely that the man's role in reproduction was so mysterious that few people could have thought it up for
themselves. 'Perhaps it's just a fairy tale handed down from mother to
daughter, one that everyone believes because it seems reasonable to
attribute some function to the man as well.' On the other hand, it is of
course remarkable that the Trobriand islanders were aware that animals
propagated their kind by sexual reproduction. The refusal to apply this
biological knowledge to human beings places mankind on a mythical
pedestal, nearer to the gods than to the beasts. In that framework, the
possibility of a virgin birth, for instance, has a spiritual function.

Ree tried to share these philosophical musings with the women who
would often assemble in his front room to discuss life and its problems:

> They are still childless and go on all the time about the ways in which
> this unseemly condition can be changed. For the sake of good manners
> I move the pieces about on the board while I listen to them. They talk
> about the new methods, such as the laboratory or the nice bystander
> who does not insist on lapsing into an old-fashioned role pattern. But
> most of them are living respectably with a man and talk about how they
> could just forget to take the pill without his noticing. That would seem
> to be quite easy; men never notice anything.

The men thus promoted to fatherhood might have worries about their future. Might fatherhood not interfere with their life's work on Babylonian weights and measures? But they'll come round all right, they always do. Ree himself, when he joins in their conversation towards the end of the pleasant get-together, has his perceptive observations smartly interrupted by

> the one who's the sweetest of them all, and very practical as well . . . : 'It would be nice to take you for a God, but you've completely forgotten that you've got an appointment tomorrow for a fertility test. Look, I've bought you a magazine, you can take that with you. And now please just go to the back room and play some chess, or look at some photos or something, because we still have a lot to discuss, and with that silly chitchat of yours we'll never get anywhere.'

In the twenty-first century, biological knowledge of reproduction seems to be reasonably complete. Even children are believed to be able to face the hard facts, so that all those old wives' tales about storks, cabbage patches and gooseberry bushes will finally come to an end. Ree assumes that spiritual needs may well keep some myths and mysteries alive, but most Catholics nowadays seem to be able to come up with a personal spiritual interpretation of their Saviour's virgin birth. Even so, one now and then hears tales suggesting that the subject of 'reproduction' can still lead to the strangest delusions.

Thus it was reported in September 1996 that British women could insure against fertilization by extraterrestrial beings. In the space of a week, 300 women took out this policy, and, encouraged by this success, the insurance company extended the cover to virgin conception by an act of God. The representative of the company let it be known that, partly as a result of the approaching new millennium, there were good reasons to expect a repetition of the New Testament story.

There is a kind of natural link between religiosity and naivety in this area, as countless folk tales bear out. A fourteenth-century German example was called *The Monk's Punishment*.[2] A young monk is initiated into the secrets of Venus by an experienced woman, and because of his clumsiness she adopts the upper position. The monk is rather worried the next morning and consults his servant:

> 'I have often heard that when a man and a woman have been together, children are born. But tell me, by your faith, which of the two bears the child?' – 'I will tell you everything,' replied the servant. 'It's the one underneath.' – 'Woe is me,' thought the monk, who was starting to

realise the extent of his misfortune. 'Alas,' he said to himself, 'whatever can I do? What a disaster! I was the one underneath. I'm going to have a baby! My honour is lost. And if the abbot notices, how will I live? For the monks will run me out. Death is better than their contempt.

In the recent past, sex educators in Dutch middle schools compiled a list of current misconceptions about fertility. Their comendable aim was the prevention of unwanted pregnancies with the help of factual knowledge. Adolescents 'knew' that you could not get pregnant the first time or if you 'did it' standing up. In the 1970s, girls had many good reasons for seeking reassurance, as reliable contraception had not yet become a matter of course. Nowadays, if a woman goes onto the pill – and she starts according to the instructions on the first day of menstruation – then she can count on perfect reliability from her first pill onwards. That piece of information has been printed regularly in all the leaflets for many years, and has been disseminated in the advice columns of girls' and women's magazines as well. Yet it transpires that there are still women who 'know' that the first month of being on the pill is not safe. Here the story seems to have been reversed: these women deny a certainty that they can absolutely count on. Perhaps some women find it intolerable that their precious fertility can be switched on and off so easily.

Some anthropological writers have doubts about whether fertilization is a single process. Is one ejaculation at the right moment all that is needed? The Gros Ventre American Indians of Montana and the Chiricahua Apaches of Arizona shared the conviction that several acts of coition were needed for a single conception.[3]

> When a man has intercourse with a woman, some of his blood (semen) enters her. But just a little goes in at the first time and not as much as the woman has in there. The child does not begin to develop yet because the woman's blood struggles against it. The woman's blood is against having the child; the man's blood is for it. When enough collects, the man's blood forces the baby to come.

Another Apache estimated that if a man and a woman had intercourse three times a week, it would take two to three months for the baby to be formed. But if a woman made love several times in one night, then it could of course take much less time.

A similar story with quite a different slant can be found in the *Decameron*. A man learns that his neighbour's wife is pregnant, and he also knows that the neighbour will be away on business for a considerable time. He puts on his most sympathetic expression and asks whether the woman is not afraid that the baby might be less than fully developed at birth. During the first few months of pregnancy, he tells her, intercourse is of great importance for completing the child's growth. The little ears in particular use up a lot of energy. The neighbour's wife gets into a panic and is only too happy to accept the man's offer to stand in temporarily for her husband. For nights on end, they work away fanatically on the little ears, until the husband eventually comes back home. The mother-to-be reproaches him bitterly, and the husband, who is less naïve than his young bride, is naturally outraged.

If we look critically at the many stories in which fertilization is said to be dependent on repeated coitus, then it becomes clear that the role of the man and his products is greatly overestimated. In the earliest medical writings, this bias was even more pronounced. There were times when men saw women as nothing more than the field in which the male seed could bear fruit. Hippocratic texts, however, made early reference to the union of male and female seeds as the source of new life.[4] Very graphic ideas on the subject were held, and one practical consequence was the presumption that conception was contingent on the woman's orgasm. That meant, among other things, that women who fell pregnant after being raped could not be telling the truth. They had clearly not been raped, but seduced, and were thus accomplices. This belief was very long-lived. Yet Averroës (Ibn Rushd, 1126–1198) had reported an early case history of a pregnancy that did not involve coitus but impregnation by sperm in warm bathwater.

The essentials of reproduction

Some women about to go on the pill are eager to know precisely how it works. They learn that there are three biological effects, each of which is fairly reliable in itself. First, ovulation is inhibited. Secondly, the uterine wall becomes inhospitable to fertilized eggs. Thirdly, the cervical mucus becomes less viscous, and so impenetrable to sperm cells. When doctors give this information to their female patients, it may be the first time that the women realize how complicated the reproductive process really is. Not every woman is interested in her own biological apparatus, and it is mainly those unlucky ones who, frustrated by their failure to conceive, find themselves compelled to look more closely at the subject. All the same, doctors are asked many questions that could be answered more comprehensively had the questioners a better knowledge of the basic facts of reproduction.

A woman's cycle has two phases. In the first, one ovum matures in the ovary. The resting ova are surrounded by a layer of covering cells that grow upon maturation into vesicles filled with fluid. These were first described by the physiologist and histologist Reinier de Graaf in 1672, and are named Graafian follicles after him. In the translation of his Latin work published thirteen years after his death, we read:

> In these I have observed something resembling small bladders, filled with water or an aqueous Moisture, sometimes yellowish, sometimes lighter and pellucid, and swollen.[5]

During the growing phase of the follicle, the three human oestrogens are the hormones present in the bloodstream in the highest concentration. In a four-week cycle, ovulation occurs on days fourteen, fifteen or sixteen (counted from the first day of menstruation). The lining of the follicle bursts – see the illustration overleaf for what follows[6] – and the ovum is expelled. Next, the emptied follicle grows into a solid yellow body, the corpus luteum, and the cells in it start to produce progesterone. If pregnancy occurs, then the corpus luteum remains active during the early phase. At around twelve weeks of pregnancy, production of progesterone is transferred from the corpus luteum to the placenta. In the absence of pregnancy, the function of the corpus luteum ceases during the next menstruation. The follicle degenerates and all that remains of it is a small scar in the ovary.

In human beings, ovulation is an autonomous process. This distinguishes us from rabbits and cats, which only ovulate when there is copulation. It is not absolutely certain that coitus has no influence on ovulation in humans. Thus it has been alleged that rape leads to an unusually high percentage of pregnancies, even when the chances of pregnancy ought to be small in accordance with the rule of periodic abstinence. German studies of this phenomenon go back to before 1950,[7] which means that the women examined were unable to opt for the morning-after pill.

Women differ widely in the extent to which they are aware of their own biological processes. Some women can feel when they are ovulating. Every month they have a slight abdominal cramp, and some are able to tell if ovulation that month has taken place in the left or the right ovary. Some women also suffer minimal blood loss from the cervix at the time of ovulation, usually referred to as mid-time spotting. Many women want to know as accurately as possible when their ovulation is taking place – sometimes because they want to get pregnant, but more often as part of periodic abstinence for contraceptive purposes. This method was formulated in a fairly reliable manner by Hermann Knaus and Kyusaku Ogino at the beginning of the twentieth century. According to them, temperature is the crucial indicator – in each cycle (provided an ovulation occurs, which does not always happen), the morning temperature rises slightly after ovulation. In other words, the oestrogenic phase has a somewhat lower temperature than the progestogenic. Peak oestrogen levels herald ovulation, and a slight rise in temperature for three consecutive days indicates that ovulation must have taken place shortly before. After the three days, sexual intercourse can be undertaken with a reasonable sense of security. Body temperature is, however, a fairly unreliable guide, because so many other factors can come into play, such as a virus or a disturbed night's sleep. For that reason another method, called Persona, has recently appeared on the market. Persona makes it possible to determine the hormone levels in urine at home, and then a small computer decides whether or not intercourse is safe.

Another observable cyclical factor is the consistency, or rather the viscosity, of the cervical mucus. A speculum inspection on the days preceding ovulation will reveal clear, transparent mucus running from the cervix. Fertility experts speak of red-carpet mucus, across which the sperm can make their gala entry. This is the kind of mucus in which spermatozoa can move readily, and women who are on the pill never produce such hospitable cervical mucus. This sign of fertility is easily detected by women; in developing countries the instruction to use periodic abstinence in conjunction with that sign is advocated as the simplest and cheapest contraceptive method. Most women will be able to tell the change in the discharge if they wipe themselves after urinating with toilet paper and examine the result. The most effective method goes like this: insert a finger deep into the vagina, find the cervix and wipe it. Press this finger lightly against a finger of the other hand and then move them apart. If a thread of mucus measuring a good 20 cm remains between your fingertips, you may take it that you are in your pre-ovulatory days.

Women can also infer the two-phase nature of the cycle from a number of other phenomena. Oestrogens are nice hormones by and large. They make people feel fit and happy, and sometimes amorous as well. As the progesterone level rises, more negative phenomena come to the fore. Some women experience fluid retention, which can often be told from the bathroom scale. Constipation is also common, and anyone with a tendency to acne can get very annoying spots during the last cycle days. Most complaints, however, are about mood changes: people become lethargic, down in the dumps, temperamental, weepy, argumentative, and so on. If the complaints are so severe that you can no longer func-

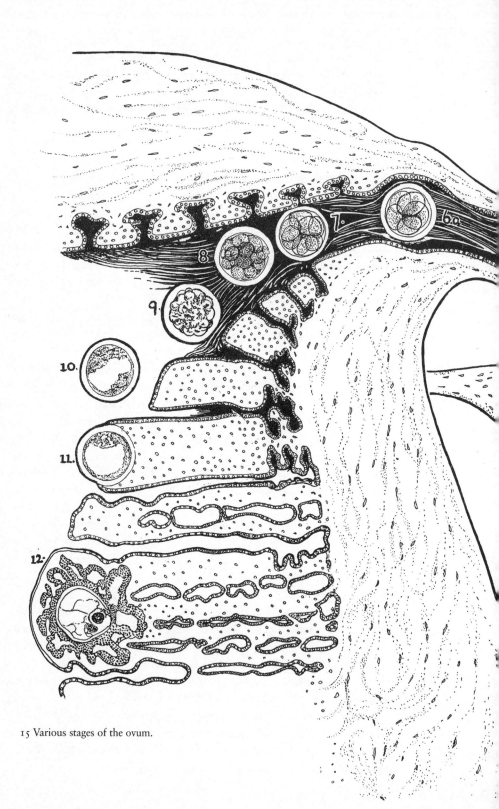

15 Various stages of the ovum.

1. Follicle bursts
2. Ovum with adherent granulose cells
3. Sperm penetrates ovum
4. Male and female nuclei
5. Fused nuclei; fertilization completed
6–7. First division
8. Morula stage

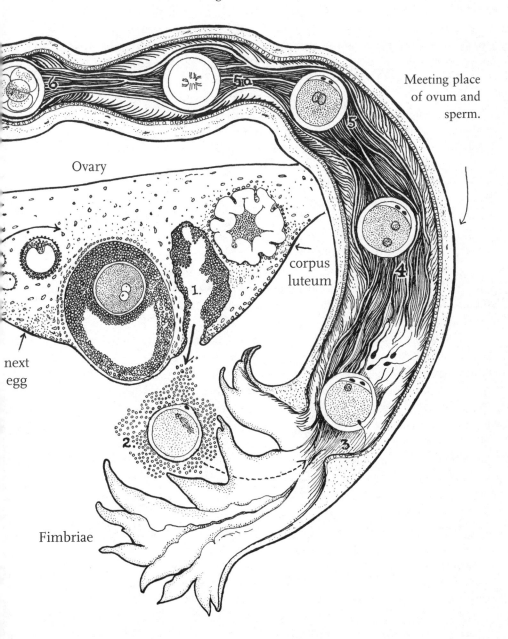

Meeting place of ovum and sperm.

Ovary

corpus luteum

next egg

Fimbriae

tion properly, you are said to suffer from 'pre-menstrual syndrome' (PMS).

Women thus release one, or at most two, ova every month. In men, the testicles are engaged in the continuous production of spermatozoa. Men do not have a menstrual cycle; at most one can speak of a diurnal cycle, inasmuch as the testosterone level is always highest in the morning. The sperm are produced in the testis, and allowed to mature a little longer in the epididymis. There they can be kept in good condition for a considerable period, and if no spermatozoa are released for a long time, they are broken down on the spot. The same thing happens after sterilization (vasectomy), when the way out is blocked. On the release of sperm, the muscles round the epididymis and the seminal duct (the vas deferens) contract, transporting the contents of the epididymis to the urethra. There, just below the bladder, lie the outlets of the prostate and of both seminal vesicles, and from there the glandular products are expelled rhythmically by contractions of the urethral muscle layer. Freshly released semen is not yet properly mixed; it can be compared to a newly laid egg, the white of which is also not of homogeneous composition. If the semen is collected in a small glass jar we see an aqueous, transparent substance, in which thicker, mucous and opaque parts can also be detected. If we examine it three minutes later, the fluid has been evenly mixed, thanks to the presence of an enzyme produced at the same time. When women are given instructions about self-insemination, they are always advised to wait a few minutes before introducing the semen, allowing dispersion to take place first.

While spermatozoa are still inside the body of the male, they do not have to provide any energy themselves but are forced out by the tubes. After arrival in the vagina, however, they have to rely on their own power (see illus. 16 for their route from testis to tube). The fertilizing sperm cell has to cover some fifteen further centimetres. It swims into the uterus via the cervix on its way to the oviducts, and only at the beginning of an oviduct – that is, close to the ovary – does fertilization take place. In a much-quoted study made in 1973,[8] D.S.F. Settlage introduced spermatozoa high in the vaginas of a number of women under an anaesthetic, and it was found it took just five minutes before the first sperms arrived in the ovary.

There has been endless speculation about whether the uterus itself contributes anything to speed with which the sperm reach their target. Medieval physicians intuitively described the uterus as a seed-slurping animal, but nowadays we can actually measure the activity of organs and these measurements give confusing results. As early as 1874, the

American gynaecologist Joseph Beck reported that he had seen the cervix of a prolapsed uterus making sucking movements during orgasm. In a diary entry that the American writer Mabel Loomis Todd made in 1875, she explained how she had tested her personal belief that orgasms affected the accessibility of her uterus.[9] She had instinctively felt that her uterus ceased to be accessible after orgasm, and hence asked her husband to postpone his ejaculation for several moments after her orgasm until she felt calm and satisfied. When she got out of bed, she felt reassured to feel a large quantity of her husband's semen spilling out. Nine months later, the birth of her daughter proved her wrong.

In the 1960s, C. A. Fox and his wife carried out a series of experiments in London. He was a physician and worked in an institute for medical technology. The Foxes acted as an experimental couple a number of times, and one of the measurements they made bore on intra-uterine pressure during coitus.[10] They first recorded an increase in pressure in her uterus during her orgasm, but a moment later a marked drop in pressure occurred. A few years ago, the biologists Robin Baker and Mark Bellis made a film using modern endoscopic methods, registering, inter alia, the movements of the uterus that might help fertilization.[11] The cervix, which during arousal is raised high, dips into the sperm pool after ejaculation. They fail to tell us if they made more than one observation. Results using just one couple do not of course carry great weight. Fox himself also knew that there were many families with a number of children in which the women did not experience any sexual pleasure. Moreover, D.S.F. Settlage has already shown that the transport of spermatozoa is also possible without involving any activity by the female anaesthetized body. On the other hand, intercourse for the express purpose of becoming pregnant naturally lends the process a quite different significance. In a Texan study of the nursing staff of a military hospital it appeared that the greater the wish to fall pregnant, the greater the chance of the woman having an orgasm after her partner's ejaculation.[12] This bore out Theodor van de Velde 70 years after he published his well-known book (referred to earlier), namely that the expulsion of the sperm towards the cervix is the strongest means of helping a woman to cross the orgiastic threshold. And evolutionary biologists will be inclined to assume, at least for the time being, that such behaviour must have sprung from the survival of the fittest and hence have proved its effectiveness.

The Gros Ventre Indian who believes that a woman's blood ('seed') struggles against conception and hence is in conflict with the male blood, is not entirely mistaken. The vaginal secretions are acidic, and therefore

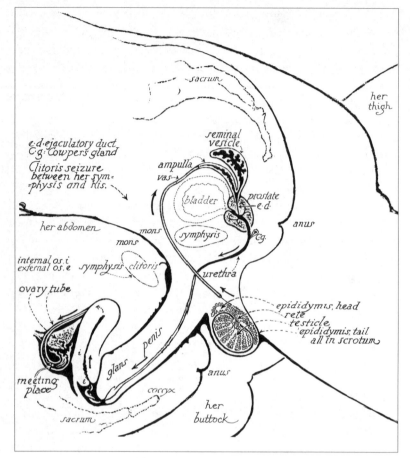

16 The route of the sperms from the testicle through seminal duct, urethra, vagina, uterus and tube, to meet the ovum.

a hostile environment for spermatozoa. Sperm thrive best in a neutral or slightly alkaline environment. Here the sexual response of the woman plays some part. When she is excited the vaginal pH rises (which means that the vagina becomes less acidic), because the extra fluid leaking through the wall has a diluting effect. Fertile sperm are moreover capable of neutralizing the contents of the vagina independently. Semen is a chemical buffer that retains a neutral pH for a considerable period of time. Spermatozoa thus have enough time to swim into the uterus, where the acidity is again safely neutral.

For women, the sperm effect on the acidity is not a boon. For hours after ejaculation her acidity remains altered, so that protection against the 'wrong' kind of microorganism is less effective. Extra vaginal fluid has to be produced to wash out the sperm. Women who are highly susceptible to vaginal infections often have the feeling that sperm is not good for them, though that is not a common reason for eschewing

17 The route
of the sperms
from testicle
to ovum.

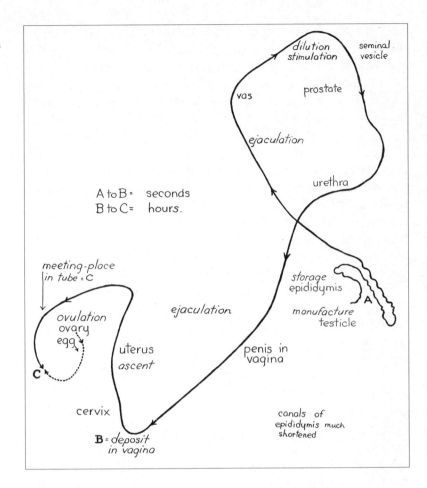

intravaginal ejaculation (that is, for using condoms, coitus interruptus or
non-coital sex). Yet the use of all sorts of vaginal medication could well
decline if women found it easier to ask for their partner's understanding
in this matter.

Spermatozoa can survive for a considerable time in the uterus
(and more particularly in the mucous glands of the cervix). The egg,
however, dies after ovulation if no fertilization takes place within
twelve hours. Any woman anxious to conceive should therefore realize that it is better to be a day or two too early than a few hours too
late. Just one sperm needs to enter the egg. Then a change takes place
in the egg wall as a result of which the fertilized egg becomes inaccessible to other sperm. Immediately upon fertilization a process of cell
division starts, and at about the time that the cell reaches the uterus
through the oviduct (the Fallopian tube), it has already become a
small lump of cells. The journey of the fertilized ovum through the

oviduct takes about three days and then in the uterine cavity again three days will pass before the amniotic sac surrounding the foetus makes contact with a suitable spot in the mucous membrane.

The endometrium (the inner wall of the uterus) grows considerably thicker during the first half of the cycle when oestrogen predominates (and the endometrium is said to be in the proliferation phase), an extensive system of tubular glands having developed in it. After ovulation, under the influence of increasing progesterone blood levels, the glandular structures enter the secretion phase. The uterine cavity needs to contain enough nourishment for the freely floating embryo, and the tubular glands supply this 'uterine milk'. On the sixth day, the embryo plunges into the endometrium, and then the intricate interaction between embryo and mother begins, leading to the development of the placenta. Through it, mother and child exchange oxygen, nutrients and the waste products of the foetal metabolism, but the placenta is also a producer of a large number of hormones and proteins. Pregnancy calls for ample progesterone, which is originally produced by the corpus luteum, but soon after implantation the placenta takes over. The exceptional growth of which the uterus is capable will also become clear after implantation.[13]

A minor miracle in the whole process is that the embryo is not attacked in utero by the woman's immune system. After all, half of the embryo's genetic material is not her own: if that woman were later to undergo a kidney transplant from her child, then every remedial measure would have to be taken to prevent rejection. The most common pathological symptom during pregnancy, high blood pressure, is probably due to an immunological reaction. In any case it is clear that it is during her first pregnancy that a woman runs the greatest risk of hypertension. In further pregnancies, the maternal body evidently becomes inured to foreign proteins. The complex of symptoms consisting of high blood pressure, oedema (swollen ankles) and protein in the urine is called toxicosis, and it can quickly get out of hand just before and during childbirth, with convulsions as the most frightening phenomenon. The medical term for this life-threatening condition is pre-eclampsia.

Recently, a Leiden research team tried to find an explanation for the striking blood-pressure differences during pregnancy and tested the hypothesis that some women are more successful in building up tolerance to their husband's proteins than others. They discovered a surprisingly high correlation with oral sex; in particular, when the woman is in the habit of swallowing her husband's semen her chances of having toxicosis are greatly reduced.[14] Most women are vaginally exposed to their partner's proteins on numerous occasions, and if this is not the case (for instance when donor sperm is used), then the risk of toxicosis is greater. However, other processes are involved after gastrointestinal ingestion, and tolerance develops more quickly after oral, than it does after vaginal, introduction of sperm.

Extra-uterine pregnancy is a relatively common exception to the usual pattern. It is astonishing that so many pregnancies should end up obligingly in the uterus, since both the egg and the sperm have free access to the abdominal cavity. The mechanism by which the fertilized egg nevertheless finds the correct path is not yet entirely clear. Medical literature gives some striking illustrations of the accuracy of our internal navigation system. A woman who has been deprived of her left ovary and her right oviduct (or vice versa) by an infection or an operation can still sometimes fall pregnant. There is the story of an ectopic pregnancy in part of the oviduct not connected to the uterus, close to an undescended ovary,[15] and thus much higher in the abdomen than where an ectopic pregnancy is normally found. Not many women will be aware that the millions of sperm cells searching for the ovum do not keep to the uterus but explore the entire abdominal cavity.

If the fertilized egg becomes implanted not in the uterus but earlier along its route, the oviduct is the usual site. The oviduct cannot, however, keep up with the embryo's growth. Sooner or later, there will be symptoms arising from the strain on the tissue. If blood vessels tear so that there is bleeding into the abdominal cavity, then an acute, life-threatening situation may well result.

Oddly enough, the most pathological situation, pregnancy in the abdominal cavity, is slightly less dangerous.[16] Although in that case too the placenta is formed on a substrate not designed for the purpose, such pregnancies can be brought to full term. The pregnant woman generally presents a number of symptoms that invariably call for surgical intervention, but in developing countries, in particular, the correct diagnosis is almost never made before the abdomen is opened. The search for a perforated appendix then suddenly turns into a Caesarean section. A child born as a result has a reasonably good chance of survival but congenital defects are quite common. The mother is in much greater danger, for how are the placenta and the foetal membranes to be removed? In the most favourable case the growth has invaded an organ that can be surgically removed (for instance the outer surface of the uterus, or the omentum majus, a fat-containing fold of peritoneum covering the intestines), but it sometimes has to be accepted that the placenta cannot be removed completely, which makes it feel like a time bomb.

The strangest discovery one can make is of a dead and mummified or calcified foetus in the abdominal cavity. In medical literature this is referred to as a lithopedion.[17] The patient shown in illus. 18 had advanced cervical cancer, and was psychotic when the x-ray was taken. Members of the family reported that she had been pregnant 28 years earlier and that the embryo had died in the uterus. Nothing else was known about her medical history at that time. Thirteen years before this x-ray plate was taken, an abdominal scan had shown something unusual, but the patient had refused treatment at the time. The possibility of bringing an abdominal pregnancy to term makes it theoretically possible that one day a man will be able to bear a child.

Wanted and unwanted

The course of fertilization is so complex that it is astonishing how easily most pregnancies come about. Unwanted pregnancies are sometimes the result of a woman's personal intuition that 'it' will not happen to her; some women have a completely unfounded personal conviction that they are not particularly fertile. On the other hand, doctors regularly dispense morning-after pills to panicking girls and women who actually have run extremely small risks. Unwanted pregnancies continue to be a highly emotive subject, though modern options have rendered the drama more manageable.

Abortion (and spontaneous miscarriage) has from ancient times been a subject familiar to medical science. Every doctor who takes the Hippocratic oath swears not to induce abortions. Elsewhere in the writings of Hippocrates, however, you will find advice for procuring a miscarriage, which is taken as proof that Hippocrates was not one person, but that the writings were collected over a long period by several scholars on the island of Kos. During the first half of the twentieth century, there was a whole series of tricks that a woman could resort to in order to bring about an abortion. She could, for instance, ride on the back seat of a friend's motorcycle across a railway track, or jump repeatedly off a chair. A very old report on this method of relying on the force of gravity can be found in Hippocrates' *The Diseases of Women*.[18]

The author was consulted by the owner of a highly-prized flute player, whose value would decline dramatically were she to be pregnant:

When I heard about it, I ordered her to kick her heels against her
buttocks. When she had already leapt for the seventh time, the seed

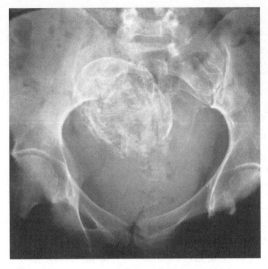

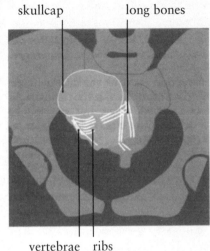

skullcap   long bones

vertebrae   ribs

18 x-ray
photo showing
an abdomen
with the calci-
fied foetus in
the right side of
the abdomen.

19 Drawing of
a mummified
foetus.

flowed down upon the ground and made a noise. The flute-girl looked at it and was surprised.

The girl had been keeping a careful eye on things, and the author gathered from her that the act of impregnation had taken place six days earlier. He described the product of this miscarriage as an egg with the hard shell peeled off.

Motives and methods change: the history of the morning-after pill is a good illustration of how fear of pregnancy has evolved. At first there was just one method: a prodigiously high dose of oestrogen on five successive days (in the early years it was a hundred times the daily oestrogen dose contained in the contraceptive pill of the time; at present there are pills containing just one two-hundred and fiftieth of that dose). So much oestrogen makes a person feel dreadful and most women were aware of that. A woman in need of a morning-after pill came into the consulting room looking positively green with misery, having previously weighed up carefully whether the risk really justified the step she was taking. In the 1970s an alternative was introduced in the United States, the 2x2 method, described by Dr Albert Yuzpe. Two old-fashioned (that is, high-dose) contraceptive pills are swallowed, and twelve hours later another two, the total hormone intake amounting to roughly that taken during one week on the pill. Most women are better able to tolerate that, and the image of the morning-after pill changed accordingly. Gradually the girls grew younger and the reasons for taking the pill less pressing. 'Going to get a morning-after pill' became scarcely more serious than buying a packet of chewing gum. The risks were sometimes wholly imaginary, and partly for that reason it took a long time before it became clear that the 2x2 method is only partly effective. Women at maximum risk (full unprotected intercourse in the pre-ovulatory days) continue to be at a considerable risk after 2x2, and, consequently, abortion clinics derive a certain percentage of their patients from failed morning-after pill treatment.

There was therefore good reason for taking the old method out of mothballs, but it is not easy to have to choose between a kill-or-cure remedy that works reasonably well and a less heavy-handed method that removes some but by no means all of the dangers. Most women had a hard time when, fully informed about the pros and cons of both methods, they had to choose one of the two. Since that time, most doctors in Dutch sexual health clinics got the impresion that women were more scrupulous in avoiding risk after their first morning-after pill experience. Which implied, as it was once metaphorically painted in a medical journal, a choice between blowing up ten trees at random because a bird was thought to be in one of them, and shaking the trees (perhaps chasing away nothing but spectres).[19] There has, however, been some good news about the morning-after pill. In 2000, a new method was put on the market, a 2x1 cure based exclusively on progesterone. It is, according to the American literature, almost as reliable as the 5x5 method, and has very few side-effects.

In morning-after consultations it always emerges that although most women have some knowledge about variations in fertility over their monthly cycle, they know practically nothing about the average chances of pregnancy. With completely unprotected sex on the day of ovulation, the chance is still less than 20 per cent, but most women come up with a much higher estimate. For couples waiting impatiently for a pregnancy, the limited chances of success are galling, so it is not at all surprising to find that over the centuries there should have been a desperate search for methods aimed at increasing the chances of fertilization. Some women, counting on help from the force of gravity, favour standing on their heads. A study in Montreal of women having undergone intrauterine insemination has shown that if they walked out of the clinic immediately after the intervention, the result was appreciably worse than when they were allowed to lie down for ten minutes.[20]

Perhaps other physical activities also interfere with the fertilization process. In his novel *The Prize Bull*, Esteban López describes the love life of Mink, a girl who never uses contraceptives and never falls pregnant because she invariably bursts out laughing when a man ejaculates inside her.[21] Occasionally a lover feels insulted by her reaction and if she then does her level best to control her laughter, she has coughing fits instead. This proves extremely annoying when she eventually decides that she would like to become pregnant. Her lover, the novel's narrator, then has the bright idea of roaring with laughter himself during his orgasm, and Mink is so taken aback by this that she forgets to laugh herself.

In the Middle Ages, there used to be lively conjecture about which coital position was the most conducive to reproduction.[22] Albertus Magnus maintained that when the couple lies side by side the sperm finds it harder to make its way to the uterus, and if the woman lies on top of the man, then the uterus is turned upside down, which surely works against conception. He preferred to remain ignorant about the whole business:

> Whether the man should lie underneath or on top, stand or sit, or whether the union should take place from the front or from the back . . . , such shameful matters would never be discussed, were it not that the strange stories one hears in the confessional nowadays force one so to do.

Pity the father confessors! How tragic that their office should force them to pester their sheep with such questions. For the Holy Roman Church, procreation is the only acceptable purpose of coitus, and for Albertus Magnus that meant that the above-named positions were against nature and hence sinful. St Thomas Aquinas was particularly interested in the hierarchy of sexual sins. If sex was patently the result of lust rather than the desire to procreate, then it was sinful, and so deviant positions, bestiality and homosexuality were all in the same category and had equally to be treated as punishable offences.

Rome still wrestles with this belief, which sometimes leads to hilarious situations. In 1987, the Sacred Congregation for the Doctrine of the Faith found that artificial insemination and IVF were forbidden to Catholics, even if the sperm was the husband's. The sticking point was less the medical intervention by which the sperm was conveyed to the right place as the impossibility of finding a sinless way of 'harvesting' the sperm. Plainly the assembled scribes realized that their point of view was at loggerheads with the clinical reality, and so the subject had to be mulled over until a way was found for running with the hare and hunting with the hounds.

Now consider this, and marvel. A well-known method of collecting sperm is sex with a condom (needless to say without the use of spermicides), but the condom is a contraceptive, that unholy invention, and has been proscribed by the Church. However, if a few holes are pricked in it, the condom is divested of its objectionable nature. The illusion that coitus with such a leaking condom might lead to a natural pregnancy is balm for the conscience. If the pricks are made carefully, there will certainly be enough sperm left over in the condom for the gynaecologists to do their job.[23]

Catholics also had their hands full with Theodor van de Velde, whose international best seller *The Ideal Marriage* came out in 1926. Van de Velde's aim was to pay sexual pleasure the attention it deserves, so the book was naturally placed on the Index in Rome. Pope Pius XI clearly had Van de Velde in mind with his encyclical *Casti Connubii*, which described certain approaches to marriage as 'perfect harlotry'. In 1929 Van de Velde wrote another book, entirely devoted to fertility in marriage, in which he set out in detail what coital positions he believed furthered or impeded fertilization. In the twenty-first century his arguments do not sound very convincing. His views have certainly not been verified empirically.

In general, we still do not know precisely why man, compared with other species, is so infertile. When couples are examined for infertility, no clear cause can be found in a great many cases, although the development of test-tube fertilization (in-vitro fertilization or IVF) has as a by-product brought many remarkable facts to light.

During the early years of IVF, doctors were prepared to take fairly drastic steps to increase the chances of success. The ovaries were stimulated with high doses of hormones in the attempt to harvest as many ova as possible. If the fusion of eggs and sperm led to three fertilized eggs, all three were implanted in the uterus, so that those early years were characterized by a large number of twins and triplets. This hormone treatment has many sorts of untoward side-effects, and in recent years a growing number of neonatologists have protested about the minimizing of the health problems associated with multiple births. Progressive IVF centres now advocate a return to the most natural form of IVF, which entails minimum intervention in the natural cycle and making do with just one egg per cycle.[24] In such cases, the woman is less laden with hormones, but for 'fine-tuning' she has to visit the clinic more frequently to undergo ultrasonic checks of the follicle size. This careful observation of the natural process has yielded new knowledge. Thus a long-term collaborative project between a Japanese private clinic and a Danish laboratory group has thrown fresh light on the influence of the corpus luteum on the developing egg.[25]

The Japanese were struck by the fact that an egg that was retrieved by puncturing an ovary that had been at rest during the previous cycle had a much better prognosis than an egg from an ovary that had also been active during the previous month. The follicular phase, that is, the growing phase of the egg, was shorter if it matured in an ovary that had missed a month. If the previous two ovulations had come from the other ovary, then the egg proved to be of the highest quality. The chances that the puncture would supply an egg in the first instance were greater, fertilization ensued in practically all cases, the first divisions ran a smoother course and there was an excellent chance that the egg would be implanted. The most obvious explanation is the following: if a follicle develops in the ovary that has also supplied the previous egg, then direct hormone influence from the nearby corpus luteum still continues at the beginning of follicle maturation. Age also plays a part: young women have a more reliable left-right alternation than older women.[26] Fukuda tested the hypothesis that the negative influence of a recent ovulation could also be eliminated by a short period of inhibited ovulation (say, by the contraceptive pill), and that study too provided encouraging results. His patients took the pill for two months, and the next, but it was especially the second month after that that the eggs available for IVF proved to be of the highest quality.

Fukuda's study has confirmed a vague suspicion that doctors working in birth-control clinics have harboured ever since the introduction of the pill. The first generation of pill users in particular was very afraid of fertility loss after stopping the pill, and it happens quite regularly that women, after going off the pill, have to wait for some time before their cycle is back to normal again. This problem, incidentally, occurs mainly in women whose menstrual cycle was already not particularly regular before they went on the pill. Of those women who returned to their old rhythm at once, we always had the impression that they were slightly more fertile than normal during those very first few months after stopping the pill.

Recent developments in the practice of IVF are likely to give critical observers the feeling that disproportionately heavy artillery is being used by a large group of gynaecologists. IVF is a field in which much glory and fame can be won, which may mislead those involved into using means and accepting risks that are not entirely in keeping with the objectives. Severino Antinori, the Italian embryologist, found a way of helping women who were long past the menopause to become pregnant (with the help of donor egg cells), and began to investigate the possibility of cloning in 2001. That takes him into competition with the Clonaid company, which is linked to the Raelian sect. In 2003, this sect circulated the news that cloned children had been born but failed to produce any evidence. The first uterus transplant was carried out in Saudi Arabia in 2002. After two months, the transplant had to be removed, but the organ had menstruated for two cycles! The authors stress that this operation can only be accepted in cultures unequivocally opposed to surrogate motherhood.[27] Clients, too, often work under the assumption that everything that can be done is always acceptable. In the feminist magazine *Opzij* of March 2000 the readers were introduced to a lesbian couple who planned to have two children using IVF. The fertilized egg of one of the women would first be implanted in the other, and next time it would be done the other way round. These plans were inspired by their desire to have children in a way that implies mutuality, and the two women considered going abroad for the purpose. Dutch IVF clinics were not prepared to meet their wishes. A later television documentary showed the same couple visiting a Flemish IVF clinic, but the Flemish specialists, too, had reservations about the project.

A fierce debate took place in the United States concerning the wishes of another lesbian couple. Both were deaf from birth and insisted on having a deaf child, to which end they deliberately sought a donor with the same hereditary form of deafness.

For couples wanting children, it would appear that no method is too demanding or too risky. Prepared as they are to do anything to get their way, they remain perhaps somewhat uncritical about their chances and postpone facing the inevitable for as long as they possibly can. That, too, is an old story. In his latest book on medical frauds and fallacies, Cees Renckens recounts the life and work of 'Dr' James Graham, who made the treatment of infertility his speciality.[28] From 1779 to 1784 he ran the 'Temple of Health' in Adelphi Terrace, just off the Strand in London. Graham offered advice on hygiene and provided mud baths, electric shocks and magnetization, but the holy of holies in his temple was the Celestial Bed. It was luxurious in form; 28 crystal pillars supported the canopy, and it also naturally incorporated a great many electric currents and magnetic fields. For a couple using the bed the highest form of ecstasy was attainable, so conception was assured. And so it should have been, since the use of the bed cost £100 a night.

More pragmatic was the method applied by Egyptian sheikhs and mullahs when infertile women applied to them for an amulet. Nawal el Saadawi heard tales about such amulets in Kafr Tahla, the village in which she was born, and gathered that many of them were nothing more than a small tuft of wool.[29] Women were told to carry the amulet about in the vagina, and it was claimed that many women did in fact fall pregnant soon after they did so. El Saadawi became convinced that some of the mullahs had allowed their own sperm to follow the tuft of wool on its peregrinations. In so doing they helped to solve what was a grave problem for these women, for as usual, failure to conceive was never blamed on the male partner. The situation is reminiscent of the doings of the gynaecologist Cecil Jacobsen, who used his own sperm for artificial insemination by donor (AID), a historical event that inspired Arlene Sanford's TV film *The Babymaker* in 1994. Furthermore, on the Arabian peninsula this way of tackling the problem is in keeping with a pre-Islamic tradition, the *istibdaa*. In this type of marriage, husband and wife were allowed to have a child fathered by another man who was generally of a higher social class.

There has been growing uncertainty about fertility during the past few decades, especially among men. Newspapers and journals regularly publish alarming reports on the quality of our sperm. Environmental pollution is often blamed, but for quite a long time there has also some anxiety about the dangers posed by tight-fitting clothes. Most men realize that there are good reasons why the testicles are found hanging freely on the periphery of the body. For optimum sperm production, the temperature in the testicles must be lower than the average body temperature. If boys with undescended testicles are not treated, they will never be fertile. Recently, disposable nappies have been condemned, not least because of their plastic layer, which may impede ventilation. A minor research project has confirmed that the temperature of the scrotum is one degree higher with disposable nappies than it is with cotton nappies.[30] At a later stage in life, tight underpants and jeans, hot baths and saunas fall under suspicion. But what threat do these cultural boons really pose to our continued existence? In Maastricht, an investigation was carried out to establish whether the harmful influence of tight underpants was fact or fiction.[31] Volunteers, who had to promise to refrain from using saunas, hot baths and electric blankets for a year, wore tight briefs for six months and boxer shorts for another six months, in arbitrary order. Although quite a few men backed out, the results on the whole were convincing. When wearing boxer shorts the same men produced almost twice as many spermatozoa per millilitre of ejaculate, and the percentage of vigorously moving sperm was found to be greater.

If several sperm samples are taken from one and the same man, considerable differences will be found, and that, too, is hard to explain. Quite a few men believe that better sex leads to better sperm – that greater excitement and better orgasms improve sperm quality. In fact, a number of studies have shown that the quality of sperm released during coitus is better than masturbation sperm. This subject, too, was examined in 1996.[32] The subjects were patients and sperm donors from the same fertility clinic. They handed over their sperm samples together with the answers to a questionnaire about their sexual feelings during the masturbation sessions in which the sperm had been produced. With one group of low-fertility males the investigators tried to determine whether watching an erotic video during masturbation had a positive effect. The results were negative: though the subjects found masturbation with a video more exciting, the sperm quality did not improve. In healthy donors, too, differences in sexual excitement did not seem to lead to a difference in sperm quality.

People with an intense desire to have children are not normally concerned whether the outcome of their longings will turn out to be a boy or a girl, but there are of course many couples who do have a marked preference. Some cultures are not neutral either. According to Leviticus 12:2–8, a woman is unclean for seven days after the birth of a man child, but for fourteen days after the birth of a maid child. In Morocco, the birth of a boy is greeted with three shouts of joy by the women, while the birth of a girl is greeted with just one shout, or none at all.[33] A Pakistani midwife never tells the mother immediately after the birth if her child is a boy or a girl. If he is a boy, the mother's joy can be so overwhelming that the placenta becomes impacted; if it is a girl, the mother's despair may have the same effect. The placenta must be expelled first and only then may the mother be confronted with her (mis)fortune.

In Bombay the proportion of women to men is just 774:1000. That suggests that selective abortion is practised on a fairly large scale. Throughout India, the traveller can see huge advertisements by small clinics which offer ultrasound investigations and, if necessary, abortions.[34]

Prospective parents will generally welcome some indication of the sex of the baby inside the mother. Hippocrates claimed that, with a daughter, the mother often feels more unwell, and recent epidemiological research in Sweden has confirmed that view.[35] Women who are admitted to hospital for excessive morning sickness are more likely to give birth to a daughter.

Do we know how the sex of the child is determined during its conception, and can the couple influence the result? In the Middle Ages, medical writers still adhered to the Galenic view that the uterus had seven chambers.[36] Galen's authority was so great that the oldest anatomists (for instance Mondino de Luzzi, who published his anatomy in 1316) invariably discovered seven chambers in the uterus of the bodies they dissected, and that, of course, is impossible. Galen had decreed that the three chambers on the right contained male foetuses only, the three left chambers being reserved for female ones. The seventh chamber was reserved for hermaphrodites. Some authors therefore considered it obvious that the right ovary released 'women's seed' that was male, and the left released female 'women's seed'. This view is incompatible with twentieth-century knowledge, according to which the child's sex is determined by the sperm that fertilizes the egg. Half of these sperm cells have an X-chromosome and the other half a Y-chromosome, and if the sperm with an X-chromosome wins the race, then the child will be a girl.

In later centuries, too, much was written about sex selection, including by Marie Antoinette's obstetrician.[37] There were times when it was a genuine disaster for parents to have too many daughters and too few sons. The family capital was frittered away, large sums had to be spent on dowries, and if no marriage was in prospect, much time had to be spent on finding a respectable vocation for the daughter. A convent was often the sole option. Scholars who dwelt on the art of producing sons all came to more or less the same impracticable conclusion: if only the act were performed with the right person, at the right moment and in the right manner, then the couple's piety was bound to be rewarded with the birth of a son.

The Davenport method seems somewhat more scientific. In 1900, this Irish physician put forward an elegant theory.[38] If none but boys were born in a family, then Davenport found that the health of the mother was significantly better than that of the father. If all the children were daughters, then the father was healthier than his wife. Nature thus ensured a restoration of the balance between the male and female influences. If the couple wanted a more balanced composition of their family, then they had to pay heed to a readjustment of their respective states of health.

A spontaneous experiment then took place. A man who had emigrated to Australia because he was in poor health, married a strong woman there, who bore him eight sons in succession. The woman then contracted an illness for which she needed an operation. At the same time the husband worked on improving his condition under medical supervision with the help of a diet and medication, and, indeed, the next child was a daughter. Encouraged by this case, Davenport built up the weaker partner in 39 couples and weakened the stronger with a meagre diet, denial of sleep and exercise, and bromide. In 4 of these families no pregnancy ensued, but in 32 of the remaining 35 the desired result was obtained.

Davenport had no followers, but the work was continued. Quite a few striking observations were obtained, but none with a practical application. Thus we know that in the world as a whole more boys are born than girls (approximately 51 per cent as against 49 per cent), but during major disasters the sex ratio is reversed.[39] After the London smog in 1952, the flooding in Brisbane in 1965 and the earthquake in Kobe in 1995, girls accounted for 51 per cent of all births. Danish health care is so comprehensive that it was possible to establish whether or not medical mishaps (hospital admissions, cancer or heart attacks in the expectant mother or father or in their existing children) had occurred with the more than 23,000 births recorded between 1980 and 1992. Approximately 15 per cent of the pregnancies had involved one medical setback or another. In this group, 51 per cent of the births were girls, as against 49 per cent in the group free of medical complaints.

The dioxin disaster at Seveso in 1977 was a similarly unwanted medical experiment. It showed that men exposed to dioxin have a smaller chance of fathering sons, particularly if the exposure occurs before they are eighteen.[40]

In the twentieth century it was still quite often assumed that the age of the spermatozoa played a critical role, coitus well before ovulation being more likely to result in boys than coitus on the day of ovulation. If you want a son, then you must have sex well before ovulation, but not afterwards, so the story went. Recently, the whole subject has been investigated methodically. In particular, an attempt was made to establish how many days before ovulation the fertilizing coital act had taken place.[41] The chances of pregnancy were in any case not very great if there were three to five days between intercourse and ovulation, but the chances of survival after fertilization were no smaller, and the ratio of girls to boys had nothing to do with the interval. The Belgian child rapist Marc Dutroux, who wanted, for the most despicable of reasons, to have a daughter after having fathered four sons, believed that 'old' sperm had a better chance of producing girls, and he inseminated his wife with sperm he had preserved for a few days in a condom. His fifth child was a girl.[42]

In the West, there has been a lengthy discussion of the ethical aspects of becoming involved in sex selection. There is, however, one case in which medical men have long recognized the value of sex selection. If the family of the prospective mother can be shown to have a sex-linked genetic defect (the best-known of which is haemophilia), the gynaecologist can readily help in ensuring that girls alone are brought into the world. The oldest, simplest but also the most questionable method is the selective abortion of boys. As soon as ultrasound scans or amniocentesis show that the foetus is clearly male, the pregnancy can be halted and in the next conception the chances are 50-50 again. The crudeness of this method cries out for alternatives, and at a time when IVF is becoming more widespread and successful it seemed obvious to perform diagnostic investigations after fertilization but before insertion. This method is proving successful but does involve a form of treatment that decreases the chance of conception.

Veterinary surgeons had begun much earlier to separate X from Y sperm cells. Of the many methods tested, cytometric separation has proved to be the most successful. In it, sperm, after the addition of a fluorescent medium, is forced at great speed through a very narrow tube, so that a laser beam can pick up a reflected signal from every individual sperm cell. The male spermatozoon differs slightly in shape from the female and hence reflects a slightly different signal, so that it becomes possible to give the speeding sperm a positive or a negative charge with lightning speed. The sperm is then passed through a magnetic field, and at the end two sex-differentiated portions remain. The process is admittedly very time-consuming and not very economical, because normally scores of inseminations are performed with one ejaculate. In human beings, intrauterine insemination is the common practice, and this helps to offset the marked drop in the number of sperm. In 1999, Edward Fugger and his colleagues at the Genetics and IVF Institute in Virginia published their findings with human beings. Selection favouring girls seemed more successful than selection favouring boys: 39 married couples wanted girls and in 37 cases their wish was granted, while of 15 pregnancies where a boy was fervently hoped for, 4 led to the birth of a girl.

Pregnant virgins

For sexologists, too, reproduction is an important subject, since problems of fertility sometimes arise from sexual problems. In mediaeval impotence trials, the issue was not the sexual but the procreative frustration of the woman. Divorce was banned by the church, but a woman could obtain a divorce if an expert jury found that her husband was unable to fulfil his marital duties. It might be that the man could not produce an erection capable of penetration and extreme forms of premature ejaculation also impeded procreation.

Women's problems, too, can interfere with reproduction, but if a woman cannot tolerate sexual penetration, many alternative methods can be employed. Vaginismus can prevent penetration, but C. T. van Schaik reported in 1975 that he had performed several abortions on girls and women who had certainly not conceived during sexual intercourse. We know about the Virgin Mary's immaculate conception, but history speaks of many other virgins falling pregnant, deliberately or otherwise. Evidently it is not difficult to hit upon the idea of introducing sperm with a finger. In 1909, the French gynaecologists Faure and Sireday reported that they had examined a woman who had borne four children, though she had never had sexual intercourse.[43] I myself once interviewed a married couple and found that neither husband nor wife remembered how they had come by their eight-year-old daughter. It was certainly not by coitus, since both of them found that repugnant.

A famous example of a virgin birth is discussed at some length in John Wells's 'anecdotal history', *The House of Lords*, published in 1997. He cites the case of Christabel Russell, Lady Ampthill. During her first pregnancy she was accused by her husband, 'Stilts', of adultery, because he had never had sexual intercourse with her. For some time before and during her marriage, Christabel had been a woman with a dubious reputation. Her mother, a colonel's widow, had brought up her two daughters in London and Paris, and Christabel had earned her living in Paris by giving tango lessons. When she returned to London society at the outbreak of the First World War, she quickly became one of its most sought-after women. Stilts Russell, the future Lord Ampthill, who had served on a submarine during the war, fell head over heels in love with her, but had to wait a long time before she made up her mind. On their wedding night she made him swear a solemn oath that there would be no question of children for at least a year. During the long separations imposed by his naval service, news reached him with alarming regularity about the rollicking nights out she was spending with numerous old and new admirers. She was completely indiscreet, and both Stilts himself and his parents kept being put in an embarrassing position. Just as divorce was being seriously considered, Christabel appeared to be pregnant. Stilts was suspicious, but Christabel mollified him with a story about finding him sleepwalking one night and taking him back into her bed. While the prospective father was prepared to believe the story, for his mother it was the last straw.

The divorce must have been a hilarious high-society event. The sleepwalking story was quickly brushed aside, yet the Ampthills' lawyer was unable to convince the court that Christabel's countless indiscretions had in fact led to an adulterous consummation. Christabel's reputation was in tatters, but Stilts was reportedly caught quite frequently dressed as a woman. His social career amounted to a series of failures, while Christabel had proved to be a successful businesswoman. Her strongest trump was her hymen: several physicians declared that though she was certainly pregnant, she had never been penetrated by a man.

Christabel gave a graphic description of 'Hunnish scenes' in her bedroom, and Stilts could not deny that he had made sexual advances to her. It was hinted that semen had been spilled during 'incomplete' intercourse. The jury was undecided. A retrial was ordered, and the Ampthills tried desperately, throwing in all their financial resources, to prove that Christabel had had adulterous relationships. Quite a few detectives made good money from the case. In the end, the Ampthills won, the court found that there had been one adulterous relationship, the marriage could be dissolved, and Geoffrey, who had since been born, was declared a bastard.

A few years later, Christabel scraped together enough money to appeal to the House of Lords. There, her arguments were viewed in the light of an eighteenth-century judgement concerning the 'bastardization of issue born after marriage'. The law was clear that a father or mother was not allowed to say after marriage that they have 'had no connexion and therefore the offspring is spurious'. Christabel was vindicated, and was able to give her son a decent education. The Ampthills for their part had been reduced to penury.

When Stilts died in 1974, a son from his second marriage tried to reopen the case, relying on the modern possibilities of genetic blood tests. The Lords refused to hear him, the worthy opinion of their predecessors weighing more heavily with them than some crude material procedure. Geoffrey became the fourth Baron Ampthill, and Christabel, 80 years old by then, sold her country estate in Ireland and set off on a world tour. She bought a second-hand camper van and drove to Australia. Halfway home on the return journey, in Central Asia, the vehicle was found to be neither taxed nor insured and Christabel to have no driving licence.

For some women (and men) intercourse is rendered impossible for psychological reasons, and medical help is then sought. Fertility specialists have a vast range of technical possibilities, but sometimes no more than modest help is needed. If a man and a woman want to have children but prefer to abstain from penetrative sex, then artificial insemination is the logical solution.[44] For that, the doctor needs only to procure the material and to issue the necessary instruction. For the rest the couple can be left to their own devices. This procedure has also been adopted by larger groups, albeit because many lesbian couples prefer to find sperm donors without the intervention of doctors and also like to be in control of the insemination. With heterosexual couples there is sometimes a sense of shame about their inability to engage in 'normal' reproduction. I know one couple in which the husband was so nervous about his reproductive role that ever since his wife stopped taking the pill he had unreliable erections and also had difficulties in ejaculating inside her vagina. With masturbation, every-thing was much easier, so they were prime candidates for self-insemi-nation. When that was suggested to them, the wife burst into tears, and reported that they had gone to a university clinic for IVF. That struck her as being much more acceptable than self-insemination, despite the cost and the less promising prognosis.

Virgin births are thus anything but miracles; most experienced midwives have helped a virgin to give birth. Remarkably, after such a birth nothing is changed for most women in respect of their inability to tolerate sexual penetration. The gynaecological literature contains one famous story about a pregnancy that may almost be called a mir-acle.[45] It concerns a fifteen-year-old girl from Lesotho who, during an argument she was having with her boyfriend and a former boyfriend, was stabbed in the abdomen (she was, incidentally, not the only one to be injured since all three were wounded during the argument). An operation showed that the wall of her stomach had been perforated. Her stomach was empty, so the operation was straightforward, and ten days later she was discharged. But 278 days later she returned to the hospital with acute stomach pains, and appeared to be on the point of giving birth. When she was examined to find out if dilatation had begun, it was discovered that she had no vagina. A Caesarean sec-tion was performed and after a healthy boy was born, an investigation through the open cervix was conducted to see how her organs were connected from the inside. A short stretch of vagina wase present, but then it stopped.

When asked, the girl said that she knew she had no vagina; it was for that reason she had taken up oral sex. The stabbing had occurred straight after her new friend had ejaculated into her mouth; the fury of his predecessor was so violent because he had caught them in the act. Perhaps it was at this very moment that she had her first ovulation, for there were no traces in the abdomen of previous menstruations. Gastric acid must be fatal to spermatozoa, but with malnutrition the production of gastric acid decreases, and saliva also has a basic alka-line pH. The abdominal cavity was washed out with a saline solution during the operation but not even that had been able to stop the one spermatozoon.

In the short term the story had a happy ending. The natural father accepted his role and the families rounded the marriage rites off with the usual gifts. Two attempts were made to create a neo-vagina, but proved a failure each time. The girl suffered much abdominal pain, undoubtedly as a result of menstruation into the abdominal cavity. For that reason high doses of an injectable contraceptive were used to suppress her menstrual cycle, but that too was no more than partly successful. Two and a half years later a hysterectomy could no longer be avoided.

Pregnancy denied

The girl discussed above had been admitted to hospital with labour pains, but in her case it was understandable that she could not believe she was pregnant. Denial of pregnancy is quite common, even when all the symptoms are unmistakable. In past centuries, plain ignorance was often the explanation. In 1899, two denied pregnancies were reported, the women concerned being firmly convinced that they had done nothing that could possibly have made them pregnant:

> One of the patients had actually been tempted into sexual intercourse
> with a fellow employee at her place of work. He had put her mind at
> rest with the likely story that what they were doing together was entirely
> different from what normally led to the birth of a child.[46]

Undiscovered pregnancies have quite possibly become more common recently because many women on the pill have stopped checking to see if they are pregnant. On the one hand, they are totally unprepared for pregnancy, and on the other hand they have become used to very light bleeding and sometimes even to no bleeding at all. Moreover, during the first weeks of pregnancy hormone fluctuations can still cause a slight loss of blood. There are situations, however, in which it must take a considerable mental effort to keep a number of unmistakable symptoms of pregnancy out of one's conscious mind. Naturally, the women concerned include cases of serious psychiatric disorder associated with a poor grip on reality. On the other hand, some cases are incomprehensible, and sometimes the entire social network (partner, parents) seems to underwrite their illusions. In the case of an Australian baby stillborn in a lavatory, the mother and her partner insisted that they would have been very happy to have a child.[47] Ignorance is not always the full explanation. A German research team, for instance, reported the case of a woman who had had five trouble-free pregnancies, but who for no apparent reason denied the sixth.

The German sexologist K. M. Beier distinguishes between concealed and repressed pregnancies.[48] A woman who has an unwanted pregnancy can be, sometimes with good cause, terrified of being rejected or ostracized, or of the financial problems involved. Readers of classical romantic literature will be familiar with the story of the innocent woman made desperate after being abandoned by her seducer. Don't we all understand that she should do her utmost not to own up? She will give birth to a child in seclusion and then she has only two alternatives: to kill the child or to abandon it. To obviate this horrible dilemma, France has the 'accouchement sous X' institute, where women can give birth in complete anonymity. Moreover, some French maternity clinics have a 'tour' – a kind of hatch – in which babies can be left.[49] In 2000, anonymity became the subject of debate. Some of the mothers bitterly regret what they have done, and many anonymously born children want the chance of tracing their mothers. In France, there are many adopted children whose mother (let alone natural father) is thus unknown. In Antwerp, the Moeders voor Moeders (Mothers for Mothers) building has recently made provision for future reunions. A sign bears the inscription 'Mother Moses' Basket', and behind the hatch lies paper and a stamp pad, so that the desperate mother can take a print of the baby's hand or foot, in case she ever has regrets.

By comparison, women in the Netherlands can be delivered at state expense and have their child adopted, but in such cases the maternity clinic records essential data about the mother. A number of poignant law cases have been brought by adopted children trying to force a clinic to disclose such records. So far, none of them has been successful.

It is probably not all that unusual for the whole affair to escape notice. Beier collected data from 1980 to 1989 all over Germany, and of the 213 infant autopsies following suspicion of unnatural death, one third of the mothers was never identified. There was an adequate amount of information about 98 mothers on the way they had dealt with their pregnancy. The picture of seduced and deserted innocence was certainly not confirmed. Most of these women were under twenty, it is true, but two thirds had steady relationships with the father, and one third had had a previous pregnancy. In 42 cases, it was impossible to speak of 'concealment', as the mothers seemed to be in complete denial. That meant that these women had turned a blind eye to all the symptoms of pregnancy that they experienced and did nothing to stop being found out. They went on swimming as before, for instance, continued to buy new clothes in a normal store, and visited their GP with their back pain. If they had a partner, they slept with him as often and in the same positions as before, and if they were accustomed to using condoms, they continued to do so. They failed completely to prepare for childbirth, and when they had labour pains, they explained them away as stomach cramps.

Phantom pregnancy

In the Edward Albee play *Who's Afraid of Virginia Woolf?* (1962) we meet the opposite of denied pregnancy. Nick and Honey had had a shotgun wedding, but as it turned out, there had been no need:

> Nick: She wasn't really. It was a hysterical pregnancy. She blew up, and then she went down.
> George: And while she was up, you married her.

Later that night George was to misuse this confidence during a game of 'Get the Guests'.

Phantom pregnancies must sometimes be treated as psychotic delusions and sometimes as attempts at manipulation, but a genuine phantom pregnancy (the medical term is pseudocyesis) gives rise to a large number of physiological symptoms reminiscent of normal pregnancy. The condition is, of course, fascinating and sensational, so we need not be surprised to learn that Hippocrates thought it worth mentioning.

Man is not the only mammal to have phantom pregnancies. Dog lovers will know that bitches quite often have phantom pregnancies as well. Biologists have discovered how this condition can be produced experimentally. In rats, it seems to appear when the nasal mucosa are dabbed with lunar caustic (silver nitrate), a substance often used to stop persistent nose bleeds. The same result can also be attained by local anaesthesia, and by the surgical removal of a ganglion (the ganglion sphenopalatinum) which stimuli from that region have to cross before they reach the brain. These interventions may owe their effect to the elimination of the vomeronasal organ. In an experiment written up in 1955, phantom pregnancies in mice were induced by extremely simple methods.[50] When small groups of females were crowded together and males were kept away from them, the concentration of female smells, and the absence of male urine smells, proved a reliable stimulus for inducing phantom pregnancies. The females showed a number of genuine pregnancy symptoms, such as the suspension of the ovarian cycle and the persistence of the corpus luteum, just as happens during a real pregnancy. A small amount of male urine put an immediate stop to this reaction. In general, therefore, we may assume that phantom pregnancy in rats and mice is a pheromonal process.

The most famous historical phantom pregnancy was that of Mary Tudor (Bloody Mary).[51] She was Catherine of Aragon's first living child after Catherine had undergone no fewer than six pregnancies. Although Henry VIII would undoubtedly have preferred a son, his daughter was very dear to him. The marriage, however, foundered, and Mary was sent away to live with relatives. Between the ages of nine and seventeen she hardly saw her parents. The king wanted a divorce, and believed he could persuade Pope Clement VII to annul the marriage contract on the grounds that Catherine had first been married to his late brother Arthur.[52] Using this argument must have taken some temerity because he had asked for, and obtained, a dispensation for that marriage from Pope Julius II. Julius ought never to have granted it, Henry now maintained. Leviticus is quite clear on the various aspects of the prohibition of incest: 'And if a man shall take his brother's wife, it is an unclean thing: he hath uncovered his brother's nakedness; they shall be childless.' The Pope had therefore exceeded his authority, the marriage was incestuous, and by Catherine's many miscarriages the Almighty had clearly let it be known what He thought of that papal decision. And then finally the affront of her giving birth to a daughter . . . . In short, Mary was a bastard. Naturally, she took her mother's side in the divorce disputes. Her father broke with the Holy Roman Church because of the Pope's refusal to legalize his second marriage (to Anne Boleyn) but Mary remained a faithful Roman Catholic. After Anne Boleyn had fallen from favour, there followed a reconciliation between father and daughter; Mary even became godmother to her half-brother Edward (from Henry's third marriage, to Jane Seymour).

The giving away of highborn daughters in marriage was not plain sailing in those days. Mary was introduced to this or that foreign prince whenever another new coalition was in prospect, but it was only when her place in the succession (after Edward) was finally restored that she again become a serious candidate. Henry died and Edward was crowned, but he too died a few years later. When, after several skirmishes, Mary finally seized the crown, she at last had the power to restore the authority of Rome. Marriage with the most powerful Catholic suitor seemed the obvious solution. That suitor was Philip II, the Spanish crown prince, nine years her junior and chiefly interested in her material worth. Everybody was against the marriage, but she had her way and from that moment on Protestants were persecuted with the fervour that earned her the nickname of Bloody Mary.

History repeats itself. Mary could not ignore Philip's indifference to her, and like her mother 40 years earlier she set her hopes on pregnancy.

She was 38 when she thought that she was with child. The date of the expected confinement passed and Mary reassured her husband with the declaration that she must have miscalculated the event by a month. A month later her husband and friends pressed her to consult another physician. Mary refused, offended, and withdrew to her quarters with just one maid to look after her. She apparently fell into a deep depression, and not for the first time; life had indeed given her good cause.

Philip left England, angry at the deception, and for the next few years Mary was plagued with suspicions about his possible escapades on the continent and made desperate attempts to win him back. He did return, but the gulf between them proved unbridgeable. It was rumoured that Philip was casting a covetous eye at Elizabeth, who had the same dynastic rights as Mary. In these bloodthirsty years, Mary undoubtedly thought of eliminating her Protestant half-sister, but Philip stopped her. That was a serious political misjudgement on his part, because Elizabeth was to become his most powerful enemy. When, shortly before her 42nd birthday, Mary announced that she was pregnant again, nobody really believed her. Four months later she herself had to face the hard truth. Philip left, and her political position became increasingly untenable. She retired to the countryside, again accompanied by a small retinue, and died later that same year. After her death everything she had striven for so passionately was wiped out at a stroke.

Another famous phantom pregnancy has come down to us in heavily veiled form, from the early years of psychoanalysis.[53] In 1895, Breuer and Freud published their *Studies on Hysteria*. The first case in that work was the treatment of Anna O. by Breuer during the years 1880 to 1882. At the time, the patient was twenty and Breuer was her general practitioner, but closer contacts began when she complained of a sore throat. Soon afterwards she developed various hysterical paralyses and seemed to fall spontaneously into a hypnotic trance every day. Breuer found himself so involved in her troubles that his wife became jealous. Remarkably enough, it proved possible with some persistence to reconstruct the origin of every one of Anna O.'s symptoms. There had invariably been a more or less traumatic event, manifesting itself via an unconscious route in a physical phenomenon.

Once the cause of a hysterical symptom had been discovered and discussed, it disappeared by itself, Anna playing at least as great a part in developing this methodology as Breuer himself. Freud heard from Breuer about his interesting experiments, and thanks to Freud the story has been preserved for posterity, for Breuer himself was not inclined to publish this episode from the nursery of psychoanalysis.

Freud must have been very insistent. Breuer's reluctance to publish his findings undoubtedly arose from the dramatic events that took place at the end of the treatment. When Anna's condition had appreciably improved, Breuer decided to put his marriage first and announced that he wished to conclude the treatment. That same evening he was summoned to Anna's bedside, where she was in a kind of epileptoid state, apparently due to her belief that she was about to give birth. It then emerged that for quite some time she had been under the delusion that she was pregnant by her beloved doctor. Breuer was not equal to this situation. Somehow he found a way of calming Anna by hypnotic suggestion, whereupon, bathed in a cold sweat, he left the house.

Freud reported later that the Breuers had immediately left for Venice on a sort of second honeymoon, during which their last daughter was said to have been conceived. This version is, however, contradicted by the known facts, the Breuers' youngest daughter having been born before the termination of Anna's therapy.[54] As for Anna, things did not go well with her afterwards. She spent quite some time in a psychiatric hospital, and Breuer is reported to have sighed that he honestly hoped death might put an end to her misery. Hence it is not all that surprising that Freud had to keep prevailing upon him to publish this case history, which finally appeared in what proved to be a rather self-aggrandizing paper. The less than satisfactory outcome to the case was omitted from the first publication, and it was not until much later that Freud himself disclosed the erotically charged dénouement. Incidentally, Anna O. (whose real name was Bertha Pappenheim) later played a fairly prominent role in the feminist movement.

The most striking feature of a genuine phantom pregnancy is that it gives rise to a number of genuine pregnancy symptoms. Menstruation fails to occur, but that is not all that uncommon. The abdominal girth may increase, and a pelvic examination may show that the uterus is slightly enlarged. Sometimes the breasts grow, and there may even be stretch marks. The patients claim that they can feel the child move, but that sensation is of course subjective by definition. Occasionally there are also unusual objective phenomena. A woman with diabetes who had, during previous pregnancies, found that her insulin input had to be reduced (which is unusual, since generally the need for insulin increases during pregnancy), had the same reaction during her phantom pregnancy. When told that she was not pregnant, she was able to revert to her normal dose. In another case, toxicosis was reported at the end of nine months: high blood pressure, albumin in the urine and swollen ankles. In this patient, too, all the symptoms disappeared once she was apprised of the true situation.

Pseudocyesis is generally considered a form of hysteria, and Anna O.'s clinical picture fits into this tradition. Hysteria is associated with such physical symptoms as paralyses and blindness (conversion hysteria). There may also be a link between pseudocyesis and dissociative disorders – the clinical picture in which various parts of one's personal experience are split off, and of which multiple personality disorder is the most spectacular and best known example. Multiple personality is sometimes associated with striking physical phenomena, for instance when one personality needs to wear glasses and the other(s) do(es) not. Finally, psychiatrists are familiar with the Münchhausen syndrome: the fabrication by a malingerer of a clinically convincing simulation of disease for the purpose of getting medical attention. Medical literature on this syndrome reads like a novel. A clinical account published in 1987 involved four persons whose case histories were a powerful illustration of the wide variability of the syndrome.[55] At the end of the account, the authors made the striking disclosure that the four patients were in fact one and the same person who had knocked at various hospital doors with different stories. Though the patient himself will have gained nothing in the wake of his hospital experiences, he cost the health service an average of £70,000 a year. A British article on pseudocyesis deliberately carried a photograph of another patient under discussion, to stop her from misleading further hospitals with her phantom pregnancies.

As an explanation of phantom pregnancy, reference is sometimes made to its link with depression, and it is quite certain that the phenomenon is more common in societies that judge the value of women by their fertility. In some cases, in which it was shown irrefutably that there was no genuine pregnancy, the patient's family helped her to maintain her illusion. The most remarkable case was that of Joanna Southcott, the leader of an English sect. At the age of 64, she announced that she was carrying the new Messiah, and many people believed her. Of the nine physicians who examined her, six declared that she had symptoms that, in a younger woman, would undoubtedly have indicated pregnancy.

In the West, the frequency of phantom pregnancies seems to be decreasing, thanks largely to better public knowledge and easier diagnoses. It must be harder to maintain that you can go to a pharmacy for a pregnancy test or ask for an ultrasound.

There exists a belief in Islamic countries that, in a sense, is akin to phantom pregnancy. It is the story of the *ragued*, the child that has fallen asleep.[56] The origins of the story are ancient: the second caliph, Omar I Ibn-al-Khattab (who reigned from 634 to 644), was consulted by a visitor who could not understand how the wife he had married four and a half months earlier could possibly have given birth to a child. She had been married before, but had kept the obligatory period of sexual abstinence – of that the man was convinced. The caliph sought the advice of the wise women, who declared that the woman had been pregnant at the time her first husband passed away. Her second husband's sperm had simply awakened the sleeping child. Caliph Omar concluded that a child could easily have slept for four years inside the woman. After him many mullahs took an interest in this question. Some schools argued that two years was the maximum, but other scholars maintained that a *ragued* could sleep for seven years before waking up and seeing the light of day. *Moudouwana*, the Moroccan family law governing marriage and divorce, stipulates that a pregnancy cannot be shorter than six months, or longer than a year.[57]

In men, too, phantom pregnancies sometimes occur. In most cases, they are part of a serious psychiatric disorder, that is, of a psychotic, delusional nature. The most detailed case history in medical literature starts with a doctor's visit to treat a swollen belly, with nausea coupled to an increased appetite.[58] The distended belly was an objective fact, so the doctor looked for possible liver disorders. When nothing abnormal was found, the man told the doctor about his suspicion that there was some 'life' in his belly. In later conversations with a psychiatrist, the man confessed that he suspected that he was a 'woman in a man's body' but had no wish, unlike a transsexual, to change his appearance. He too felt that his pregnancy was a religious experience; although he was not a churchgoer, he felt sure that a higher being must have had a special intention for him through this miracle. He was a solitary man, the only child of an aloof father and a mother who had died soon after he was born. When he was sixteen, his father was declared an alcoholic and stripped of his parental powers. The boy was more or less adopted by a widow who became his landlady. He served in the Navy during the Second World War, and later became a merchant seaman. He had positive sexual experiences with both sexes, but as he grew older he leaned increasingly towards homosexuality. For someone with so obvious a pathological condition, he was remarkably 'ordinary', and after two months of therapeutic discussion both his delusion and his physical symptoms disappeared completely.

Couvade

Anthropology has familiarized us with cultures in which the partner of a pregnant woman is treated as if he were bearing the child. This custom is called couvade, and Marco Polo has left us a memorable account of it. His observations were made during the thirteenth century in the Chinese part of Turkestan. No sooner had a Turkoman woman given birth to child than she was up and about again and able to return to her normal activities, while her husband kept to his bed for 40 days solemnly receiving childbed visitors. That same century, Henry of Aachen wrote the romance *Heinric en Margriete van Limborch*, in which he related that:

> Pauca the queen, whose fame is known,
> a woman of Pauca who,
> followed by VIII M women,
> all their husband's masters are;
> and bear little pain,
> for when these women recover
> from childbirth, the man lies down
> and the women, I have heard say,
> must serve him until the term is up.
> The cornet has peace,
> and the women must go to war,
> as the man cannot bear the pain.[59]

In the Dutch colonies, the sailors made similar observations. Wouter Schouten could not hide his indignation in the seventeenth century:

> The black woman who has given birth to a child does not keep to her bed but goes directly with her newborn to the river, and having cleaned it together with its swaddling clothes, she goes back to her work; everything then turns out well. Beyond that I was told that when black girls come from the island of Buru to bear a little one, they make the lying-in man look quite ludicrous and sickly, and pamper him so that the poor fool is spoilt even more than usual. And meanwhile the weak woman has to prepare tasty dishes for this man-in-childbed so that the feeble fellow can get back on his legs again.

Schouten's Calvinist rancour still comes across in the twenty-first century, but couvades are sometimes part of a wider ritual involving less saccharine behaviour.[60] Writing about couvades in Martinique, J. B. du Tertre explained in 1654 that a period of 40 days of 'illness' with fasting and a strict diet was followed by a ritual by which the father was transformed from 'an imaginary into a real patient'. He was taken from his hammock and his skin ripped open in various places with the teeth of an agouto, whereupon the wounds were rubbed with a kind of pepper. It goes without saying that he was not allowed to make any sound during this ordeal. After that he was free to move about again, but not allowed to eat meat or fish for many months.

The significance of these rituals is difficult to fathom, but the vegetarian diet might well be an expression of the fact that the child is part and parcel of the father and that the father must therefore take no food that the baby cannot digest. With some tribes, the couvade ritual goes hand in hand with the belief that the child, the product of the male seed, has merely used the mother's belly as a fertile field. The bloody character of the ritual can, however, also be intended to scare off evil spirits, for if an evil spirit has invaded the body, it is often found in the blood.

In sixteenth- and seventeenth-century Britain, the symptoms of the husband of a pregnant woman were often blamed on witchcraft. Midwives in particular were suspected of having the power to transfer their patient's pains to the husband. When Mary, Queen of Scots, was due to give birth in 1566, one of her ladies-in-waiting tried to assuage her pains by passing them over into another royal attendant. She was not entirely successful: the queen had labour pains like every other woman, but the royal attendant did share some of them.

The couvade is closer to us than we tend to think. The French physician Gustave Cohen reported that on a visit to Staphorst in the Netherlands during the First World War his wife had seen a woman who had just given birth standing up making pancakes while her husband, dressed in his Sunday best, wearing a top hat and decorations, received the visitors in bed.[61]

The couvade is a ritualized illness, but even today men come down with such classical pregnancy symptoms as morning sickness and back pains during their wife's pregnancy.[62] During the Second World War, American soldiers stationed in Europe had more than the average number of medical disorders if their wives had been pregnant when they left home. Toothache was also a common complaint and in popular mythology a man's toothache was often treated as a sign of the wife's pregnancy. Emotional problems such as anxiety and depression are nowadays mentioned more often than physical symptoms. Sometimes this leads to inappropriate behaviour. In a study conducted in 1966 of a number of men who were under psychiatric investigation following a recently committed offence, it was discovered that those whose partners happened to be pregnant at the time were far more frequently arrested for sexual offences (especially exhibitionism and paedophilia).

Choice of partner and paternity doubts

The woman who wants a child must find a sperm ready to fuse with her egg. Nowadays a whole gamut of possibilities is at her disposal, but the most usual is still her search for a man with whom she can share the child's upbringing. The family continues to be the cornerstone of society, and in addition marriage plays an important role in the wider social and economic framework. All over the world there are still societies in which the forging of family ties is subordinate to the laws of capital distribution. Thus descendants are part of the property on which husband and wife base their existence, and in certain circles couples used not to get married until the prospective bride was pregnant. This placed greater pressure upon monogamy, for the man who wants to have no doubts about whether or not his capital will be handed on to his own flesh and blood must be certain that he has sole access to his wife's vagina.

That was the function of the chastity belt. It was introduced in Europe at the time of the Crusades, but some American Indians, including the Cheyenne, were also familiar with this device.[63] In the Middle East, the wife, having obtained her husband's consent to visit a woman friend, was usually escorted by a eunuch as a chaperone. If no chaperone was available, then the Arab husband too had recourse to a belt, in this case equipped with a round wooden rod that filled the vagina.

In the Middle Ages, the cunning and calculation of women was a standard cultural theme, which explains why chastity belts gave rise to a widespread cycle of picaresque tales. The locksmith's profession was the subject of countless jokes: how much money did these craftsmen make on the side through the sale of duplicate keys? The print of a woman with a belt (illus. 20) dates back to the sixteenth century; the banners read as follows:

> The old man: Money and goods I shall lavish upon you / Will you but live the way I desire / Pick what you want inside my pockets / The lock I'll leave in your good hands.

The woman: No lock can withstand a woman's guiles / There is no trust where love has flown / That's why I'll buy the key I want / And make you pay for it, to boot.

The young man: I have a key for locks like these / Albeit many shake their heads / He truly wears a dunce's cap / Who true love tries to buy.[64]

In our age, too, some women still wear chastity belts. A newspaper of 4 December 1999 carried a short report of a court case heard in Munich in which a woman accused her boyfriend of assault and forcible restraint. He had attached a chastity belt to piercings in her labia. It was just a game, the man said in his own defence. Some erotic photographers now and again portray their models wearing a chastity belt.

Fear of a cuckoo in the nest is a powerful cultural theme. In his play *The Father* (1912), Strindberg portrayed the mental distress of a man who doubts his paternity and is subtly led on by his wife. But the subject continues to be topical. In 1991 a Campari commercial showed a Sleeping Beauty in her next life phase, presenting her newly born baby to her youthful Prince Charming. A single glance is enough: this roly-poly midget could not possibly have sprung from his loins. And in a corner of the room we see a portly prelate sniggering as he looks the other way. That sort of story can be told in twenty seconds by implication only and everyone knows what it is all about.

How often does it not happen in real life that the proud husband is not the genetic father? The Belgian newspaper *De Morgen* of 14 March 1998 carried a report about the work of the Ghent Centre for Medical Genetics, which does some 2,000 DNA analyses every year. The reason for a DNA investigation is generally the fear of genetic disease, but the results also allow conclusions about the genetic relationship between father and child. Of the children investigated, 15 per cent could not possibly have been sired by their putative fathers, a figure that was considerably higher than had been expected. (To restore the moral balance: data about extramarital sex by men during the pregnancy of their wives reflected roughly the same results: 12 of the 79 husbands interviewed by Masters and Johnson about sex during their wife's pregnancy admitted adulterous relationships.[65])

The use of donor sperm in cases of male infertility during the last 50 years could have explained some of the Ghent results, but in view of the reasons why this group consulted the Centre, this information would not have been withheld. Of the fathers who asked for a DNA test precisely because they had doubts about their paternity, one in four applicants was shown to have had justified fears. In a number of states in the

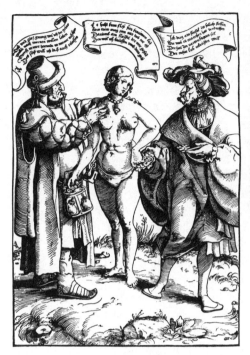

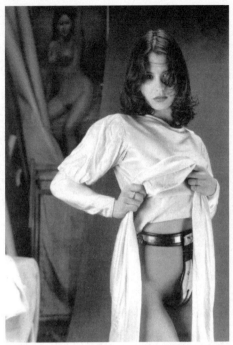

20 *Left*:
*Woman with
chastity belt*.
Woodcut,
c. 1540.

21 *Right*:
A wearer today.

United States it has become standard practice to demand paternity tests in divorce cases so as to avoid later legal disputes.

Animal research has led to similar discoveries. Some primate species live in small colonies, and normally both males and females have a strict hierarchical order. The higher the female is in her hierarchy, the more exclusively she belongs to the top male, certainly during her fertile period. Chimpanzees are fairly promiscuous but it has long been believed that they keep to their own group. However, paternity tests in 1997 have shown that the DNA of some of the young could not possibly have come from males in the group.[66] The investigators were surprised because they had no idea that the females occasionally left their group, nor had they ever got a glimpse of the sneaky assaulters of the group's honour. But there was no escaping the facts: adultery was rife in what seemed to be so cohesive a society, and the females were plainly too clever for the males.

In the human world, various factors can lead to paternity doubts. Karel Glastra van Loon's novel *The Passion Fruit* revolves round this subject. The main character has a son, becomes a widower, and many years later it emerges in a new relationship that he is infertile, and, moreover, for an unquestionably congenital reason. Another fictional illustration of this dilemma is highlighted in the film *Irren ist männlich* (*To Err Is Masculine*) of 1995, Sherry Hormann's amusing and stylish comedy. A happily married man with two children has a mistress who yearns to have a child by him. However she does not become pregnant and on investigation it is discovered that the man is infertile. How is this possible? The cuckold turns detective and recalls two possible candidates whom he somehow manages to track down and invites to a party. He tries every trick in the book to get hold of a sample of their blood, but all his efforts prove of no avail. In his plight he pours his heart out to his brother, a priest, so used to listening to confessions of all kinds. In the next scene we see this brother in earnest deliberation with the wife. We come to understand that all those years ago she had decided to use the brother to solve the problem discreetly, thus sparing her husband the humiliation of a donor insemination. The two of them now dream up a cunning solution: the brother swears to the husband that fertility clinics occasionally slip up, and that a second opinion would therefore not be money wasted. Brother and wife prepare a small phial of the priest's sperm and are about to call the clinic's courier service clinic and to switch phials, but a mistake of unprecedented improbability ensures that neither phial reaches its destination. With Plan B, the mistress has to be made privy to the plot. The mistress is a good sport who knows perfectly well on which side her bread is buttered. Once she has her pregnancy, her lover's emotional equilibrium is restored in no time. Next, we make a jump forward to her child's christening, with the brother naturally conducting the ceremony and the wife playing the part of godmother. She has apparently meanwhile become the bosom friend of the mistress, of whom she knows officially no more than that she wanted to be a single mother. Despite the multitude of deceptions, the scene is heartwarming, and the spectator is not at all surprised to hear the husband whisper in his wife's ear that there is room in their family for a third child. Over his shoulder, the wife meets the glance of his brother, who is cuddling one of the children. The film ends with an unspoken confession by the brother before the image of Christ in his parochial church. There is much, it is clear, that shall be forgiven him, including this time.

Nowadays testing for blood relationships is a simple matter. If any woman wants to know if her father is her real father she need only go on the Internet and call up www.Bsure and follow instructions.

Paternity doubt has again come into prominence in the press, so much so that Ronald Plasterk, professor of developmental genetics, advocated on 22 October 1999 that the subject be used in a reality-TV programme. After *Big Brother*, he understood what the public really went for, and suggested the title *Father Yes, Father No*. The proposal went as follows: three pairs of fathers and children are questioned by a perceptive and witty panel, and after the first round, panel and public decide which son or daughter is the bastard, and which father the cuckold (the nail-biting mother is naturally also on camera). After the name of the first couple is revealed to be the wrong choice, voting is resumed and when the truth finally comes out, the sobbing mother can be questioned about her lapse, we can see how bravely father and child deal with the blow, and as the credits appear we are shown the pictures of the three families who will be put on the rack the following week.

Sperm competition

Animal behaviourists have a great deal of influence on human social psychology. In 1993, the biologists Robin Baker and Mark Bellis published the results of their investigation into human sperm competition. In 1996, Baker processed the results for the public at large and his account proved to be a bombshell.[67] The final conclusion was that the evolution of man was helped if women have firm ties with male partners who are caring, faithful and non-aggressive, even if these men do not necessarily provide the best genes. The biological nature of women causes them to make unconscious choices, which lead them to share their bed readily with another partner at the exact time of their ovulation. A recent investigation published in *Science* confirmed a definite fluctuation in women's evaluation of men.[68] It was discovered that at about the time of their ovulation women are more strongly attracted to faces with pronounced masculine features. Since sperm can survive in the uterus for five days, it frequently happens that there are two populations of sperm lying in wait for the next ovulation. Baker and Bellis have calculated that in 4 per cent of all fertilizations two sets of genes have in theory an equal chance of success.

For eugenic reasons, the woman is not neutral: she wants the macho sperm to win the race. The survival of the fittest thus not only applies to the millions of sperm released by one ejaculation, but also to two armies of sperm that encounter each other in a woman's body. Baker describes an ejaculate as a kind of colony of ants in which every one of the various sperm has its own rank and function. Only a small elite makes straight for the egg; the fighters in the group remain in the uterus and the small mucous glands in the cervix, whence they are able to colonize the area for at least five days. If individuals from a different tribe pass by they are recognized by chemical signals, leading to a fight by exchanges of cytotoxic material. A third group of sperm cells is known in sperm analysis as unfit because their heads are too heavy and their motility is poor. Baker assigns them a passive function: they are said to block the tight channels in the chemical structure in the mucous membrane of the cervix. A woman's white blood cells serve the same function.

The man who wants to restrict his sexual partner to his own genetic material has to ensure that he has enough sperm to offset the effects of possible adultery. In a small group of volunteers, Baker and Bellis have measured the size of the ejaculate, determining the total number of sperm and the number of sperm that flow out after coitus. They discovered that, without being aware of it, men ejaculate larger quantities of sperm if they have little control over their partner. If their partner is in their vicinity during the greater part of the day, they can permit themselves the luxury of deploying smaller forces.

The role of the female body must not be underestimated either. The woman determines whether she keeps the major portion of the sperm inside her or if most of the sperms are expelled; unbeknown to her, her sexual organs adopt a stance of their own. Differences in sperm retention have not been discussed at greater length in the medical literature, but in the Hippocratic writings we do find relevant observations, for instance in the story of the pregnant flute player mentioned earlier:

> The flute-girl had heard the kind of things which women say to one another – if a woman is going to conceive, no generating seed exits from her, but it remains inside. She understood what she had heard and she always watched carefully; when she perceived that the generating seed did not leave her womb, she mentioned the fact to her mistress and the story came to me.

This story does not consider the flute player's orgasms, but Baker and Bellis are among the believers with respect to the female orgasm's role in the retention of sperm. In their series of experiments the backflow was low if the woman had had an orgasm from one minute before to 45 minutes after the ejaculation. In the wake of these conclusions, other investigators interviewed a group of women about the timing of their orgasms while having intercourse with their partners on the one hand, and the urgency of their desire for pregnancy on the other hand.[69] They confirmed that women who mostly have their orgasm after ejaculation were most certain about their wish for a child.

Orgasms between intercourse with men also play a part. Because of the increase in the fluid content of the vagina and of the uterine cavity the mucous plug in the cervix can be manipulated. After an orgasm without ejaculation the acid contents of the vagina content are sucked in, and sperm cells present there will succumb to the acidity. If a woman is looking forward to a secret tryst with her lover and consequently treats herself to an orgasm, she unconsciously clears the path for his sperm. The humidity of the mucous plug also helps to open up the small channels, so that a high percentage of sperm can be preserved.

At a time when Baker and Bellis were still relatively unknown, I heard them present their ideas at a meeting of the International Academy of Sex Research, and was particularly struck by the cheerful reception of their somewhat tall story, particularly by the women in the audience. The idea that their own love organ also served as a battlefield obviously appealed to the female imagination. Anyone active in sexual health and contraceptive advice services is bound to have heard stories from women who made peculiar choices when it came to taking risks with the 'wrong' partners. I have a very distinct memory of one, who had been attending a fertility clinic for some time in order to conceive at long last in her childless marriage, had intercourse with her lover on the day of ovulation, and deliberately abandoned her extramarital routine by not using a condom. She then regretted her decision, decided that a morning-after pill was called for, and opted deliberately for the 2x2 method, fully recognizing that in her case the risk was maximal, and hence not completely eliminated by this type of morning-after pill.

The research by Baker and Bellis attracted a great deal of attention and it is debatable if that was entirely due to the quality of their work. The original publications reveal that they used relatively few experimental subjects, and that a great many complicated calculations were needed to arrive at their conclusions. The adaptation Baker addressed to the public at large is highly romanticized, a sort of mixture of soft porn, tabloid gossip and science fiction. It may be stimulating, but for the time being I consider the book to be on a par with *Were the Gods Cosmonauts?* A small dose of scepticism seems indicated, particularly since the results follow on so seamlessly from the age-old stories about the wiliness of women.

The theory of evolution has given birth to even more remarkable freaks. In Matthijs van Boxsel's *Encyclopaedia of Stupidity* we are told about the intellectual contribution of Patrice J. J. van der Vorst, lawyer and engineer.[70] She postulates an evolutionary outward displacement of the clitoris, as a result of which the human female is the one and only subject in which the separation of reproduction from pleasure is not only possible but inevitable. The human female is puzzled about her lack of satisfaction during intercourse, and that is the origin of logical thought. 'Eve' discovers masturbation, the pleasure option. She demonstrates her discovery to 'Adam' and he has to interpret the mystery of her behaviour in his turn. 'Does she want me to touch her in that way as well? Why, and how do I set about it?' His newly acquired powers of thought are thus at once in the service of ethics, of altruism; he discovers that in addition to pleasuring oneself it is also possible to pleasure another.

So female bisexuality (in the Freudian sense) is the source of abstract thought as well as of ethics. This is a wonderful concept. The clitoris is then in fact 'the origin of culture'. But why does Patrice van de Vorst think that the clitoris has ever been found more deeply inside?

The physiology of pregnancy, childbirth and breastfeeding

The body of a pregnant woman is capable of exceptional achievements. In the Dutch textbook *Obstetrics and Gynaecology*, the changes in heart and vascular function during pregnancy are compared with the condition of endurance sportsmen. The other organs must also increase their output.[71] The uterus itself becomes twenty time as heavy within nine months, and, which is perhaps even more remarkable, after the birth of the child it takes just three weeks for the mother's uterus to return to its old weight. The strongest effect on the shrinking of the uterus is exerted by oxytocin, a hormone that also plays an important role in childbirth. The expansion of the vagina during the descent of the child's head is a stimulus to which the pituitary gland responds with the release of oxytocin, and this strengthens the contractions. This is called Ferguson's reflex after its discoverer.[72] After birth, oxytocin boosts the flow of milk during lactation, following stimulation of the nipple. When the mother offers her breast to the baby, the baby's sucking stimulates the pituitary gland to release oxytocin, which rapidly reaches the breasts and causes the 'led-down' reflex, encouraging the flow of milk. At the same time, oxytocin also acts on the uterus: many women feel contractions of the uterus while the baby is sucking. That may be accompanied by an enjoyable feeling of sensuality, with some women being shocked to discover that contact with their newborn can act as such a strong erotic stimulus. Conversely, many women make use of the oxytocin response to nipple stimulation in their sexual repertoire. Some sexologists are convinced that women who have a liking for intensive penetration ('fisting', for instance) are essentially making erotic use of Ferguson's reflex.

In the Middle Ages a link between the uterus and the mammary gland was identified and by way of an explanation it was assumed that a blood vessel ran straight from the uterus to the breast.[73] The female seed (menstrual blood), which during pregnancy did not come out in the normal way, was diverted to the breast and changed into mother's milk. This explanation goes back to Hippocrates. Empirical research failed to adduce any evidence in favour of this explanation of milk production and it is thus mentioned very tentatively in late mediaeval anatomical texts, but in a frequently reproduced drawing of copulation by Leonardo da Vinci the blood vessel running to the nipple is clearly shown.

Oxytocin thus promotes the contraction of organs, but the production of milk is stimulated by prolactin. This hormone, too, is produced in the pituitary gland, and quite early on in pregnancy its level begins to increase sharply. The placenta then ensures that the breasts do not produce milk too early. The milk-stimulating levels of prolactin and oxytocin are offset by an excessive production of oestrogen and progesterone. Only when the placenta is born do the lactating tendencies get the upper hand.

The blood of a pregnant woman has far higher hormone levels, something she can tell from numerous phenomena. A high progesterone content can, for instance, lead to drowsiness, while a high oestrogen content has a mood-lifting effect. Couples sometimes find it difficult to understand why the pregnant partner, with all her irksome symptoms, can nevertheless remain so radiant. Some pregnant women have an irrepressible craving for certain kinds of food, of which pickles are a classical example. It used to be thought that these cravings reflect the needs of the child, but nowadays it is thought more realistic to blame the tempestuous developments in the hormones. Something in the pregnant woman's perception of taste and smell changes, but this does not provide an adequate explanation of the whimsical shifts in preferences and aversions. The precise reasons for the cravings have not yet been established.

Another hormone to manifest its presence more strongly is the melanocyte-stimulating hormone (MHS), produced in the pituitary gland. Melanocytes are cells that are, essentially, capable of causing pigmentation of the skin. The increase in MHS can be detected through the intensification of the colour of those skin areas that are always somewhat darker than the rest. Everyone knows that the nipples grow darker and, moreover, considerably larger. The labia are also pigmented, and can become very dark, almost black. A narrow line running from the navel to the pubis can equally contain many melanocytes and become very conspicuous. Partly due to exposure to the sun, the face can bear what is known as the pregnancy mask, with the upper lip in particular turning darker in colour. In the early years of the pill, when the dose was much higher than it is today, the pregnancy mask was one of the most common complaints resulting from the use of the pill.

The skin also reacts strongly to the stress hormone cortisol produced by the adrenal glands, the visible effects of which are stretch marks (striae). The connective tissue of the skin is weakened by cortisol, and in the places in which the skin is stretched most (the abdomen and the breasts), the tissue is so unevenly drawn out that in the stretch marks the underlying layers rich in blood can show through. During pregnancy the striae are bluish in colour. After childbirth, that is, after normalization of the hormone level, scarring occurs and the result is a white stripe.

The enormous increase in hormone levels during pregnancy leads to yet another skin change, namely impairment of the tactile sense. Compared with other pregnancy symptoms, this is a little known phenomenon. In 1977, Robinson and Short published the results of a study of the sensitivity of the skin surrounding the nipple (the areola) and in the rest of the breast.[74] The test revealing the clearest differences in touch sensitivity was the two-point discrimination test. This is a very simple experiment requiring equipment that is no more sophisticated than a pair of compasses with two needle points. The blindfolded experimental subject is touched gently with the two points and asked to say if there are one or two pricks (to increase the objectivity the subject is occasionally given a single prick). The aim is to discover the smallest distance that can still be experienced as two pricks. Boys and girls before puberty have the same two-point discrimination, but after physical maturation boys became less sensitive in the breast area and girls more sensitive. The effect of the menstrual cycle can be demonstrated: the greatest sensitivity occurs during menstruation (or shortly before) and ovulation. In pill users, this cycle disappears almost completely. During pregnancy, and particularly shortly before childbirth, sensitivity has lessened so significantly that the areola is too small for the subject to differentiate two separate pricks. Within twenty-four hours after childbirth normal sensitivity is restored, and increases to far above the normal level. With the compasses that these researchers used, the points could not be brought close enough together for the subjects to feel them as a single prick. Sensitivity to pain also increased slightly immediately after childbirth.

The writers concluded that changes in sensitivity at about the time of childbirth play an important role in the regulation of the milk flow. If there are high oestrogen blood levels, then stimulation of the nipples does not lead to prolactin production, and the breast remains at rest. As long as the baby is in the uterus, the sucking mechanism is not needed, but afterwards an intensive interaction between baby and breast has to be built up. Once prolactin has set milk production going, oxytocin causes ejection: the let-down reflex in the mammary gland. The quick response of the breast to the baby's mouth is a reflex that is easily conditioned by all the other stimuli coming from the baby. Thus a great many breastfeeding women notice that their breasts start to leak when they hear their baby cry.

The baby cannot do many things straight after it is born, but it is almost invariably able to find the nipple. It is probable that its sense of smell guides it there. In one study, mothers had one of their breasts washed with a neutral soap immediately after birth, and when their babies were given the choice most of them chose the unwashed breast.[75]

After childbirth many things in the mother's body changes. Hormones in particular need time to return to their old levels, and women who breastfeed their babies differ in this from those who use a bottle. During the period of breastfeeding, the mother retains high levels of prolactin and oxytocin, while the mother using a bottle quickly returns to normal. During the suckling period oestrogen and progesterone levels are temporarily so low that the situation might be compared to that prevailing after the menopause. This may come to the woman's notice when she resumes sexual relations with her partner and her physical excitement lags behind her mental excitement. She may notice that her vagina is fairly dry during intercourse, and if this is ignored, coitus can turn into a painful affair. That last is an ever-present risk with women who have been cut or torn during childbirth.

The period of pregnancy, childbirth and breastfeeding is so marked by hormonal revolutions that it seems obvious why attempts have been made to draw conclusions from this phase of life about the influence of the various hormones on the emotions. This is a fairly recent departure in biological research. The physiological effects of hormones have been known for quite some time, but on closer investigation most reproductive hormones also seem to have central, emotion-controlling effects. Theresa Crenshaw's book *Why We Love and Lust* (1996) is devoted to this very subject.

The case study with which she starts her book revolves round the problems of a married couple while the wife is breastfeeding her baby. The high doses of prolactin seem to lead to complete disinterest in sex;

in the most striking cases an exceptionally low level of male sex hormones makes a further contribution to the lack of sexual initiative.
However, if husband and wife adopt a positive attitude to the unilater-
al character of the sexual initiative, then the difference can be entirely
compensated, for arousal response to erotic interaction is undisturbed,
and orgasms too do not suffer from overdoses of prolactin. Thus while
the physical excitement can lag behind the mental, a little patience and
possibly a lubricant as well may help to find a way round the problem.
The crux of Crenshaw's message is that husband and wife ought to realize that breastfeeding renders the woman more sexually passive but no
less receptive.

There are undoubtedly many married couples who lack information about the changes in sexual experience during the lactation
period, but that is equally true of the experts who are expected to
advise them on the subject. Medical literature has long paid attention to the question of whether or not women need sex during
pregnancy, but the general assumption is that the woman's desire is
an autonomous process, the role of the man's sexual desire being
brushed aside together with the interaction between the partners.[76]
In general, it can be asserted that in almost all couples the frequency
of coitus decreases towards the end of the pregnancy, and the resump-
tion of intercourse after childbirth comes later in couples in which
the wife breastfeeds her baby or needs stitches after giving birth.
However, the individual range is considerable. In the past, doctors
undoubtedly admonished their patients far too often to be careful
when there was no real need. Perhaps in so doing they were unconsciously delving into our Christian heritage, since as coitus during
pregnancy cannot of course lead to pregnancy it necessarily has a
sinful air.

The other lactation hormone, oxytocin, has the psychological effect
of fostering a sense of togetherness. The sucking baby gives his mother
an oxytocin high, as a result of which she becomes more and more
bonded with her baby. Again, when a woman is touched by her lover,
her oxytocin level rises, and that adds to the pleasant feeling of togetherness with the partner. And as mentioned earlier, oxytocin makes a
contribution to orgasmic contractions during sexual intercourse.

The hormone most closely related to oxytocin is vasopressin,
which acts directly on the blood pressure and the kidney function. If,
due to a congenital aberration, the body does not produce vasopressin
then the kidney is unable to concentrate the urine, which means that
the patient passes enormous quantities of water and has to drink a
great deal. This illness is known as diabetes insipidus. Nowadays vaso-

pressin is made synthetically and administered by a nasal spray. The spray can also be used to treat bed-wetting: if the intake of liquid is limited in the evening and a small puff of vasopressin is taken before going to bed, then the urine production at night will be reduced enough to prevent the need to urinate.

Vasopressin seems to have been considered as a rather inconsequential substance by the medical world, but biologists claim that it also plays a part in the life of hibernating animals. The vasopressin level must drop before hibernation can begin. Even more revolutionary have been the findings by animal ethologists studying prairie voles.[77] It was known that the males of this species are monogamous and make excellent fathers; while gentle with the litter, they are fiercely aggressive if another male approaches the burrow. That is in marked contrast with the behaviour of other voles, in which the males care little about pair formation or care for the young. Young, sexually inexperienced males have excellent social contacts with fellow males. The new behaviour of the male begins the first time he copulates. That first sexual encounter is also of unprecedented intensity, for copulation can take a good forty hours.[78] It would appear that this experience leads to changes in certain parts of the brain in their response to vasopressin. During the 'wedding night' new receptors are formed, and these provide the stimulus for good paternal behaviour throughout life. The researchers provisionally concluded that while oxytocin refines maternal behaviour, vasopressin refines paternal, protective behaviour. For the rest, the character changes brought about by the first copulation are so incisive that, by comparison, every other copulation is over in the blink of an eye.

Pregnancy in a cultural context

People cannot remember their own birth. Everything they know about it is hearsay. Nor shall we be able to say anything about our deaths. Hence the moment when a man and a woman bring new life into the world is the only existential drama at which we can be consciously present. No wonder then, that for almost everyone who has experienced it, it is one of life's most significant events.

What precisely determines the beginning of a confinement is still not absolutely clear, but it is indisputable that different cultures react differently to that event. From anthropological writings we know the stories of pregnant women who go unobtrusively into the bush and return a little later freshly washed and with a baby. That contrasts sharply with the behaviour of the Western woman with her many options. In the Netherlands, a large section of the population holds the view that childbirth is more of a celebration if it takes place at home and with as little medical intervention as possible. In the United States it used to be the rule rather than the exception that the child was delivered under anaesthetic and it is not unusual for there to be an arrangement with the obstetrician that the birth take place on, say, the Fourth of July or on the anniversary of a much missed grandmother. If that means a Caesarean, it is hardly considered a drawback. In any case, American tradition treats childbirth as a medical matter, in which the new mother plays no more than a subsidiary role.

Medical involvement in childbirth is under increasing attack: in some parts of the United States it is almost impossible to obtain obstetric help because midwives and obstetricians can no longer afford the enormous premiums demanded by insurers for claims for professional negligence. In Russia we find the other extreme. There, the expectant parents have no say, and fathers are not allowed in the maternity wards in case they introduce bacteria. While preparing to give birth, the women sit together on an open toilet by a large shared enema syringe. There is no personal attention and the child is delivered quickly and then taken away at once. This situation was uncritically turned to account in a commercial for mobile telephones: the fathers are shown standing outside the clinic after the birth while the mothers, holding their babies up at the window, chat eagerly on their mobiles so that they are at least sharing their excitement verbally. The richest women can go to private clinics, but anyone able to afford the fee generally prefers to make for the West.[79] The less affluent have to make do with primitive alternatives. In May 1999, an American journalist working for the *Moscow Times* wrote an article about two pregnant women who had planned their confinement in a camping site far from the inhabited world, without medical help. Their previous deliveries had been so traumatic that they did everything they could not to end up in a maternity clinic again.[80]

In the West, women and their partners have had great freedom of choice during the past few decades in deciding how to plan one of the greatest moments of their life. At home or in a clinic, lying down or squatting in a birthing chair, even under water – all these are possibilities about which people can nowadays decide for themselves. In some European countries, doctors and midwives by and large agree that childbirth should involve a minimum of medication, which explains why pregnancy exercises and courses for painless childbirth are so popular.

Most couples stop having sexual intercourse towards the end of pregnancy, though coitus may well be considered a good way of bringing confinement a little closer.[81] Orgasms are believed to render the contractions more goal-directed, and touching the cervix can serve as an extra stimulus. The Japanese now use a special vibrator to stimulate the cervix, thereby speeding parturition. Two substances gynaecologists normally use for inducing confinement can be produced naturally. Erotic excitement, and especially nipple stimulation, produces a high oxytocin concentration in the blood; the synthetic variant (Syntocinon) is the most commonly used method of inducing contractions. Sperm contains a great deal of prostaglandin, and synthetic prostaglandin (applied vaginally) is also used to bring on contractions.

During birth, a number of elements are identical with the sexual response, and it is undeniable that sexual excitement and orgasms have a favourable effect on contractions.[82] During the Ninth World Sexology Congress held in 1989 in Caracas, Galdino Pranzarone from Salem University, Virginia, drew attention to certain alternative obstetric practices that had begun to regain ground in the United States during the eighties. These were then incorporated into a communal lifestyle in which reverence for nature determined all human activity. Thanks to Alice Walker, this approach also found its way into the novel:

> I had the most sought-after midwife in France – my competent and funny aunt Marie-Thérèse, whose radical idea it was that childbirth above all should feel sexy. . . . My vulva was oiled and massaged continuously to keep my hips open and my vagina fluid, I was orgasmic at the end. Petit Pierre practically slid into the world at the height of my amazement, smiling serenely even before he opened his eyes.[83]

Childbirth is a very special event; hence it is not surprising that people with a spiritual bent should through their very intense experience discover their own personal set of beliefs. They want childbirth to be something beautiful and transcendent, and if everything goes well, childbirth undoubtedly does provide a satisfaction that is beyond compare. That birth was accepted as a spiritual experience is an old tradition. Disappointments are sometimes unavoidable, for unpredictable things can happen and for these nothing can prepare us. And there have been quite a few recorded aberrations in which the desire for childbirth as the individual expression of an individual emotion no longer serves the needs of the infant. The flower-power movement has been made fun of in the British television series *Absolutely Fabulous,* which pours scorn on the treatment of childbirth as a fashionable happening. In a flashback, Patsy, the alcoholic best friend of the leading character, Edwina, relives her own birth. Her exhibitionist, extravagant mother brought her into the world in the glory years of the hippie movement. Her confinement was witnessed by a host of friends, and she believed that this act had been her most ultimate performance. The baby itself was an affront to her artistic eye.

Childbirth is a complex event, and many of its facets have a touch of ritual. What should be done with the afterbirth? In some large maternity clinics, the placenta is placed in a large freezer and the contents regularly handed over, against payment, to a pharmaceutical concern that uses them to make dermatological and cosmetic products. Some mothers, including those who during pregnancy volunteered to provide urine samples for Mothers for Mothers to make into fertility-enhancing hormone preparations, do not like the idea of their placentas ending up in a pharmacist's jar and would far rather give them a ritual burial, just as our ancestors used to do. In *The Amazon Army,* published in 1999, Willem de Blécourt writes about the work of healers from 1850 to 1930, and it would seem that maternity nurses in particular were intimately familiar with the ancient rituals. Maternity nurses were in any case very close to the new mothers. Doctors and even qualified midwives were a little suspect because they were of a higher social rank than the patients. The afterbirth had to be buried and the maternity nurse knew best how to do that. The most favoured burial place was close to a window, because then one could quickly intervene should a dog start digging the placenta up not too close to the side of a ditch, because the child might play nearby later on. If you lived in an upstairs apartment, then you could not bury the afterbirth outside, but had to cut it into small pieces and flush it down the lavatory. Swaddling the newborn child was a special art. The best maternity nurses were those who swaddled the baby most tightly. That seems quite uncalled for to us today, but the medical literature recently published a discussion about whether or not fewer hip dislocations occur in peoples who swaddle their babies with outstretched legs.

Modern obstetricians will sometimes find that new parents have their own ideas about what they want to do with the afterbirth, but that is unusual. Dog owners occasionally have their pet lick and smell the placenta to foster bonding between dog and child.

Yet another choice the modern mother is free to make is whether to breastfeed or bottle-feed her child. This is a question on which emotions sometimes run high. Formula manufacturers have come under severe attack because of their advertising campaigns in developing countries in particular. In the West, opting for breastfeeding sometimes means expressing milk for use during periods when mother and child are separated, and that is a time-consuming business. It is of course possible to buy electric suction pumps, but until recently very little technical common sense has been applied to this problem. In 1996, a father in Florida was so shocked by the antediluvian equipment his wife had to resort to that he used his technical expertise to devise an instrument that for one thing fits so snugly that it can be worn undetected under a roomy cardigan. Moreover the sucking power of the pump can be varied in such a way that the milk throughput can be built up gradually. There are quite a few mothers (and babies), it appears, who start off slowly and tolerate stronger suction only after some time.[84]

In the past the choice used to be between feeding the child oneself and employing a wet nurse. The way in which a wet nurse was chosen is graphically shown in *La Balia* (*The Nanny*), a film by Marco Bellocchio (1999) based on a short story by Luigi Pirandello. One can of course rely on one's eyes and choose the fullest breasts among those on offer, as the father does in the film. But appearances are deceptive. Are there other factors that ought to be taken into account? In 1899, a journal dwelt on the question of whether a woman who had started to menstruate again should be rejected as a prospective wet nurse.[85] The journal recommended the choice of a wet nurse who had given birth six to eight weeks earlier. She might have started menstruating again, but if that had not led to a decrease in her milk secretion, she could be counted on being able to breastfeed a child for some considerable time. In France, however, there has been a law since 1874 according to which the child of the wet nurse must be at least seven months old, or itself have been fed by a wet nurse. The local mayor was expected to supervise compliance with this law.[86]

The Church also had views on the choice between breastfeeding and a wet nurse.[87] It was plain that a woman was impure after childbirth until after her lochia, the vaginal discharge of mucus, blood and cellular debris following childbirth. In the church's view, the postnatal period is identical with menstruation. In a letter written in 731 by Pope Gregory I to an English bishop, the Vicar of Christ included breastfeeding among the taboo periods. For that reason he was most suspicious of the habit in higher social circles of delegating breastfeeding to a wet nurse. Had he realized that breastfeeding also meant a deferment of fertility then his view might well have been seen in a different light – a woman who delegates the feeding of her child to another may fall pregnant again more quickly. Later, the reason given for abstinence during breastfeeding was reversed; there was then a firm conviction that sexual intercourse addles the mother's milk.

Most children receive no other milk than their own mother's, but in Morocco it is not unusual for women to exchange babies.[88] Besides natural brothers and sisters, Moroccans can also have suckling brothers and suckling sisters. The hope is that, as a result, the families of suckling partners will have greater respect for one another's children, and for daughters in particular. Girls are normally strictly separated from their male contemporaries, but are allowed to have close relations with a suckling brother. Marrying a suckling brother or sister is treated as a form of incest.

chapter eight

Women's Sex Problems

Marketing managers know that sex always sells. If sex were a trademark, then no advertising would be needed, since its brand recognition is universal and its prestige largely unassailable. Do you want to be cool? Sex! Do you want to be sure you're not missing out in life? Sex! For both young and old: sex! And in this heady atmosphere sex is made out to be simple and straightforward. Sexologists, however, are chiefly consulted by men and women who are unhappy about their sex lives.

'Not feeling like it'

Feeling like sex, a spontaneous urge for physical intimacy and sexual pleasure, is seen by most people as something perfectly natural. If you are healthy, the need for sex bubbles up spontaneously every so often, much like hunger and thirst if you have not eaten or drunk enough. Sexual need is considered to be an instinct, a drive. Freudians speak of 'libido', and if there is no libido then the layman is likely to blame it on 'frigidity' (at least with women; a male version of this word doesn't exist).

Sometimes the problem is more than an absence of sexual appetite. Some women (and some men) have a downright aversion to sex, and sometimes to everything connected with the lower part of the body. And in sexological practice we also come across couples in which one of the partners is willing enough but so much less so than the other that their sex life is a source of constant friction and a great deal of tension.

People worried about their lack of sexual appetite often experience it as a purely physical shortcoming. They feel less healthy and vital, are afraid that something may be seriously wrong with them, and often ask their doctor if hormone imbalance has anything to do with it. Many questions are also asked about the influence of the pill on sexual desire (especially in the early years, when progesterone used to be administered in such high doses as to have a decidedly dulling effect), and during the menopause, too, general practitioners will be asked frequently about the relationship between hormones and the libido. The role of sex hormones has been referred to earlier. Some women are in fact aware of the influence of their menstrual cycle on their sexual impulses, and many are not happy with that idea. If a woman has a ravenous sexual appetite during menstruation or during ovulation, she may be brought up against the instinctive, animal aspect of her nature. The same is true of women who feel especially eager for sex during pregnancy.

On the other hand, if there is never any spontaneous sexual desire, that too is disagreeable. It can be in sharp conflict with one's self-image ('I'm not really like that') and can lead to a lopsided relationship. Having a relationship, after all, often determines the situation to be a problem. Unattached men and women rarely consult a sexologist because of lacking sexual appetite.

Interest in sex is a brain activity, and lack of interest is actually a symptom of depression. Psychopharmaceutical preparations include quite a few with a damping effect on the spontaneous sexual drive. Anyone emotionally burdened, for instance by the illness or the death of someone close to them, can temporarily lose their sex drive as a result and no one finds that odd. Again, if physical fitness is seriously below par, then erotic needs generally decline to a minimum. Patients undergoing dialysis, asthmatics, MS patients, but also heroin addicts and alcoholics, all run the risk of having their sex drive drop low on their list of priorities.

However, the physical, that is, the biological side of the problems involved in sexual desire, is often overestimated. Thus the belief that men, by virtue of their nature, their more insistent hormones, are always more interested in sex than women is certainly an oversimplification. One or two psychological factors are often brought into play as well. The case histories of women who come for sexological treatment have certain elements in common. The sex education given by parents to their daughters is still far too often associated with the instillation of fear and the playing down of pleasure. The example many parents set their children is often less than inspiring, and shockingly large numbers of women have in addition been confronted occasionally as children or teenagers by deviant sexual behaviour that violated their boundaries. In some families disparate messages are given to boys and girls, often making girls feel inferior to their brothers and to boys in general. The combination of a poor knowledge of sex with a low self-image can prevent women from objecting to their partner's sexual demands.

The interaction between the partners can also involve a dynamic by which the desires of one partner are conveyed to the other in such a way as to make his or her life more difficult. The power struggle into which some sexual relationships degenerate sometimes looks comical to an outside observer. That does not apply to heterosexual couples only, since disagreements over the frequency of sex also occur in lesbian relationships.

Most relationships are riddled with conflicts of interest. Thus while one partner may want to go for a walk in the woods on a Sunday afternoon, the other may insist on watching Wimbledon on TV. If there are many such conflicts then the couple has a problem, albeit an identifiable, not to say normal one. When it comes to differences in sexual preferences the pressure to be normal is a complicating factor, and that applies to the frequency as well as to the quality. If one of the partners desires the other infrequently, that can cause particular difficulties. The worrying question is: 'Don't I love him/her any more?' If one partner feels a regular need for 'spooning' (lying in bed like two spoons), but is frustrated by the other, who feels there is little 'hard' sex in such behaviour and wants to stretch the frontiers all the time, then it will not take long for the first partner to give up his or her desire for physical intimacy. If the couple goes to a sexologist, the problem is usually presented as: 'I think we're having too little sex, and it's all your fault.' The fact that the accused partner is often experiencing too little physical contact as well scarcely registers with them.

Differences in the sexual needs of male and female partners can manifest themselves in distinct ways. Sometimes the conflict is dwelt on and fought over tooth and nail, but there are of course all sorts of ways of dealing considerately with situations in which one partner needs sexual release and the other requires a different kind of intimacy. The sexual revolution has generated so much tolerance that in many beds it is no longer thought odd that husband and wife should lie next to each other feeling close and safe, the one nodding off fully relaxed while the other sees to the desired sexual relief on his or her own. That strikes me as an improvement, compared with the classical scene in which the plaintiff keeps nagging the accused to please, please make love. A tacit ground rule during such debates is that sex can take place only if both partners are involved, from foreplay to intercourse and orgasm. Consequently, the gridlock can often be broken only by a sordid shagging, leaving one partner feeling coerced and used, and both unsatisfied and unable to fall asleep.

Perhaps the reader will have filled in the sex of the plaintiff (male) and the accused (female) in the scene sketched above, but the choice has deliberately been left open. If the division of roles does indeed reflect that sex stereotype, then everyone can see that this couple is having a hard time, but there is also something familiar, something reassuring in the picture. It confirms an ancient world view; the man does indeed feel rejected, but can console himself with the thought that 'women have always been like that', and that things are not all that much better with the neighbours. He can in any case make in-jokes on the subject with his friends and colleagues, and perhaps he also has one really good friend with whom he can share his disappointment, anger, sorrow and uncertainty. The woman will probably feel guilt-ridden, but she knows that all men have sex on the brain, and that quite a lot of women succumb to their pressure. And she too will have no difficulty in sharing her feelings with a few confidantes from whom she can expect loads of sympathy and support. They are likely to confirm that, if women have other worries, sex must take its place in the queue (and that men will never understand this).

The woman who is desirous and is frustrated by her partner has a much harder time of it, because her situation is abnormal; in fact it shakes the foundations of our basic beliefs. She will feel instinctively that this is a subject she had better not discuss with anyone or risk ostracism. The situation requires an explanation, but the answers seem fairly ominous. Perhaps the whole thing is her own fault. Is she unattractive? Does she say all the wrong things? Does she have a bad smell? Is her vaginal discharge (which her doctor told her during her last visit was normal, and yet . . .) the reason for his aversion? Or is he in love with someone else? Is he gay perhaps? Is the way she makes her wishes known perhaps too forward for him? The same holds for the man: he will talk to no one about it, since it is bad enough that his wife wants to discuss it all the time, which merely increases his misery and impotence.

The only book to deal with this situation is called *What To Do When He Has a Headache*, and the answer given by the American psychologist Janet Wolfe is somewhat depressing.[1] She stresses that the situation in which a woman craves sex more than her male partner is so unusual that it calls for the utmost subtlety and understanding from her. Men cannot read Janet Wolfe's book without a vicarious sense of shame. It does not become them that women must permanently pamper their fragile self worth by assuming a non-threatening position; and it does not become the women to pretend that they are satisfied with so patently unequal a situation. The book is part of the American tradition of which John Gray is the leading proponent (*Men Are From Mars, Women Are From Venus*). This literature cherishes a romantic love ideal in which everything unpalatable in a relationship is viewed from the firm conviction that both men and women have the very best of intentions and only get in each other's way thanks to ignorance and naïvety. The fact that relationships also reflect a good measure of anger and thirst for power is not reported in these books, and nor is the fact that from an emancipatory point of view some question marks should be raised about the division of tasks (factual and emotional) in many heterosexual relationships. The same subject has been discussed by the Austrian sociologists Cheryl Benard and Edit Schlaffer with considerably greater depth and sarcasm in their *Leave the Men Alone*.[2]

In conclusion, here are a few figures: in an interview research project about ten years ago in the United States it emerged that one woman in three maintained that she had too little desire for sex, while in men that ratio was one in six. Twenty years ago, sexologists used to be consulted mainly by couples in which the woman complained about feeling less like having sex than her partner, but in the last few years there has been a swing the other way. Nowadays sexologists are mainly consulted by inhibited men. Obviously, there are quite a few couples now in which husband and wife, with the help of emancipatory information from the media, are able to handle their desire discrepancies without professional help, while men who disappoint their partners are increasingly less reluctant to ask for help.

Arousal problems

The excitement phase in the sexual response cycle of Masters and Johnson is characterized by the parallel course of a mental phenomenon (excitement) and a physical phenomenon (blood congestion in women, felt as swelling of the labia and of the clitoris, and vaginal lubrication). During this phase we meet the most prevalent sexual problem of men: the inability to have an erection. An erection is a very complex response, and there are a large number of diseases, post-operative conditions and drugs that interfere with man's ability to have an erection even with optimum mental excitation. Nevertheless, lack of excitement plays a part in the largest group of men with erection problems, even when there is some physical cause, for if the body shows little reaction the result is often uncertainty and that leads to a loss of concentration during sexual arousal.

In women too, illness and drugs can lead to a disturbance of the links between mind and body. After the menopause, when the body is less influenced by oestrogens, the vaginal mucosa alters in such a way that the vagina lubricates more slowly even during considerable arousal. In the early years of the pill, when the progesterone dose was still very high, pill users sometimes complained of a dry vagina. That was, however, usually the result of reduced arousal.

Sexologists see few women who complain about lack of arousal, but general practitioners and gynaecologists are often consulted about pain during intercourse, and undoubtedly there are also women who come to their doctors with a pseudo-complaint because they find it difficult to talk to them about sex. There are many non-sexual vaginal complaints they can use as a presenting symptom: discharge, itching, pain in the abdomen and menstrual disorder. General practitioners, who have been trained to ask about possible sexual difficulties when confronted with this type of problem, will often discover that arousal difficulties are at the heart of the complaints.

Medical help is needed because problems during the arousal phase are difficult to fathom by the men and women burdened with them. People are generally much more aware of the physical aspects than of what happens simultaneously in the emotional sphere. If both the man and the woman allow themselves to be guided by their feelings during sexual intercourse, then one of them might well come to think after a while: I'm not really being turned on tonight, I'm a bit unenthusiastic, I'm not on the same wavelength. There are all sorts of ways of conveying that to one's partner, and if he or she should happen to be in a state of high excitement, then the situation is somewhat disappointing. It is as if your partner doesn't think much of the book that completely bowled you over. Talking about the difference in appreciation can, however, lead to the restoration of a close relationship.

That is how things would be if both partners gave free rein to their emotions, but most people with problems do not. A man and a woman begin to make love, and the atmosphere becomes worrying if, after a time (the time that for him counts as normal foreplay), he has no erection. On enquiry it will sometimes emerge that he had not been very keen to begin with, but felt obliged to initiate sex because they had not had it for a long time, or because the partner wanted it so much, or because the man thought it reflected badly on his manhood to let any opportunity for sex slip by. For such men, 'I want sex' (cognition) is tantamount to 'I desire sex' (emotion), and once this logical error has been committed it is quite understandable that the failure to have an erection should be seen as a physical problem.

If a woman makes love regardless of her emotions, she will probably fail to realize that she is not aroused, and if the couple then perform 'the act' in the accustomed way, small wonder if it proves a difficult business. There are women who have become so used to doing what is expected of them at such moments that they may suffer significant physical pain. Some women go so far in following this pattern that their mucous membrane becomes damaged.

Pain during sex is a matter of degree. If a random group of women were asked if they had ever experienced pain during intercourse, the score would undoubtedly be more than 50 per cent. This includes such situations as the first time, intercourse while suffering from vaginal thrush, as well as intercourse without arousal.

Occasionally a woman will ask for help for a 'genuine' arousal problem: she makes love with great passion, becomes highly excited, but the expected physical satisfaction fails to materialize (wholly or partly). The cause can be deduced from our knowledge of physiology and our much greater knowledge of erection problems in men. With a low oestrogen level (that is, after the menopause, or after an ovariectomy, or following dialysis in kidney disease), the vagina can react much more slowly than normal to a given stimulus. Sometimes the blood vessels (which must dilate to effect physical arousal) have become sclerotic. This will usually go hand in hand with high blood pressure and nicotine addiction. Diabetes may contribute to the malfunctioning of the blood vessels; moreover, women with diabetes are appreciably more susceptible to vaginal infections (which also can give rise to vaginal pain). The nerve signal setting off the vascular reaction can be interrupted in such diseases as MS and lesions of the spinal cord. Some major operations to the pelvis minor cannot be performed without damaging nerves terminating in the vagina; the most common of these operations is removal of the rectum in cases of cancer (an operation that usually calls for an artificial opening in the colon, a stoma). And finally, some drugs inhibit the physical manifestations of sexual arousal by their effect on the nervous system. In this area, too, we have far wider knowledge about men than about women, but we may take it that the substances inhibiting an erection in men will also interfere with the vaginal responses of women.

Orgasm problems

An orgasm demands well-focused stimulation, that is, a certain degree of concentration, and begins with an understanding of one's physical apparatus. There are subtle differences between the learning processes of girls and those of boys, so that it is fairly easy to explain the differences in the orgasmic skills of men and women. In general, nearly all boys learn to masturbate, and they nearly all reach their first orgasm unaided. Among women, too, a majority come to their first orgasm through masturbation, but there is a large minority who owe their first orgasm to a partner, and there is a significant percentage who will never resort to masturbation after that. The timing, too, is different: in a very large percentage of boys, the first orgasm occurs between the ages of ten and sixteen, but in girls the distribution is much more dispersed. It is relatively unusual for a boy not to have had an orgasm before he is twenty, and his counsellor will have to bear in mind that this situation reflects powerful inhibitions and neurotic conflicts. With a twenty-year-old girl who has not yet had her first orgasm, there is less need to look for complicated psychological motives. In the 1970s, the American psychologist Lonnie Barbach therefore saw fit to replace the term 'anorgasmia' with the more optimistic 'preorgasmia'.[3] Today that term may cause raised eyebrows in some quarters because it smacks of political correctness.

Women who seek help for problems with their orgasm fall into two groups: those who have never had any kind of orgasm, and those who were quite content about the role of orgasms in their lives but are content no longer. In the second group (the secondary anorgasmia group), the problem usually arises in a relationship. Couples still come for advice to therapists who take the Freudian view that there is an orgasmic problem when the woman does not climax in response to exclusively vaginal stimulation. Sexologists make it a rule of thumb that secondary anorgasmy involves both partners, while primary anorgasmy needs a predominantly individual approach. Lonnie Barbach designed a form of group therapy for preorgasmic women based on the belief that these women can best come to grips with their own orgasmic responses if they take control of their sexuality by masturbation. At the time, this was considered a provocative assertion, because the group with orgasm problems included women who clung to the idea that sexual growth must necessarily occur in the context of a relationship.

In the 1990s, however, the proportion of anorgasmic cases in sexological practice declined appreciably. Some centres did apply the group approach to women's sex problems, but the participants had less uniform scale of problems. While the number of anorgasmic women has reduced, the complexity of their psychological problems has increased. Sexologists are now regularly confronted with orgasmic difficulties that no longer confirm their earlier optimism. In women, too, a complex combination of fears and inhibitions can lurk beneath the cloak of this problem.

With men, the main orgasmic problem is premature ejaculation, and it is striking that there is no female counterpart of this condition. Whatever may have been changed by the sexual revolution, a woman still does not have to exert control over her climaxing, while men do.

Many men assume a responsibility for controlled releases, while women by and large are expected to behave with blissful abandon.

Afterglow

This period is called the resolution phase on Masters and Johnson's curve – the organs involved in the sexual responses come to rest again. That much is clear, but little scientific attention has been paid to the emotional aspects of this period. *Post coitum omne animal triste,*[4] said Aristotle. That all animals (except women and cockerels) are sad after intercourse is a dictum that comes from a time when animal ethologists were still by and large groping in the dark; as for human sexual emotions, scientists had ideas before the nineteenth century that suprose us today. Albertus Magnus, dean of the University of Paris (and thus by definition a priest), came out with pronouncements in his *De coïtu* (On intercourse) that were fairly tolerant for his age, but he was unable to answer a then topical question: Why, of all animals, is man the only species that during copulation utters no sound at all.[5] The question may strike as inadequate, one that could only be raised by scientists living a celibate life and adhering to biblical precepts. Maybe Albertus Magnus also believed that women have one rib fewer than men.

Problems during the resolution phase are unusual. Occasionally we are told by couples living in sexual discord that men and women can have distinct sexual habits. If one makes for the shower within seconds while the other likes to savour the breathlessness, sweatiness and stickiness of the moment, then that can be difficult. If there is a marked difference in sexual need, the excitement of the sexually more active partner can seem a censure of the other. 'You were enjoying it just now just as much as I was, so why don't you want to do it more often?' Some people experience their sexual ecstasy as an exceptional state, and after intercourse they slip quickly back into their normal, respectable and controlled self. If one partner habitually re-enacts the event in his or her mind, and wants to share this pleasure with the other, who has already switched off, then the two are not on the same wavelength.

Women sometimes consult their doctors about persistent pain in the abdomen, which continues after intercourse. This is a complaint that is hard to explain. In some cases there seems to be a link with a persisting high level of excitation (and hence blood congestion in the pelvis minor), in the absence of orgasm. Persistent congestion may well lead to an oxygen shortage in some women, and an orgasm, with the associated muscular activity, ensures a speedy return to the normal flow of blood in the vascular system. Some women are able to end a period of intense sexual activity without feeling the need for an orgasm, but can finish up with physical problems. The only way to find out is to try having an orgasm. Women sometimes have difficulty in forcing themselves to climax when their mind is on other things. Some people have headaches after sexual intercourse, a complaint that is difficult to treat.

Vaginismus and dyspareunia (pain during sexual intercourse)

There are two distinct problems associated with sexual penetration. We speak of vaginismus when a woman feels so strong an aversion to sexual intercourse that she blocks (or almost blocks) entry, and of dyspareunia (difficult or painful sexual intercourse) when penetration is possible but causes pain.

The classical picture of vaginismus goes as follows: a young woman who is rather ignorant and reserved when it comes to sex, notices during her first attempt at sexual intercourse that she is unable to admit her partner's penis into her vagina. If the lovers keep trying then she feels pain, and even if she is willing to put up with that, her vagina is so tightly 'locked' that her partner cannot enter her. Sometimes there is so much muscle resistance even before the genital organs make contact that this point is never reached. The whole endeavour is quite bewildering for the woman – she may be more than willing, but when it comes to the point, her legs suddenly clamp tightly together, she arches her back and thrashes about so wildly that no penetration can take place.

If the couple consult their general practitioner, he or she is likely to propose a physical examination, and then the same thing often happens on the examination couch as happens at home in bed. The GP is familiar with the phenomenon and can therefore explain to the couple that it is not that the woman is too narrow inside, but that she has a reflex spasm of the muscles that causes her vaginal sphincters to contract. Sometimes after this explanation, if the doctor is patient and the woman has enough confidence, it is possible for an internal investigation with one finger to be made. This can bring great relief, for it demonstrates that if she can become more aware of these muscles she may learn to abandon herself to her partner during lovemaking.

As early as 1948, the American gynaecologist Arnold Kegel devised exercises for the pelvic-floor muscles. At the time, Kegel worked mainly with women suffering different problems following difficult deliveries. Urinary incontinence is quite common, and prolapse of the uterus, too, often causes severe discomfort. The muscles in the pelvic floor that provide a solid foundation to the abdominal cavity may have lost their tone, something that can often be detected by an internal examination. Kegel taught women how to retrain their muscles, and with some women that meant becoming aware of muscles they knew nothing about. It did not prove easy to detect the new sensation, and for that reason a small pressure gauge was devised to provide an objective record of the effect of the contractions. It did not take long for Kegel to attract a number of enthusiastic patients, despite the fact that it was imperative to exercise regularly if good results were to be obtained. Later, all sorts of electrical stimulation devices were marketed to produce the same results without any great effort on the part of the patient. Another aid was the 'trainer', a set of small conical weights that the woman could keep in her vagina. The shape and weight were such that the trainer continually threatened to fall out and the muscles were thus permanently challenged to prevent that from happening. One of Kegel's first patients surprised him with the report that a strengthened pelvic floor also had very pleasant sexual consequences for both partners. That news spread quickly among doctors and laymen.

After the Sixties' sexual revolution, many women strove to attain a high sexual energy level, and Kegel's exercises became part of a new lifestyle. In a small book on vaginal muscles and sexuality published in 1982, three case histories are presented of women who were determined to learn how to have orgasms without clitoral stimulation. Their progress was meticulously documented by the researchers during a course of pelvic-floor exercises.[6] A remarkable feature of the book is the detailed nature of the medical observations. The female researcher performed an internal examination at every check up and recorded precisely where she thought the muscles were unable to contract adequately as well as her view of the quality of the tone of the muscle at rest. The progress with Patient 1 charted here (illus. 22) is impressive. This way of mapping the vaginal sphincters has not been repeated, but in a recent self-help book the exercises recommended for women are again very ambitious.[7] The women are guided in such a way as to help them concentrate separately on the lower, middle and upper layers of the pelvic floor.

The Kegel exercises are thus designed to give women a better muscle tone, but part of the learning process involves conscious awareness of the pelvic floor. And that is what women suffering from vaginismus lack, or such was the impression of the investigating physicians. It was only logical to devise a variant of the Kegel exercises, in which aware-

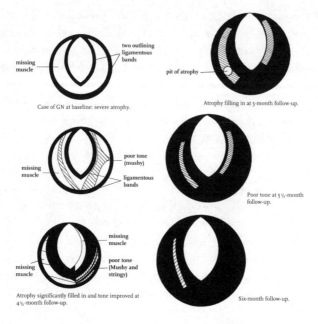

two outlining
ligamentous
bands

missing
muscle

Case of GN at baseline: severe atrophy.

pit of atrophy

Atrophy filling in at 5-month follow-up.

poor tone
(mushy)

missing
muscle

ligamentous
bands

Poor tone at 5½-month
follow-up.

missing
muscle

poor tone
(Mushy and
stringy)

missing
muscle

Atrophy significantly filled in and tone improved at
4½-month follow-up.

Six-month follow-up.

ness of the vaginal sphincters would lead to relaxation. In the treatment
of vaginismus, relaxation exercises have always played a part, but it was
not until 1999 that a serious attempt was made to determine objectively what was happening to the pelvic-floor muscles, and the woman's
ability to contract and relax the pelvic floor deliberately. Janneke van
der Velde, a psychologist at the University of Amsterdam, discovered
that women suffering from vaginismus had a higher resting tone in the
pelvic floor, but did not differ from the control group in their ability to
contract their pelvic-floor sphincters deliberately.[8] There was, however,
a significant difference if the patients also had complaints about urinating and defecating. That is a quite common combination. Quite a few
women with vaginismus also suffer from constipation and often hold
back their urine so long or pass urine so inadequately that they will have
bladder infections quite often.

Tension in the pelvic floor proved to increase in threatening situations. This was established in the investigation by the use of video
extracts: a rape scene and a scary non-sexual situation. The sphincter
muscles reacted in the same way to sexual and non-sexual threats, even
with women in the control group, and not only in the pelvic floor –
other muscles were also put in a state of heightened tension (the measurements were made on a muscle in the shoulder area). At the end of
her thesis, Janneke van de Velde concluded that the role of relaxation
and awareness-raising exercises in women suffering from vaginismus

should not be overestimated, and that attention should therefore not be confined to the muscles.

In the classical picture of vaginismus, the woman is still a virgin. She may have tried 'it', but failed. There are, however, women who in fact succeed now and then in keeping their defence reactions so tightly under control that penetration is possible. Some of the women who come for therapy already have one child or more, which means that their determination, underpinned by their desire to have children, has been so great that they were able at the time to distance themselves mentally from what they were doing. Psychologists then speak of dissociation: during emotionally fraught moments part of the consciousness, for instance awareness of one's own vagina, can be split off.

In dyspareunia the picture is far more variable. During coitus the woman feels pain. Sometimes this happens from the first contact of penis and vagina, in which case the pain is mostly felt in the entrance to the vagina. That type of complaint is fittingly referred to as entry pain. If the pain is deep in the abdomen, it is called thrusting pain. In some women lovemaking starts without unpleasant sensations, but after a while pain sets in and sometimes persists for quite some time after coitus. The pain is described in a variety of ways: burning, raw, rough or spasmodic (as in menstrual cramps). The emotional impact of the pain also varies greatly. There are women who accept the pain as part of sexual intercourse, and others who suffer a kind of panic, a fear that something might be damaged inside. The feeling is sometimes described as 'a bit like being raped'.

Dyspareunia can be due to a variety of causes. Entry pain is a normal side-effect of vaginal infections such as candida (thrush) and trichomonas. Among sexually transmitted diseases, herpes is generally associated with pain. Women with infections of the bladder and the urethra usually have to stop having penetrative sex, and some painful conditions of the rectum can also be provoked by the penis. Childbirth, too, makes heavy demands on the opening of the vagina, and the scars from cuts (epis) and tears (ruptures) are a regular cause of dyspareunia. Thrusting pains can be a result of diseases of the uterus or the ovaries, since with deep thrusts organs that are normally inaccessible can be moved about. The uterus is rather loosely placed among the other abdominal organs, so that in principle it can be shifted slightly by the penis. Some women like the feeling that results, while others dislike it intensely. After childbirth, the internal positioning of the organs can be altered so much that the pleasant feelings in the uterus disappear (for the most part temporarily).

Abdominal infections (for instance in a Fallopian tube or the intestine) can be the foci of pain, and the infected region can sometimes be touched during intercourse. After removal of the uterus, the vagina can be so shortened that penetration can no longer take place without pain, and after the menopause, too, the vagina often loses some of its depth and elasticity.

The causes of pain we have mentioned so far fall into the category of 'diseases', and their treatment follows the classical model of diagnosis and prescription. Unfortunately, things are not always that simple. Some women complaining of pain are found to have nothing wrong with them. Occasionally a woman finds it hard to relax during a gynaecological examination, and when asked she will sometimes recognize this response as a problem during lovemaking. With some women who feel pain during intercourse the cause is the same as that responsible for vaginismus, though less pronounced. We have already suggested that pain is probably the most common expression of some problem bound up with sexual arousal. Some women know perfectly well that their vagina is not lubricated during sex, but see no reason to refuse to have intercourse. Sometimes the lack of arousal is explained entirely by a total absence of sexual desire, intercourse only being conceded because the partner 'cannot do without'.

A typical story concerns the married woman who asks her family physician to rid her of the pain she feels when performing her marital duties, but who is pleased and perhaps even a little proud because all these goings-on have never really touched her. Every GP must have heard the claim 'I have never turned my husband down', and for some women that is the normal interpretation of the 'act of love'. So it is only reasonable that they should expect solutions that do not alter their emotions in any way.

The other, more modern sounding extreme is the woman who makes love with great pleasure, has a partner who is receptive to her wishes and desires, who only has intercourse if she herself wants it, who proves to be in perfect health during medical examinations, and yet feels pain when she has her lover's penis inside her. If there is no obvious cause of the pain, then this is one of the most difficult of all the conditions sexologists are asked to deal with. It is more than likely that such women have had medical treatment (in particular vaginal medication for fungal infections), and often more than once.

Crested symphyses

The question 'Am I really sick then, or is it all in my mind?' worries many women, and sometimes they are driven from pillar to post between gynaecologist and psychologist. There is an anatomical peculiarity that can cause entry pain and that has remained virtually unrecognised by physicians and sexologists alike.[9] This involves the width of the symphysis pubica, that part of the pubic bone a woman can feel at the front of her vagina if she presses down on her mons veneris (see illus. 23). The variation in its width is considerable, and the volume of the symphysis determines the position of the vaginal opening. A wide symphysis means a vagina that lies fairly far to the back. In some women, this phenomenon is so marked that the opening of the vagina lies midway between abdomen and back, which conflicts with the image held by most women (and men). Parents speak of the 'front bottom' and girls and boys grow up with the idea that the 'little hole' can be found just round the corner from the mons veneris.

Coen van Emde Boas, the first Dutch professor of sexology, was one of the very few to draw attention to this cause of dyspareunia. In 1941, he described this form of 'pseudovaginismus'.[10] He had seen a number of newly married couples who had met with unexpectedly severe pains during their wedding night, and he had the impression that the inexperienced husbands aimed too high with their penis and caused abnormal friction in the area of the urethra. Even when they penetrated their wives successfully, the women still felt pain in this region. After coitus, urethral friction left some women with a feeling that resembles that of a bladder infection. The mucous membranes in this area are thin and vulnerable, and lie flat against the hard bony pelvis, and in some cases the symphysis has a somewhat sharp edge on the inner side (whence the term 'crested symphysis'). Van Emde Boas's solution was pragmatic: there is room enough for a penis in the minor pelvis, but it does not give at the front. Muscles can give, but bones cannot. He advised his patients to draw their legs right up and to place a firm pillow under their buttocks. Rear entry helps to spare such a sensitive area.

Van Emde Boas was famous in his day, but the medical world did not take this subject seriously. The gynaecological literature does mention a few related conditions. Some doctors assume that some women have an opening of the urethra that is too low (the technical term is hypospadias). The consequence is that the opening is pressed inwards during coitus so that the penis chafes against it all the time. That might be an explanation of the pain, and Van Emde Boas's advice would

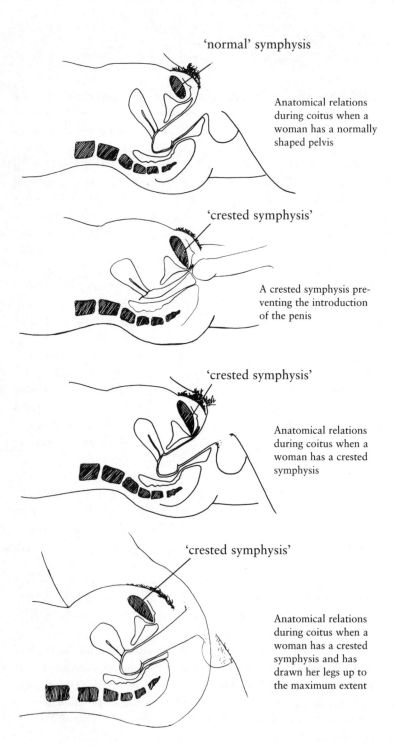

'normal' symphysis

23 Crested symphysis: a reappraisal in the 1980s.

Anatomical relations during coitus when a woman has a normally shaped pelvis

'crested symphysis'

A crested symphysis preventing the introduction of the penis

'crested symphysis'

Anatomical relations during coitus when a woman has a crested symphysis

'crested symphysis'

Anatomical relations during coitus when a woman has a crested symphysis and has drawn her legs up to the maximum extent probably be helpful to these women as well. Women with this kind of anatomical variation often have unsatisfactory encounters with therapists and others. The doctor investigates and finds nothing abnormal (no infection, no abnormalities of the mucous membrane, no vaginismus), and advises the woman to consider her problem a psychological condition. The psychologist or sexologist who then deals with her will very quickly be at a loss. The existence of such problems is a powerful argument for the multidisciplinary approach in sexology.

The variation in the width of the symphysis can be demonstrated if the woman is examined in the classical gynaecological position. The placing of the vagina varies, something that is hardly referred to in the textbooks. Dickinson alone mentioned older German anthropological opinions in 1949, according to which the vagina of primitive people lies closer to the anus.[11] That is understandable in the light of the cultural premises that held sway at the time: the more primitive a tribe, the greater the chances of their copulating like animals.

In ancient Chinese love manuals a distinction is, however, made between a high, a middle and a low vagina. Love manuals were very popular in China from the fifth century BC onwards. The Ming period (1368–1644) was unusually discreet by Chinese standards, and love manuals were less frank. The extract given below comes from the only extant manuscript published at that time. It is written in the form of a dialogue between the Emperor and the Plain Girl. Like the Victorian authors of erotica, Robert van Gulik, the sinologist who made Western readers familiar with this type of Chinese literature, invariably translated the most explicit language into Latin:

> The Emperor asked: 'Wherein lies the difference of high, middle and low vulvae?' The Plain Girl replied: 'Bonitas vulvae non in loco, sed in usu sita est. Vulvae et alto et medio et infima loco omnes possident utatur. Mulier cui vulva in medio sita est [i.e. medio inter montem veneris et anum spatio] idonea est cum qua quis per quattuor anni tempore copuletur omnesque veneris figuras inducet. Nam (in mulieribus quoque) optima est aurea mediocritas. Mulier cui vulva altus in fronte sita est, frigidis noctibus hibernis idonea est. Cum illa enim vir coire potest sub pictis quadrati lecti opertoriis ei incubando. Mulier cui vulva inferius magisque in recessu est posita ardoribus aestivis praesertim idonea. Cum illa enim vir coire potest in sedili saxeo sedens sub umbra harundinum, penem a tergo inserendo, dum illa ante eum genu procubuerit positu. This is what is called utilizing the particular advantages of the shape of the woman one copulates with.'

(The quality of a vulva is not determined by its position but by its use.
The high, as well as the middle and the low vulva, is suitable for use.
A woman whose vulva is in the centre [that is, between the mons veneris
and the anus] is suited to intercourse in all four seasons, and in all
positions. For the golden mean is always the best, even in women. The
woman with a high vulva is suited to cold winter nights. On her a man
can fling himself under multicoloured blankets on a square bed. The
woman whose vulva is placed low down is suited to warm summer
nights. A man can have intercourse with her sitting on a stone seat in
the shade of the rushes, introducing his penis from the back, for which
purpose she kneels down before him.)

Van Gulik even mentioned that there were separate slang expressions in
modern Japanese for a high, a low and a medium vulva. That these
expressions exist suggests that some Japanese find the distinction important for one reason or another. The word for 'high vulva' differs in pitch
only from the word for 'refined', and the word for 'low vulva' is almost
identical with 'vulgar'; and in that way the Japanese evaluation of the
position of the vagina resembles the interpretation of the old German
anthropologists.

Oriental love manuals dwell at some length on the correct matching
and size of male and female genitals. In the *Kama Sutra* the 'yoni' and
the 'lingam' are divided into three classes: hind, mare and elephant for
women and hare, bull and stallion for men. The best coupling is between
like classes. Hare with elephant, or hind with stallion may be compati-
ble but it greatly depends on the temperament and skill of the partners.
Western sexology pays little attention to the male factor in causing pain
to women, but there is so much variation in penis width and length that
this factor cannot be neglected.[12] The subject is evidently still taboo.
If *he* is above average size, then *she* knows instinctively that she
ought to be just as proud and glad about it as he is himself. Men are
inclined to consider below average size a problem, but above average size as perfectly normal.

This was clearly demonstrated in a small survey carried out in the
United States.[13] Men were asked to estimate the size of their own penis:
average, a great deal or a little either above or below average. The same
question was asked about their feet. In the case of feet, it appeared that
the group followed the normal statistical distribution: as many men gave
themselves above average scores as came away with below average
scores, and 'average' was the most popular score of all. Not so in the case
of their penis. 'A little below average' was the top score, implying that
most men think that the average is bigger than it is in reality. We have

always known that men can be very sensitive on this subject, so much so that there are countless jokes about it. Here is the cabaret entertainer Theo Maassen:

> Porn, now there's something that makes me feel insecure. You see all those girls holding a penis in their hand and you can tell that it's almost too big for the hand. And I'm not an idiot, I know perfectly well they were specially picked for the job.
>
> All those girls with those incredibly small hands . . .

Conversely, there are women who tell their doctor they are afraid their vagina is too narrow; they rarely complain that their partner's equipment is too large.

Vaginismus: expert opinions, now and then

Vaginismus is a sexual problem first described early in the nineteenth century by the American gynaecologist J. Marion Sims.[14] This early interest is not surprising, since infertility is a logical consequence of the complaint. Vaginismus fits well into the Victorian setting. Imagine a young bride, brought up largely in ignorance of sex, and a husband who has perhaps had some experience with prostitutes, but who probably acquired little erotic sophistication in his encounters. This situation can easily lead to a wedding night on which the bride is willing to receive her new husband's advances, though she is scarcely aroused. If things do not turn out well in such circumstances, a defence reaction is only to be expected. At the time, sensibility was a highly prized feminine attribute; every home kept a small phial of Hoffmann's drops, just in case a lady felt like swooning. In those days, an oversensitive woman would undoubtedly have expressed her vaginismus in a way that fitted into the prevailing view of femininity. On the one hand, it became her, and it could not be expected that she herself should fathom the problem and solve it. On the other hand, the marriage could not be consummated, and of course that marital objective justified the most aggressive means. Sometimes the woman was deflowered and fertilized under ether, an anaesthetic that had just come onto the market. The standard interventions, however, were surgical. The sphincter muscles were cut and the hymenal area removed, after which women had to exercise daily with glass moulds to keep the surgically expanded space open. Sims was able to publish quite a few convincing accounts of his surgical successes.

In Europe doctors were clearly more conservative. In 1867 the *Wiener Medizinische Wochenschrift* (Vienna Medical Weekly) published a gentler and more modern form of treatment based on exercises.[15] Psychology was admitted into medical practice, and in 1917 a professor of gynaecology, Hector Treub, suggested that emotional problems were better tackled with understanding than with a scalpel.[16] Even so, the surgical approach was to have a long life yet. In 1987 Jos Frenken, a professor of sexology, looked into the sexological knowledge of gynaecologists, and when he extrapolated from the answers to his questionnaires how often vaginismus was still being treated by surgical means in the Netherlands (his calculations showed 117 operations a year), questions were asked in parliament.[17] Masters and Johnson had meanwhile introduced a simple behaviour-oriented treatment.[18] They bombarded married couples with positive information on all aspects of sexuality and eroticism, at the same time encouraging the woman to get used to vaginal penetration with the help of plastic dilators. By gradually increasing the thickness of these dilators, the sphincter muscles' reflex contraction could be terminated. Masters and Johnson reported a 100 per cent success rate in dealing with highly motivated married couples whom they were able to treat intensively for a fortnight. In the 1990s, a number of physiotherapists specialized in pelvic-floor problems (in addition to vaginismus, incontinence and other bladder complaints in women, and occasional prostate problems in men).

Therapists changed their ideas not least because patients were not what they had been in the nineteenth century. On the basis of vaginismus, it could be clearly demonstrated that a particular problem may be treated in many different ways, and also how much the treatment is a reflection of given conceptions about the relationship between therapist and patient. The stereotypical picture sketched above has become rare. Ever since the sexual revolution in the 1960s, we have seen more and more women who have received a positive sex education within their family circle and who have experienced their sexual feelings and orgasms without any problems, but who nevertheless, during their first, willing, attempt to have sexual intercourse, bar entry completely. It is as if their body were adopting its own attitude to penetrative sex, and this discovery strikes them like a bolt from the blue.

In the 1990s, vaginismus became part and parcel of the information with which girls grow up. It is rarer nowadays for a woman to be taken wholly by surprise by vaginismus during attempts to shed her virginity. Often she realizes that she is doing something that goes against the grain. She may for instance have tried to use tampons without success, either because she was afraid to push, or because she could not get used to the idea that a foreign object has to stay in her vagina. She may also believe that that she is unusually narrow. If women in therapy are able to talk at some length about their vaginistic reaction, most come to realize that they have a very high emotional resistance to the idea of penetration. There are still some women who are astonished when experts tell them that their pain is in their mind, but the influence of psychology has been spreading to non-professional circles for many years now.

The partners of women with vaginismus are also less ignorant than they used to be, and more sensitive. After pleading 'let's just try it once more', men are now more inclined to call it a day after subtle signs that fear and pain are imminent. Sometimes a boy and a girl have clearly got together precisely because of a certain sexual reticence. Boys, too, are sometimes afraid of penetration and anticipate that it may be a painful experience for them. And some do indeed feel pain, for instance if they are usually very careful when handling their penis. A boy who has never pulled his foreskin back completely during an erection can indeed experience pain on his first attempt at penetration.[19]

Even if vaginismus is considered a psychosomatic problem and surgical intervention is rejected, there is still much controversy about how best to tackle the problem. Vaginismus is a bone of contention in the sexological world. In the 1970s, gynaecologists and general practitioners maintained that vaginismus could only be diagnosed by an internal examination, and therefore only by a doctor. The diagnostician would have to see with his own eyes if there was good reason to speak of a muscle reflex over which women had little if any control – no treatment without a definite diagnosis. More psychotherapeutically trained sexologists insisted that women themselves were best able to tell what happened during coitus, provided they were asked the right questions. There was no need for the diagnostic examination women so dreaded.

Even so, the effects of a physical examination can be positive. If the atmosphere in the doctor's surgery is good, much information and clarification can be gleaned, and if understanding and the sense of ease can be increased during the consultation, internal investigation with one finger is generally possible, and that is very reassuring for many women. It has been suggested that the woman perform exercises on the gynaecological couch in the presence of her husband and the doctor.[20] Other sexologists consider it ethica`lly unacceptable that a woman should have to expose herself to men in this way. Most sexologically minded gynaecologists, however, have never felt particularly disconcerted by the criticism that this approach is nothing less than a kind of *droit du seigneur*.

The medico-didactic approach aims to remove all impediments to coitus as quickly as possible, and that has led to feminist objections.

The emancipationist premise is that if a woman feels reasonably certain she desires penetrative sex, but her body signals that it is not prepared for it, then it is quite wrong for her or anyone else to listen to the mind alone. The aversion the body signals has to overcome an army of coercive forces – partner, family background, society. The therapist has the task of bringing the woman into contact with her deeper feelings, and if she herself does not take her body's signals seriously, then too quick a choice of a consummation-directed approach will be much like making common cause with the enemy.

The feminists' premise then became that society subjects women to phallocratic demands, and that these can conflict with women's own interests. The aim of emancipationist therapy must therefore be to reconcile mind and body once more. However, the result may well turn out to be a victory for the (penetration-rejecting) body. That implies conflict: a clash of interests in the relationship is brought to the surface. If exercises involving penetration have to be performed, then the woman is better off using her fingers instead of dilators and vibrators, because her finger can feel if it is welcome.

Feminist demands nowadays are not always as well-supported as they were in the 1970s. Today's aggressive *grrls* (as they are called in some parts of Europe) do not criticize role models in the way that their mothers did did, but it is far from clear what they actually want. There are married couples who have had a satisfying sex life for years without penetration; they only set up an interview at a clinic when they reach the point of wanting children. For most couples that brings the whole problem to the fore once again, for people tend to feel guilty about shelving the issue. The counsellors they consult are likely to confirm this: playtime is over, now enter the world of real sex. So pressure increases, but that does not render intercourse more attractive. The woman may also have all sorts of ambivalent feelings about pregnancy, childbirth and motherhood, and these feelings may be camouflaged by her vaginismus. On the other hand, simple methods for becoming pregnant exist, a fact of which the public is well aware nowadays. Since lesbian couples have children by inseminating themselves with donor sperm at home, heterosexual couples who do not have penetrative sex can do the same.

In reality, the general practitioner or gynaecologist will usually suggest that the couple intensify their attempts at natural conception. The desire to fall pregnant is a strong motivation. At Groningen University Hospital, the sexology department did a follow-up research project into the effects of its treatment method (especially the use of dilators), and if women did not have an immediate desire for children the results proved to be modest, with only one woman in three reaching their goal.[21]

Among women who entered treatment because they wanted to become pregnant, the results were much better: three-quarters could report that there was a marked improvement. Where the problem with coitus remained unsettled, most of these women became pregnant by artificial insemination. Women who had inseminated themselves and gave birth as virgins had no more obstetric problems than women who became pregnant as the result of sexual intercourse. Giving birth does not generally help, or at best helps only a little, to overcome the fear of intercourse. There are women who have performed excellently during confinement, yet are as helpless as before with regard to erotic penetration.

The desire for a pregnancy can thus motivate women to overcome their fear, but if the only reason for seeking therapeutic help is sexual, then the behaviour therapy method is significantly less helpful. It is only logical that a simple, straightforward approach should not be in tune with problems patently caused by unconscious conflicts. It is crippling if you have absolutely no understanding of your own problem. The problem is blown up out of all proportion and the woman concerned inevitably gains the impression that she is the only person like that in the world. At the end of the 1980s, my branch of the Rutgers Foundation introduced a new format of group therapy, bringing together women who had never had an orgasm with women who had never had sexual intercourse. It proved very liberating for both groups – both the preorgasmic women and the women with vaginismus believed that their particular problem was universal. The women with vaginismus needed a great many answers before they could believe that the preorgasmic women had failed to master something so simple as climaxing, and the preorgasmic women sat there open-mouthed when they were told that the women with vaginismus had such difficulties with something to which they themselves had never had to give a moment's thought. And then there was the relief at discovering that there were other women with the same problem. In these groups, a burden shared did indeed seem to be a burden halved.

The explanation that the problem was caused by an unconscious muscle response may well be reassuring, but does not tell us what impels the unconscious. What explanation is there for the fact that these women have remained so ignorant about the inside of their bodies? The fear some women have of inserting a tampon is incomprehensible to regular tampon users. But if vaginismus is seen as a phobia, then we need not be surprised, since it is characteristic of phobias to blow up an ordinary fear out of all proportion. Sometimes the fearful woman will manage to insert a dilator into her vagina, but to do that she has to thrust the experience as far as possible out of her consciousness (this is called dissociation). This means she will not develop any confidence, which can lead her to break off the treatment. Even if the therapy does make headway, the success can sometimes be short-lived. The benefit of penetrative sex proves disappointing, the woman does not think very highly of it, and sometimes the couple simply gives up.

The odd thing about the problem of vaginismus is that, since Masters and Johnson published their findings, the professional view has been that, given the right motivation, a complete cure can be effected in a very short time, yet all practising sexologists regularly treat couples who call it a day and drop out after a good start. When this dead end is brought up for discussion, it often results in referralto a psychotherapist, but the chances are fairly good that in that case no further attention will be paid to the bodily aspects, even though the unconscious fears are deeply embedded in the body.

The role of the vagina is certainly exaggerated now and then. Vaginismus is perhaps no more caused by the vagina than anorexia is caused by the mouth, and it is therefore desirable that gynaecologists stamp their mark less heavily on its treatment. Anorexia, too, is a mysterious condition, one that nonplusses the outsider, but luckily there are women who feel the need to give voice to the motives underlying their behaviour. There are a number of biographies that air the problems of women, and anorexia is the most frequently described clinical picture. Vaginismus, alas, has inspired very few women to autobiographical writing. Linda Valins is an important spokeswoman.

Focal vulvitis, a new diagnosis in dyspareunia

Dyspareunia, too, can be a bone of contention in medical circles. Over about the last ten years, a new clinical picture called focal vulvitis has been described.[22] In some women who complain of pain during insertion of the penis, a gynaecological examination will reveal a characteristic syndrome. At the entrance to the vagina, there will be small red wounds that cause sharp and acute pain when touched. Sometimes that area can look dramatically irritated. The story told by the patients and the results of the medical examination match extremely well, but where do the small wounds come from? When routine medical tests are done, the results are negative. That is a pity, since what could provide a cure now remains mere speculation.

In the United States the condition quickly gave rise to a typical American response, namely surgical intervention. The hymenal region with a small crescent of the introital mucosa containing the wounds was excised and the gap filled by pulling the wall of the vagina slightly outwards. J. D. Woodruff, the gynaecologist who invented this method, assumed that the misery was now completely averted. However, a large group of gynaecologists, some of whom have psychosomatic training, continues to object to diagnoses that, time and again, entitle the medical profession to cut away enthusiastically at the female organs. A telephone follow-up study, in which 70 per cent of 215 women responded, concluded that only 57 per cent were entirely satisfied by the results of their surgery. An unexpected side-effect of the surgery was that the subjects became lubricated less easily during arousal.

For some, surgery for focul vulvitis is just as wrong as it is for vaginismus. Amsterdam University sexologists have researched the sexual behaviour and experience of women with the condition, and their results are illuminating. It became clear that the small wounds were an obvious result of totally inappropriate behaviour. All the women interviewed were inclined to continue having penetrative sex with their partners, despite the pain, and moreover just as often as before. Because of the pain and the prospect of the return of the pain these women made love with ever-decreasing pleasure, hence with less excitement and less lubrication. They allowed their partner's wishes to prevail so their own problems could be attributed to lack of sexual assertiveness. It is conceivable that having intercourse in this way leads to an untoward muscle response. The muscles in the pelvic floor are continuously on the defensive without the woman being conscious of it. In addition, women with this complex quite often suffer from bladder complaints as well, which seem equally to have been caused by high muscle tone of the pelvic-floor muscles. The treatment is based above all on rest (absolute abstinence from coitus) and proper care of the wound (which, in this case, means no more than covering the affected area with a thin layer of oil-based ointment). The woman has also to learn how to deal with the tension in her sphincter muscles, and to that end she is often referred to specialist physiotherapists. And finally, therapeutic discussions (sometimes in groups) are aimed at discovering the emotional motives underlying this form of behaviour. Not as many patients were treated as had been hoped. Even so, the conclusions were quite unequivocal: in the majority, an approach based on explanations and relaxation exercises with dilators worked just as well as an operation, and just as quickly. If the condition is unusually obdurate, surgical intervention can always be kept in reserve.

It seems remarkable that such a syndrome should arise quite suddenly and that it should arouse so much emotion. Every sexologist needs time to fathom how focal vulvitis comes about, but sometimes a patient will come up with a sexual biography from which the origins of the damaged areas can be inferred. For me, the eye-opener was the following story:

A girl started to masturbate at an early age by rubbing herself against her teddy bear. That gave her very pleasant sensations and explained her avid search for erotic experiences while still very young. On the road she had come across the occasional boy who was more forward in experimenting than she would have liked him to be, although she was saved from the really traumatic events. At the back of her mind, she vaguely entertained the idea that her vagina was very small, and that she would have a lot of difficulty if she ever wanted a child. She almost never used tampons; nor were tampons needed, as her periods were very light. When she moved into lodgings, she decided the time was ripe for taking the plunge with her boyfriend. She lay on top; it made her feel she was in control. However, things did not turn out as planned and she felt humiliated. Intuitively she discovered a way of making love with her friend's penis placed between her thighs as she made the same squeezing movements as she had with her teddy bear. That worked perfectly, she climaxed easily, and so did he. They never talked about it and perhaps he thought all along that he had had normal intercourse with her.

With her next boyfriend, attempts at full penetration were made from the start. Again it did not work, and she gradually felt more and more pain, which clearly originated in the small damaged area. Reading this story, we do not find it very difficult to understand why this young woman had such strong muscles round her vagina. From a young age she had been a little afraid of penetration; later her sexual pleasure was coupled to the contraction of her sphincter muscles; finally she made love for a whole year with her boyfriend's glans close to, but not inside, her vagina, which certainly increased the tension even further.

It may seem an odd comparison, but if a small child turns up regularly in the doctor's surgery with bruises and broken bones, the doctor thinks immediately of abuse by one of the parents. The child itself will deny that, for the child knows that it must not betray its parents. In the case of focal vulvitis (and actually in most cases of dyspareunia), the working hypothesis is that the woman has more penetrative sex than is good for her. She herself will often think otherwise; in particular girls who have their sexual debut at an early age are sometimes victims of immense pressure to join in. If the doctor tells her to abstain from coitus for a time, she may not comply, but may well be afraid to admit that to the doctor.

chapter nine

Clitoridectomy

The October 1998 issue of *Viva*, a women's magazine mainly for younger readers, carried a brief interview with the Somali actress and writer Yasmine Allas, who now lives in the Netherlands. In Somalia she was one of only a few uncircumcised girls, something of which she was deeply ashamed. Terrified that her friends would find out, she begged her parents to have her circumcised. It was not until much later that she came to appreciate her parents' resolute refusal.

It seems inconceivable to most Western observers that in large parts of Africa young girls should be subjected to an extremely painful ritual, the excision of their clitoris. The circumcision of Muslim boys marks their entry into the male world; Jewish circumcision reflects tribal kinship. Both fill the Westerner with less revulsion than clitoridectomy because they are patently less injurious. With clitoridectomy, it is indisputable that the woman is not only being maimed anatomically, but also that her sexual function is impaired. Worse still, nearly all analyses of the purpose of this custom show that the main motive is the subjection of female sexuality to the perceived needs of men. And if that is indeed the dominant motive, then it is very difficult to understand why women should be more fanatical than men in perpetuating, indeed reinforcing, this custom.[1]

Africa north of the equator is the cradle of clitoridectomy, the most Westernized countries (Morocco, Algeria, Tunisia and Libya) being the exception. Explanations invariably hint at links with Islam, but that seems a lame justification since clitoridectomy is not customary in the Arabian peninsula. The operation is usually performed on girls aged from five to twelve years. It is treated as a festive occasion at which only women are present. Women decide who is to be cut, when and how, women hold the girls down during their ordeal, and women wield the knife.

There are different degrees of excision. The lightest is called 'sunna' and involves no more than a small snip of the prepuce. The next variant involves the removal of the clitoris, wholly or in part. One step further brings us to the method in which the labia minora are also removed. The most radical operation is performed in Somalia and the Sudan. It involves the removal of the clitoris and the labia minora, followed by the stitching together of the labia majora, leaving no more than a small opening just above the anus. This form of intervention is known as infibulation.

Infibulation means 'clasping' or 'pinning' together. In 1993, gynaecologist M.M.J. Reyners published a detailed study of female circumcision in which he also went into the historical, religious and anthropological links of the practice.[2] He recalled the Roman physician Aulus Cornelius Celsus, who asserted in his *De medicina* that

> a bronze pin or fibula can be used, not only to keep the toga in place, but also to ensure that sexual intercourse cannot occur. The pin pierces both small labia of the woman, often a slave girl, who cannot be allowed to fall pregnant lest her sale price be lowered.

That purpose has had a long life; until the abolition of slavery, circumcised girls fetched a higher price on African slave markets than their uncircumcised sisters. Infibulation is also known as Pharaonic circumcision, a term reflecting the belief that even the most ancient Egyptian cultures practised female circumcision, something that could be verified by the inspection of mummies. Reyner came across stories of circumcised mummies in countless books and articles, but when he consulted the actual sources the indications proved to be sporadic and far from clear. Hence it is by no means certain that Nefertiti or Cleopatra were circumcised.

What happens during an infibulation is crude beyond belief, notwithstanding the fact that it is accompanied by festivities and the exchange of presents. The incision is usually carried out without an anaesthetic, sometimes with a shard of glass or a razor blade. Virtually no attention is paid to hygiene and the prevention of wound infection. It is traditional practice to use an acacia thorn for sewing up the labia majora. The girl is then swathed so that she cannot spread her legs for forty days. Most women will be unable ever again to take big steps. The opening through which they have to urinate and menstruate is so small that they must squeeze the urine out drop by drop. There are countless complications resulting from the operation itself, and throughout her life the girl will be more susceptible to infections and injuries during childbirth. Women in countries in which circumcision is the rule consider a circumcised vagina to be 'clean', in flagrant contradiction of the facts.

What happens when an infibulated woman marries? Hanny Lightfoot-Klein is an American anthropologist who did her field work in the Sudan and in Kenya.[3] The Sudanese in particular stole her heart: a people who though miserably poor are exceptionally hospitable, and, moreover, willing to discuss clitoridectomy with her with complete frankness. She describes how, after a long journey, she arrived in a village where she had been told there was a hotel. In that hotel she was greeted with some surprise ('where is your husband?'), and only after not taking no for an answer was she given a room at the end of the corridor. In the middle of the night she was awakened by piercing shrieks. When she summoned the night porter, he tried to put her mind at rest. The hotel, he told her, was a honeymoon resort and the screams she had heard were what the porter considered normal wedding-night sounds. Lightfoot-Klein packed her rucksack and left in the dead of night. Yet she might have known what to expect. She knew that it generally takes a few weeks to effect the penetration of a circumcised girl and that quite often a midwife with a knife has to be called in. Calling the midwife is, however, considered a shameful business (the man has not been virile enough), which is why the bridegroom will rather wield a knife himself, naturally without any knowledge of female anatomy and often helped along by alcohol.

Once again, it is difficult to remain neutral about a ritual that so evidently does violence to a woman's physical and psychological well-being. Yet the custom is held in high esteem by women, and most attempts to stop the worst excesses by legal means have foundered on the rocks of the tenacity of (grand) mothers and midwives. The Kenyan leader Jomo Kenyatta wrote his doctoral thesis *Facing Mount Kenya* in 1939, and in it he called the circumcision of girls and polygamy examples of Kenyan culture that Europeans would never be able to understand and which served them as an escape valve for neo-colonial meddling. When Kenyatta came to power, the old custom was reinstated. Ten years earlier, Anglican missionaries had made pupils and teachers sign a declaration that they were opposed to clitoridectomy before they could be admitted to educational establishments, and that had led to riots. An elderly nun was raped, clitoridectomized and maimed. Under Arap Moi, Kenyatta's successor, a new legal ban on clitoridectomy was issued after fourteen girls died in one year from complications following the procedure. Once the girls are seventeen, they may decide for themselves. In September 2001, twenty parental couples were fined in Nairobi for the first time for allowing their daughters to be circumcised, and on

Independence Day, Moi enjoined the police to exercise stricter control.[4]

Perhaps Kenyatta was right and Westerners will never be able to understand the significance of clitoridectomy. The cultural motives have, however, been set out at some length. What is certain is that circumcision consolidates tribal ties, and that girls who have not been circumcised run the risk of being ostracized. In the Sudan, just three categories of women are left uncircumcised: very young girls, the mentally handicapped, and the daughters of prostitutes.[5] For the normal Sudanese woman, encounters with an uncircumcised woman are as horrifying as the first encounter of the gynaecologist Reyners with a woman who asked him to 'open her up'. Hanny Lightfoot-Klein mentions a Sudanese midwife who dropped everything she was holding in her hands when she was unexpectedly confronted with an uncircumcised woman in labour. Hanny Lightfoot-Klein herself was introduced to the female paramedics in a hospital by a male gynaecologist, who asked that the visitor be told as candidly as possible about anything connected with the subject of her research. The nurses gladly promised to do so, on condition that Lightfoot-Klein would be as candid about her own affairs. In the exchanges that followed the anthropologist was clearly given to understand how delightfully lurid and outlandish some of her audience found her situation. She was also asked many times if she was sure her mother was not a prostitute.

In cultures in which circumcision is the rule, uncircumcised women will always be afraid that they might not find a husband, and without a husband and children social acceptance is hardly conceivable. Men tend indeed to reject uncircumcised women, and that is due to uncertainty about their virginity. The infibulation scar is treated as a kind of seal, the visible sign of a woman's purity. Scar tissue can grow astonishingly hard. In medical texts such tissue is said to be keloid, and keloid tissue is most common in black races. A surgeon told Lightfoot-Klein that he had had to perform an operation on a woman who was still a virgin after seven years of marriage. It was not surprising that her husband had been unable to enter her since even a surgical scalpel snapped when wielded on the hardened tissue, and it was only when the surgeon used the heaviest cartilage knife (chondrotome) that he could accomplish his work. This made a deep impression on the young surgeon, and what horrified him just as much was the haste with which the husband rushed his wife home from the hospital. He did have some sympathy for the man, however, for he realized that he had had to bear the taunts of his fellow villagers for seven long years.

In addition to the clear evidence of virginity, a contributory 'advantage' of circumcision is the woman's loss of most of her sexually sensitive organs, which is thought to provide protection against her unbridled sexuality. Here too we encounter the deeply rooted fear of woman's bottomless lustfulness. Even in the Song of Solomon, though it is a hymn to sexuality, that fear is brought home (8:8–10):

THE BRIDE AND HER BROTHERS

We have a little sister,
And she hath no breasts:
What shall we do for our sister
In the day when she shall be spoken for?
If she be a wall,
    We will build upon her a palace of silver:
And if she be a door,
    We will enclose her with boards of cedar.

This passage makes it clear that Judaism and Christianity share several roots with Islam. And time and again we come upon the image of woman as a sexless creature who undergoes a metamorphosis in her encounter with the one man who cherishes her:

I am a wall,
    and my breasts like towers:
Then I was in his eyes
    as one that found favour.

The meaning is clear: a woman's jewel must be reserved for the one man in her life. If she fails in that respect, her husband is entitled to take a second wife – the nightmare of all Sudanese women. If she is too easy to enter during defloration, she may well be cast aside, for after the wedding night the husband will be questioned by his friends and they will be only too prepared to fan the slightest spark of doubt about her virginity. Some women actually enjoy the pain they feel during their honeymoon. Lightfoot-Klein quotes a nurse who performs circumcisions and who told her that her own defloration took ten days and that she was in pain for another two weeks. 'Do you generally enjoy pain?' Lightfoot-Klein asked her, taken aback. 'No, not at all. I hate pain as much as anyone. But I enjoyed *that* pain.'

And what about the husband whom they are so keen to please? An interview with a 40-year-old hospital technician provides a whole palette of ambivalent attitudes. This man ran the risk of breaking with his mother because he would sanction the removal of no more than one centimetre of the clitoris of his first three daughters. His fourth daughter would be allowed to grow up completely undamaged; he was fairly optimistic about the future acceptance of uncircumcised women. His own wife had been infibulated; before his wedding his mother-in-law had begged him to have his bride opened up surgically, but that had been beneath his male dignity. Using great violence he had been able to enter her after three hours, whereupon she had had to be rushed to hospital because the tear was bleeding so heavily. How did he feel about this event? His face plainly shows it. 'I felt like a criminal,' he says. 'I could hardly bear to live with myself.'

His wife recovered and eventually became able to enjoy sexual intercourse. The married couple was quite open about their feelings in bed, and the husband felt sure that his wife had orgasms. He could compare the sexual sensitivity of his wife with that of uncircumcised Ethiopian prostitutes, and it was obvious that she was far more difficult to satisfy. Her confinements were traumatic, with forceps deliveries on two occasions, and it took at least two months for the tears and stitches to heal.

After childbirth, most Pharaonically circumcised women allow themselves to be reinfibulated. Before they make love to their husbands again, they have themselves sewn up much as they were before their wedding night, and that too is done because they believe it makes them more attractive to their husbands. This part of their sexual culture is the most incomprehensible of all, the more so as it is a very recent aggravation of the ritual. Women born before 1930 were never reinfibulated. Anthropologists are given contradictory replies in answer to their questions: some women claim they do it for their husband's sake; some husbands say that they do not set great store by it and blame their wives' mothers, and it is often emphasized that reinfibulations are a lucrative practice for the midwives performing them. The following is an extract from an interview with the hospital technician:

Does she have herself resutured to pinhole size after each child?
    Yes, she does and it creates many problems for both of them. . . .
But she insists on doing it for 'aesthetic' reasons and he does not stop her. He feels that she does it because she is ashamed to be loose, as she is bound to be due to the damage inflicted on her.
    'But why not a more reasonable opening?' I ask.
    He shrugs. 'It is women's business.' He does not interfere. He knows she orders the midwife to do it for his pleasure, but he feels if she were sewn less tightly it would be easier for him and easier for her.
    Why does he not tell her this?

'Women do not allow you to interfere in this,' he insists. 'It is their business, they tell you. . . . They do it because they feel it will make them sexually more attractive to their husbands, and they will tolerate a great deal of pain for this. It is a misguided act of love.' He tells me that he is losing his desire for his wife, and cannot explain this because she is a good, loving wife to him. Perhaps it is because she has no passion for him any more, and seems to have sex with him only out of a sense of duty.

How does he explain this?

He can only guess the answer, he says. Probably she has simply suffered too much.

This interview makes it clear that husband and wife can hardly influence each other once there are so many greater cultural pressures upon them. Hanny Lightfoot-Klein failed to determine the origins of reinfibulation. Westerners fully expect that customs that strike us as so archaic and traumatic will naturally die out. Sometimes that does happen: the Eritrean Liberation Front, for instance, banned the practice and within five years clitoridectomy disappeared in Eritrea. But in Uganda, where the operation used not to be practised, the elite has introduced the Pharaonic circumcision of their daughters. The ostensible reason is that it helps to strengthen the African roots of their national identity. In Indonesia, it has long been customary to give girls a near-symbolic snip, but there are reasons to assume that with the growing custom of wearing the veil, circumcision is also becoming more radical.[6] Even in the United States *The New Black Monitor* advocated the introduction of excision and infibulation at the beginning of the 1980s, the better to prevent premarital sex.

Alice Walker has written about clitoridectomy at length.[7] Tashi, one of the characters in *The Color Purple*, tells her own story in *Possessing the Secret of Joy*. Tashi grows up in Africa with her closest friend, Adam, the missionary's son whom she is later to marry. When she is a little girl, she watches her sister die from the consequences of her circumcision. Even so, she willingly undergoes the infibulation ritual herself at the beginning of her adult life, as a mark of her kinship with her tribe, the Olinkas. The inspiration for this step comes from the Olinka idol, the Great Leader, who is languishing in a colonial jail and is Jesus Christ, father, brother and perfect lover combined in the eyes of all the girls. The operation is so traumatic that she immediately represses its memory. She moves to the United States with her husband, and in her struggle with fear and despair she is helped by a number of psychotherapists, who work through the trauma of her mutilation with her. In the end, she returns to her tribe, kills the woman who circumcised her, and is sentenced to death and executed.

Alice Walker articulates the motives underlying the ritual in a conversation between Tashi and her psychotherapist:

It was only after I came to America, I said, that I even knew what was supposed to be down there.

Down there?

Yes. My own body was a mystery to me, as was the female body, beyond the function of the breasts, to almost everyone I knew. From prison Our Leader said we must keep ourselves clean and pure as we had been since time immemorial – by cutting out unclean parts of our bodies. Everyone knew that if a woman was not circumcised her unclean parts would grow so long they'd soon touch her thighs; she'd become masculine and arouse herself. No man could enter her because her own erection would be in his way.

You believed this?

Everyone believed it, even though no one had ever seen it. No one living in our village anyway. . . .

But you knew this had not happened to you?

But perhaps it had, I said. Certainly to all my friends who'd been circumcised, my uncircumcised vagina was thought of as a monstrosity. They laughed at me. Jeered at me for having a tail. I think they meant my labia majora. After all, none of them had vaginal lips; none of them had a clitoris; they had no idea what these things looked like; to them I was bound to look odd. There were a few other girls who had not been circumcised. The girls who had been would sometimes actually run from us, as if we were demons. Laughing, though. Always laughing.

And yet it is from this time, before circumcision, that you remember pleasure?

When I was little I used to stroke myself, which was taboo. And then, when I was older, and before we married, Adam and I used to make love in the fields. Which was also taboo. Doing it in the fields, I mean. And because we practiced cunnilingus.

Did you experience orgasm?

Always.

And yet you willingly gave this up in order to . . .

. . . To be accepted as a real woman by the Olinka people; to stop the jeering. Otherwise I was a thing. . . . Besides, Our Leader, our Jesus Christ, said we must keep all our old ways and that no Olinka man – in this he echoed the great liberator Kenyatta – would even think of marrying a woman who was not circumcised.

One shameful detail in Tashi's story is that after her mutilation it is only during anal sex that she can occasionally let herself go and have an orgasm again. Anal sex is a subject mentioned quite a few times in Lightfoot-Klein's interviews, but it is not made clear how often married couples use this undefiled 'secret passage'. Even so it is an important matter in the light of the AIDS epidemic, which is nowhere as devastating as it is in Africa. There, the HIV virus is transmitted as readily by heterosexual as it is by homosexual intercourse, and in that respect this part of the world differs from the West. The transmission of the virus is facilitated by damage to the mucous membrane, and the greater the friction during sexual intercourse the greater the chance of passing the virus on.

It is almost inconceivable that infibulated women should be able to enjoy sexual intercourse, and yet the answers to Lightfoot-Klein's questions about sexual pleasure covered a whole gamut of sensations. Often the question was sidestepped, or the answers were stereotypical and hence not entirely credible. However, the most challenging answer came from a woman aged about 40, who almost turned it into a comic turn. She doubled up with laughter, slapped her thighs and literally rolled off her chair. The interpreter, who did not at first grasp what all this merriment was about, quickly became helpless with laughter herself and finally Lightfoot-Klein herself joined in the hysteria, even though she still did not know the reason for all the hilarity:

> In the end, my translator calmed down sufficiently to enlighten me. 'She says,' she managed to gasp, 'she says that you must be completely *mad* to ask her a question like that! She says: "*A body is a body,* and no circumcision can change that! No matter what they cut away from you – they cannot change that!"'

This was one of the first interviews and was a great help to the investigator in asking her questions with an open mind, without preconceived Western ideas. Most discussions of clitoridectomy, after all, have a negative bias. The ethnographer Lori Leonard came across a musical rendering of the clitoridectomy story in a small village in Chad but discovered that the scientific world was hardly disposed to listen to an alternative interpretation of this kind.[8] Had her sponsor but known what Leonard was about to discover, she might never have been given a grant.

Leonard did her research in Chad, a country in which some 80 per cent of all women are circumcised, though the custom is not evenly distributed over the country. In a number of villages it is not practised at all, but Leonard found one in which clitoridectomy had not been introduced until recently. This was Myambé, a village of about one thousand inhabitants of whom one, Kékéta, was one of the first to have her clitoris excised. What an event that had been! It was no longer known exactly when it took place. People remembered that it had been during the war, because the schools were closed. Someone recalled that it had been in the dry season, and that Bamadé's wife had still been alive. After Kékéta, five groups of girls had had the same operation, but all in all they probably numbered no more than thirty. Why they had done it was something the villagers did not quite understand, but in that village there had also always been girls who had their lower incisors pulled out, and the reason for that too was not clearly understood. You could have it done, but then again you might not. It did not increase your chances of finding a husband.

The circumcised girls liked to boast about the brave thing they had done. They thought that circumcision was what Westerners call 'cool'. After the circumcision there was a kind of coming-out ceremony, when circumcised girls did not allow uncircumcised girls to join in the dancing. They themselves had institutionalized the practice, since the Nanda, the country's religious leader, was a declared opponent of circumcision, and the village elder certainly did not encourage it. But the village at large obviously approved of the practice, for the girls were given presents and money during the dance. The girls were young, from eight to ten years old, because it was considered quite unacceptable to have yourself circumcised after you had lost your virginity. There were years when there was no woman in the village who knew how to cut, but once the possibility of circumcision returned, the social pressure to have it done grew. An uncircumcised girl was called a 'sato', 'kara' or 'koy', and though no one knew what these words meant, no one could bear the disgrace of being called one. Kékéta, the matriarch of circumcision in Myambé, knew that her own mother had not been circumcised and she had never revealed what she thought about her daughter's decision. When Kékéta had her first child, her mother saw for the first time exactly what had been done to her daughter. Clearly, Kékéta had fully expected to be rebuked and was therefore doubly relieved when her child was delivered without any complications. Again, her mother said nothing.

The village elder might have been opposed to the practice, but some old people viewed circumcision as a sign of progress. If Yasmine Allas had lived in Chad, perhaps her parents would not have exerted enough influence on her to protect her from her need to suffer her destiny: to be absolutely the same as everyone else.

Clitoridectomy in the West

We associate the word 'clitoridectomy' primarily with Africa. In *Possessing the Secret of Joy*, Alice Walker reminds Americans that the Western medical world also has ample experience of this intervention.[9] Her psychotherapist introduces Tashi to Amy, a woman of about 80 whom she is treating for depression. Amy has always been able to conceal her own problems, because she had a depressive son whom she dragged from one therapist to the next almost all his life. Only when the son committed suicide at the age of 40 did his mother's own desperation come to the surface. Tashi cannot make out why she has been introduced to this woman:

> I mean, said Amy, sighing, that when I was a very little girl I used to touch myself . . . there. It was a habit that mortified my mother. When I was three years old she bound my hands each night before I was put to bed. At four she put hot pepper sauce on my fingers. At six years of age our family doctor was asked to excise my clitoris.
>
> Is New Orleans America? I asked suspiciously. For this was all I could think to say.
>
> Yes, said Amy, I assure you it is. And yes, I am telling you that even in America a rich white child could not touch herself sexually, if others could see her, and be safe.

Alice Walker goes on to describe little Amy's reaction. Her mother tells her before the operation that her tonsils are about to be removed, and Amy keeps repeating this lie.

> I was sore for a long time, she said. My mother let me stay in bed and brought me lemonade to soothe my throat – for she convinced me it was my throat in which the work had been done and therefore where I felt the pain. And I could not touch my fingers to where the pain actually was, for fear of contradicting her. Or offending her. I never touched myself – in that way – again. And of course when I accidentally touched myself there I discovered there was nothing left to touch.

Amy has to get over it somehow. She becomes a sportswoman and later sleeps with virtually every man who crosses her path. She feels no resentment towards her mother, and only when her own son dies does she establish contact with herself again. And then the memory, too, returns.

For many decades since the beginning of the nineteenth century, clitoridectomy was considered a normal surgical intervention that answered a particular problem.[10] The gynaecologists who removed the clitoris told their contemporaries precisely what their reason for the operation was, and we also know how their colleagues reacted to the idea. It was a remarkable period in the history of medical thinking. Removal of the clitoris was indicated as the most effective treatment of mental disorders, at least in the eyes of some doctors. That was, of course, before the – nowadays often disdained – separation of body and mind in medical thinking. More than a century later it is difficult to imagine, but there were heated discussions for a time as to whether hysteria was the province of the gynaecologist (with or without a scalpel) or the psychiatrist. In an appeal launched in 1855 for the extension of the women's hospital in New York, we can read:[11]

> Statistics of our insane asylums show that 25 to 40 percent of all cases
> of insanity in women arise directly from organic female disease which, in
> most cases, might be remedied by appropriate and timely treatment.

The leading proponent of medical clitoridectomy was the English gynaecologist Isaac Baker Brown. He helped to found St Mary's Hospital, where he had a distinguished reputation as a gynaecological surgeon. Many colleagues would watch him at work in the operating theatre and were deeply impressed by his expertise and daring. In 1858, his star stood so high (and his financial resources had grown so large) that he was able to open a private clinic, the London Home for Surgical Diseases of Women. In 1865 he was elected president of the Medical Society of London, and in 1866 he published a book entitled *On the Curability of Certain Forms of Insanity, Epilepsy, Catalepsy and Hysteria in Females*. The book was an enthusiastic polemic in favour of clitoridectomy. The inspiration for this operation had come to Baker Brown from the then popular ideas on the physiology of the nervous system: if the brain is in total confusion, the cause may lie in 'peripheral irritation'.

> Constantly engaged in the treatment of diseases of the female genitals,
> I had been often foiled in dealing successfully with hysteric and other
> nervous affections complicating these lesions, without being able to
> assign a satisfactory cause for the failure. . . .
>   Long and frequent observation convinced me that a large number
> of affections peculiar to females, depended on loss of nerve power, and
> that this was produced by peripheral irritation, arising originally in
> some branches of the pubic nerve, more particularly the incident nerve

supplying the clitoris, and sometimes the small branches which supply the vagina, perineum and anus.

In his two hospitals, Baker Brown had ample opportunity to see emotionally disturbed patients. The loss of mental power he observed took the following fixed and fatal course in women:

Hysteria (including dyspepsia and menstrual irregularities)
Spinal irritation (with a reflex action on the uterus, ovaries, etc., and
   giving rise to uterine displacements, blindness, hemiplegia, paraple
   gia, etc.)
Epileptoid fits or hysterical epilepsy
Cataleptic fits (a psychiatric condition involving dummy-like rigidity)
Epileptic fits
Idiotcy (*sic*)
Mania
Death

He was undoubtedly sincere in his conviction that the nervous complaints he came across must ultimately lead to the woman's total decline, and seen in this light his drastic measures become understandable. He described his work as follows:

The patient having been placed *completely* under the influence of chloroform, the clitoris is freely excised either by scissors or knife – I always prefer the scissors. The wound is then firmly plugged with graduated compresses of lint, and a pad, well secured by a T bandage.

The patient had to be carefully guarded by the nursing staff, and sometimes her hands were tied together to prevent her touching the wound.

A month is generally required for perfect healing of the wound, at the end of which time it is difficult for the uninformed, or non-medical, to discover any trace of an operation.

After eighteen pages of explanation, the author continues with a series of forty-eight case histories, the triumphant tone gradually beginning to pall on the reader. The range of complaints that, according to Baker Brown, can be subsumed under the heading of hysteria is extremely wide (something for which he cannot be blamed entirely, for the same applies to all physicians who have used the term 'hysteria', from Hippocrates to the Freudians). Quite often, the clitoris was removed the very day the patient was admitted to hospital, and she nearly always left the Surgical Home two or three weeks later, having been pronounced 'cured'. Some patients and their relatives wrote effusive letters of thanks: years of constipation gone from one day to the next; women who had apparently been barren for years fell pregnant, and even a tumour disappeared. Sometimes the operation was followed by a kind of catharsis:

> A few days after the operation this patient was observed to be occasionally very violent and unmanageable, and to have a wild maniacal look. On questioning her husband, it appeared that for several years she had been subject to fits of violent excitement, especially during the menstrual period, and that at such times 'she would fly at him and rend his skin, like a tigress'.
>
> This patient made a good recovery; she remained quite well, and became in every respect a good wife.

The surgeon as exorcist. In some case histories Baker Brown demonstrated that in his own sphere he had much the same objectives in the medical field as African circumcisers had on the cultural plane. Take case history no. 48, who

> had developed a great distaste for her husband . . . and cohabitation with him. I pursued the usual surgical treatment, which was followed by uninterrupted success; and after two months' treatment, she returned to her husband, resumed cohabitation, and stated that all her distaste had disappeared; soon became pregnant, resumed her place at the head of her table, and became a happy and healthy wife and mother.

Masturbation was sometimes mentioned as the cause of the irritation. A seventeen-year-old girl had been introduced to the habit when she was fifteen by a classmate, and ever since she had had attacks of catalepsy that had turned her into a complete invalid. Baker Brown convinced the worried parents, apparently without great difficulty, of the need to remove her clitoris.

However, his colleagues were not convinced. In a book review, one of them challenged Baker Brown's claim that he was not the only clitoridectomist in the British medical profession. Next, he exposed Baker Brown as a hypocrite. With the exception of his last case history, he had consistently concealed the true nature of 'peripheral irritation'. What clitoridectomy was really meant to cure was masturbation, and the reviewer of his book was quite prepared to grant that in that it was effective. Baker Brown was certainly not the only doctor to believe that masturbation had all sorts of deplorable consequences, and that draconian measures to eradicate it were thus justified, but why did he not say so outright? The reviewer pointed out that in that self-same year, a certain Professor Braun had written an article in the *Wiener Medizinische Rundschau* (Vienna Medical Review), the title of which – 'Curing masturbation by amputating the clitoris and the labia minora' – made much clearer what was really at stake. The article went on to point out that Baker Brown was, if anything, too thorough: he sometimes removed the clitoris without bothering to obtain the consent of the patient (or of her husband and family).[12]

Here it might be added that Baker Brown's self-glorification, not least as reported in the daily press, did not go down well with his colleagues. Within a year of the publication of his book, the Obstetrical Society decided to recommend his expulsion. That recommendation was preceded by a reprimand from the inspectorate of mental homes which was anything but pleased with this wood-chopper's method used by a doctor who was completely unqualified to treat mental patients. One hour before the crucial meeting, gynaecologists arrived from all corners of the United Kingdom, and by eight o'clock all the seats had been taken, and all the standing places as well. The report of the extraordinary meeting in the *British Medical Journal* filled fifteen closely printed pages. The complainant, Mr Seymour Haden, did not mince his words:

> But now, quackery of the present day is dangerous in this respect; that the quack of today has found out that he can base his operations upon an actual professional legitimate footing. He can obtain a degree; and from that moment, if he does become a quack, he becomes one of the most dangerous character. [*Cries of 'Question'.*]

Haden questioned the bona fides of the Surgical Home, and all institutions of that type:

> It is a 'Hospital for Women', or it is a 'Home' or something of that kind . . . Then three sets of appeals are sent out in the form of circulars, and they are of this kind. One is addressed to the middle classes, principally to women; that appeal is for money. Another is sent out to the upper classes, to the titled people, that is for patronage; that is for the long list of great names – headed in this instance by the Princess of Wales – so little do these patronesses know what they are about. The third appeal is to the clergy, and it is always couched in these words, 'for their co-operation in the good work'. [*Loud laughter and cheers.*]

Can someone who propagates such repulsive practices be trusted? Haden was an accomplished demagogue:

> . . . what wonder that some poor weak woman, or even that some weaker man should take a wife or a daughter to the Home . . . the operation is so very trifling: a mere nothing perhaps, except the cutting of a pile or the excision of a nerve. The husband remains downstairs. The patient is taken up and put under chloroform, and her clitoris cut out before she has recovered from the anaesthetic. Down comes the promoter of the scheme to the expectant victim below; invites him to write a cheque for 100 or 200 guineas, or whatever it may be, before he leaves the house. Now, if he objects to this, which he is very likely to do, I do not say that he is informed, but at all events he is made to feel this: – 'Your daughter' or 'your wife', as the case may be, 'has undergone a disgraceful mutilation, because she has been given to disgraceful practices: if you can afford to tell your friends this, and to tell the man who is going to marry her that she has had her clitoris cut out, and that for disgraceful practices, well and good; but if you cannot afford to tell them this, I think you had better pay the money and say no more about it.' [*Cries of 'No, no', 'Oh, oh', and great uproar.*] Yes. ['*No, no.*'] What! [*Cries of 'No, no', 'Chair', and great uproar.*] . . .
>
> I will not call it an operation: it is a mutilation, and it is in itself questionable, unpublishable, and therefore secret . . . I say that there are many women – ladies in this city – who are dying to speak upon the subject, and dare not for their honour. [*Hear, hear, and great sensation.*]

Baker Brown put up a successful defence against the blackmail charges, but he overplayed his hand with the claim that there were many other doctors performing clitoridectomies. He confirmed that he believed that masturbation could lead to mental disorders (a point of view no one in his day would firmly contradict), and that compulsive masturbation was therefore correctly treated by excision of the clitoris. He had never operated without the consent of the patient, or at least of her husband or parents. 'If the Society decides that clitoridectomy is wrong, then I shall never perform it again,' was how he set out his position. It proved of no avail:

> At about ten minutes to twelve, the scrutineers entered the room. The room was full, although many country members and others had been compelled to leave. As Dr. Braxton Hicks, Dr. Murray, Dr. Tanner and Dr. Parsons advanced up the room, there was a dead silence.

One hundred and ninety-four votes were cast for the motion, thirty-eight fellows voted against and five abstained. The required majority of two thirds was amply exceeded. Baker Brown was suspended, and the evening was rounded off with a unanimous motion complimenting the board on the laudable manner in which they had upheld the dignity of the profession.

One year later, the ex-president was also forced to resign from the Medical Society of London, his humiliation and downfall complete. He took legal action following the publication of certain details in *The Lancet*, but without success. Baker Brown died in 1872, and for the last two years of his life he had to depend on the financial support of a few loyal old friends. Modern readers will be astonished by his obituary. It lists in detail what cerebral defects were found during his post-mortem examination. He must have had advanced arteriosclerosis for some time, and his death was caused by a vascular disorder.

In Britain, clitoridectomy seems to have completely disappeared after the Baker Brown scandal. Only very occasionally did someone in authority still dare to say in public that the total ban of the practice was perhaps going too far. In the United States, by contrast, Baker Brown had numerous followers. According to the historian G. J. Barker-Benfield, clitoridectomies were performed from the 1860s until 1904, and circumcision of the clitoris (that is, removal of the foreskin) was advocated as a cure for mental illnesses.[13] Baker Brown's book was a source of inspiration, as appears from a report of a meeting of the Obstetrical Society of Philadelphia in 1873. On that occasion, one Dr Goodell made his colleagues privy to a dilemma: one of his patients, a 30-year-old woman, had been a compulsive masturbator since the age of fourteen and had previously consulted a surgeon when she found that her health was suffering from her aberration. The surgeon had found that her clitoris was abnormally large and had removed a part of it. Because that operation had proved of no avail, Goodell was wary of further surgical intervention, and a few alternatives were discussed. Those present were familiar with the work of Baker Brown and there were complaints that his account of the operation had been very vague, but no one referred to the ethical outcry against his work or to the suspension of the champion of clitoridectomy.

Alice Walker's Amy is a literary figure; her operation would have taken place in the interwar years. In 1929 Marie Bonaparte met a woman in Leipzig who had recently had a clitoridectomy at her own request because an uncontrollable urge to masturbate prevented her from doing her housekeeping.[14] Since the age of ten, she had had itching and burning sensations in her clitoral region. When she married at the age of 29, sexual intercourse proved to be very unsatisfactory and masturbation continued to be her main source of sexual pleasure. She had three operations. In the first, the nerves to her genital area were cut; later, her retroflected uterus was corrected. When these failed to change her sexual behaviour, her ovaries and Fallopian tubes were removed, as was the clitoris. That too altered nothing. A woman neurologist then started her on psychoanalytical therapy, but after four weeks the patient cut it short because a new surgeon had held up the prospect to her that all surgical options were not yet exhausted.

In 1941, Marie Bonaparte escaped the war by going to Egypt, where she was able to observe traditional circumcision at close quarters. She reported two long interviews with circumcised women, whose country of origin she did not reveal for discretionary reasons. She gathered that both women did in fact have orgasms during sexual intercourse, even though they needed so much time that it did not always happen. Moreover, both still had some sensation in the scar area. One of the women continued to masturbate regularly even after her circumcision. It was not quite clear precisely which region she stimulated, but it was not her vagina.

Hanny Lightfoot-Klein corresponded in the 1980s with Dr Haas, a gynaecologist who had been asked by a mother to remove the clitoris of her fifteen-year-old daughter. The daughter masturbated, and the mother herself had had a clitoridectomy at about the same age, also as a cure for masturbation. Haas refused the request, but saw the daughter five years later to give her pre-natal advice and discovered that she had lost her clitoris as well as her labia minora. A second request to Haas came from a German woman who wanted to get rid of her clitoris 'in order to improve her marital relationship'. Haas tried to get her to change her mind and thought that he had succeeded in doing so. But two years later she consulted him for something else, and during the investigation it emerged that her clitoris and labia minora had gone. In her case, we have no information about the husband; it may well be that he came from a country where clitoridectomy was the custom.

The last stronghold of clitoridectomy

Until quite recently one form of clitoridectomy went unchallenged, namely the cosmetic intervention used with hermaphroditic children and with girls who, due to hormonal imbalances, are born with an exceptionally large clitoris. Such girls are by no means rare. Certain genetic metabolic disorders (the most important of which is adrenogenital syndrome, AGS) are caused by an abnormally high testosterone level, before and after birth. Boys with this complaint have exceptionally large genitals, but there is no doubt about their sex. With girls, the clitoris can be very prominent, and the labia fused and pigmented by testosterone, so that the newborn baby is sometimes registered as a boy. The problem then is what to do about a girl who, at first sight, seems to be made like a boy. The situation is even more complicated with true hermaphroditic children. There are indeed some people who are genetically half man and half woman. In their case a choice has to be made, for a child must be registered as either a boy or a girl. Traditionally, it has always been the practice to correct anatomical aspects conflicting with the chosen sex by surgical means.[15] Since the 1950s the consensus has been that any doubts should be removed as early as possible. That, in the view of the leading authorities at the time, would create the best conditions for the unhampered development of a sexual identity, even if the chosen sex were not the genetic one.

A large clitoris was often remodelled, and genetically male children who were born without a penis were 'converted' into girls as best as possible. All these were often problem children, if only because the causal disorder sometimes called for lifelong treatment, and always because they had been operated on at an early age, and usually several times. From puberty onwards, moreover, they had regularly had to put up with taking the sex hormones their own bodies did not produce.

No one will be surprised to learn that some of these 'intersex' children suffered a real identity problem, and that they should have turned to self-help groups in which the prevailing 'standards of good clinical care' were brought up for discussion. The journal of the Intersex Society of North America (ISNA) bears the proud title of *Hermaphrodites with Attitude,* a name that proclaims their ideal: a society that recognizes that some individuals are neither men nor women. That is a viewpoint nowadays also reflected in the modern approach to transexuality. Until recently, a genetic male who steadfastly maintained that he had been born in the wrong body was only accepted for hormonal or surgical sexual treatment if he was prepared to go 'all the way'. Meanwhile, gender clinics are visited by men who, while wanting female hormones and breasts, have no objections to possessing a penis.[16] In prostitution and pornography, too, interest in intersexuals ('she-males') is growing,. Within the ISNA, AGS patients can tell their story, and recently we have been able to read about the dismay at genital mutilation even in the West. According to 'Ana':

When I was twelve, I started to notice that my clitoris had grown more prominent . . . I'm sure that it was at least three months after I had taken note that my mother caught a glimpse of me as I bathed one day after returning from the dance studio. She tried very hard not to let on how alarmed she was, but a twelve-year-old girl-child just senses such a thing. When the pediatrician examined me the next day she was also obviously alarmed.[17]

Ana was sent to a specialist clinic, where they explained everything to her:

They didn't mention the part where they were going to slice off my clit. All of it. I guess the doctors assumed I was as horrified by my outsized clit as they were, and that there was no need to discuss it with me.

Ana shut up like a clam, wrestled with depression and bulimia, and took a long time before she dared to come out as a lesbian. Sexually, she lost a great deal:

I sometimes masturbate and I do have an experience which I call an orgasm – some faint muscular contractions. But the response is unreliable, and nothing like the tremendous sensitivity and wonderful juicy orgasms I had before the clitoral surgery.

Only very late in her life did she realize that genetically she was a man, that her body responded to testosterone far too weakly (she had a congenital partial androgen-insensitivity syndrome), and that, under strong pressure from the hospital, her parents had deliberately concealed the facts from her. Probably no one had even thought that a twelve-year-old girl could be experienced in producing orgasms.

The influence of self-help movements is considerable, certainly in the age of the Internet. Information about the strangest matters can now be exchanged by those directly concerned. In the future, cosmetic clitoris corrections will probably be postponed until the child herself can understand the risks. We should not underestimate the problems involved. Parent and child will often be unable cope to with the stigma of abnormal sexuality without expert help. The parents of an intersex child sometimes wrestle for a long time with the whys and wherefores. If they continue to look for the meaning of it all, they are often trapped in a maze of guilt feelings.

Other forms of surgical intervention involving the female genitals

Medical clitoridectomy, and also the removal of the prepuce of the clitoris, are treated as marginal phenomena in the medical literature, and in medical encyclopaedias, too, we are told little about them. Other surgical treatments of the female genitals are described much more openly, in particular castration (the removal of the ovaries) and hysterectomy (the removal of the uterus). Castration used also to be prescribed for the treatment of mental disorders, and particularly of uncontrollable sexual desire leading to masturbation. The intervention was called Battey's operation after its leading advocate.[18] The sexual desires of women were considered to be pathological, which rendered the correct diagnosis of the condition all the more important. What tests could the doctor apply? Of course, he had to see the condition with his own eyes, and in the process even elicit the forbidden response by stimulation of the clitoris or the breasts. If the patient responded with signs of excitement, then that was taken as proof that a clitoridectomy or castration was called for.

The book by Barker-Benfield mentioned earlier makes fascinating reading.[19] He portrays the typical American as seen through the admiring eyes of Alexis de Tocqueville. This French politician, who during a less successful period of his career toured the United States to study democracy on the spot, used a highly romantic brush to portray the true American. The latter was a self-made man who knew how to seize the thousands of opportunities offered by that marvellous country in a strictly honest and democratic way. His spouse had to be a model of self-effacement. In the relations between American men and women there was accordingly no place for a genuine feminine sexuality. The possibility that women might enjoy sex was not categorically denied, but only allowed if the man was the motive force of her sexual experience. Sex was a difficult subject at the time, and if anything went wrong in that area, it was invariably the woman's fault. If a marriage remained childless, then there was not even the shadow of a suspicion that something might be wrong with the husband.

The life of J. Marion Sims, the most famous American gynaecologist, provides a splendid illustration of this attitude. After the bankruptcy of his father, a businessman, Sims started his career as a humble country doctor, but by the end of his life he could boast that he was the second richest physician in the whole country. A statue to his memory, initially erected in Bryant Park in New York, was moved in 1936 to its present location on the edge of Central Park, opposite the New York Academy of Medicine. The New York elite provided him with his fortune, but for the large number of guinea pigs on whom he tried out his new surgical techniques he founded the Women's Hospital, whose beds were mainly filled with penniless Irish immigrants.

Anyone studying the life of Sims is bound to feel a mixture of admiration and indignation. His name lives on in the textbooks; doctors still use Sims' speculum; vaginal examinations in the knee-chest position are said to be performed in Sims' position; in fertility research the Sims-Hühner test remained popular for a long time, and everyone using the term 'vaginismus' is following in the footsteps of Sims, for he was the first to describe this condition and to give it a name. Undoubtedly, Sims himself fought hard to ensure that all these inventions would render his name immortal. Modesty was not one of his virtues. At the end of his career he was no longer able to go on working in the hospital he had founded because he refused to accept the new regulation that no operation could be watched by more than fifteen spectators. During a European tour he undertook, things were organized so that he could perform the widest possible range of operations before the largest possible audience in just four days.

Sims was above all a 'cutting' gynaecologist; one biographer bestowed the title 'architect of the vagina' on him. Yet he had to overcome a certain distaste at first. At the end of his life he confessed that as a student he had studiously avoided examination of the female genitals, preferring to leave that to his colleagues. His first documented surgical exploit was in quite a different field: he operated on a young woman with a double-sided harelip (cleft palate and lip). The woman looked most unsightly, she had problems eating and drinking and she dribbled uncontrollably. The young doctor corrected her congenital defect in two stages, and he would have liked to perfect the result with a third operation but the patient had had enough. Sims was delighted that he had been able to turn so unprepossessing an appearance into something normal, and Barker-Benfield assumed that only after that was he able to deal with female genitals in the knowledge that he had the ability to correct all sorts of flaws and anomalies, even in that area. Specialization in his chosen field was still unusual; in the early years of his women's hospital, Sims was the only medical man in the world to devote himself exclusively to the treatment of women.

Sims was impressively inventive, but the extreme ordeals to which he exposed his patients was shocking. On one occasion, he was consulted by a woman who had serious abdominal pains after falling off her horse. Sims suspected that the pain was caused by a pro-lapsed uterus. To bring the organ back up, he asked her to rest on her knees and chest, and when he held her vagina open with his fingers he not only heard the sucking in of a quantity of air but he was suddenly able to look some way inside. He realized that he needed an implement to help him look more deeply inside, and to that end decided to bend the handle of a pewter spoon. And so 'he brought the female organs out of the darkness into the light'. In biographical accounts this moment is always described in the same kind of heroic terms as those in which Columbus's first sight of America has been immortalized.

With the first glance Sims cast into the vagina, he must have seen chiefly the anterior wall in the main, the area adjoining the bladder. That suddenly inspired him to realize for what medical treatments the speculum could be used, for the anterior wall of the vagina is always in serious danger during difficult childbirths. A fistula can quite often be formed between the bladder and the vagina so that the (generally young) patients are rendered incontinent for the rest of their lives.[20] Any doctor able to repair vesico-vaginal fistulas is bound to earn the deepest gratitude of his patients. Sims accepted this challenge and had no difficulty in obtaining patients. For the first few years, the work was largely experimental, and the most obvious target group was made up of female black slaves, of whom there was a multitude in Alabama. Sometimes Sims would buy the women from their owners, and he had a crude shelter built as a hospital in his back yard where black female slaves lived for years. The first patient on whom he performed his experiment was called Anarcha, a name that suggests to us that she fully supported her ordeal. That was probably true of all the inhabi-tants of the shelter. Since Sims's colleagues wanted to have nothing to do with his experimentations, the patients had occasionally to assist him in his work on their companions in adversity. In four years, Anarcha underwent 30 operations (with little anaesthesia, since Sims was not very skilled in that department), and time after time the sutures became infected. But after four years he could claim suc-cess: all the slave women had been cured and were continent.

Following his success with the fistula operations, Sims ventured to New York, where he was to celebrate his greatest triumphs. Here, Irish immigrants served as his guinea pigs, but in the end operations became accepted in the best circles. Sims's first vaginismus operation was on a young woman, of whom he wrote that her nervous system was in a deplorable state. On her he began to develop his method of treatment, which ultimately came down to the surgical removal of the hymenal region, the cutting of the most important sphincter muscles, and instructions to the patient to practice inserting glass moulds every day. It may be a strange comparison, but what Sims had women do bore a striking resemblance to what male-to-female transsexuals have to do with their surgically created neo-vagina. The first patient did not react well to the surgery, which meant just one thing to Sims: another operation. The girl's mother accused Sims of experimenting with her daughter's body. Sims did not deny this, but found the mother's attitude deplorable (and was supported in that by her husband, who threatened her with court action or divorce).

The alternatives were not very attractive either. Before Sims's surgical intervention, the medical profession could think of nothing better than to administer ether to the woman, after which the husband would be able to fertilize her. For reproduction was of course considered a couple's bounden duty. Sims, too, concerned himself with fertility problems, and, typically, he used a surgical approach. His theory was that an infertile woman's uterus was not permeable enough, and he accordingly made an incision in the cervix (and, in keeping with his character, often more than once). It all proved of no avail.

Barker-Benfield has painted the character of Sims, and the society in which he could flourish, in fairly sinister colours. He is described as a small, insecure man, who could only contain his fear of women and of their genital organs by taking the knife to them, and who in so doing triumphed over all other male physicians in the competition for control of the female body. 'Heroic', if necessary at the patient's expense, is a term that became attached to gynaecology when it was transformed into a 'cutting' specialty. The illustration of an ovariotomy in Rachel Maines's book captures the new experimental approach.[21] In England, Baker Brown did not hesitate to strip his own sister of her ovaries. Operations in the abdominal cavity were still experimental and fairly risky at the time. This was Baker Brown's fourth attempt in this field, and his first three patients had not survived the operation. His sister was his first triumph. Neurologists and psychiatrists had to stand by helplessly as their prospective patients submitted to treatments based on magical expectations. 'A surgeon who has performed a successful abdominal operation is like an Indian tiger which has tasted blood for the first time.'

Gynaecologists have often been accused of having little respect for the female genitals. However, women themselves were keen to go under the knife. In 1894, an American critic mocked women thus:[22]

Pelvic operations on women has become a fad. It is fashionable, and the woman who cannot show an abdominotomy line is looked upon as not

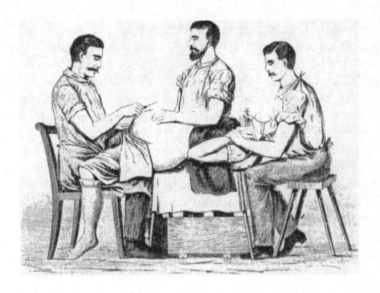

24 Three male
surgeons
performing an
ovariotomy on
a patient with
a large cyst
around 1880.

in style, nor belonging to the correct set. It is a mark of favor and considered 'as pretty as the dimple on the cheek of sweet sixteen'.

Professor of gynaecology Hector Treub (1856–1920), emphasized in
his inaugural address that he regularly sent women away with the
advice that they refuse to be operated on and thereafter for that reason
continue to keep out of the reach of the medical profession. But not
even he was always proof against the persistence of the complaints and
the resolution with which the patients pinned their hopes on surgery.
Medical historian Lidy Schoon has described Treub's minefield – pelvic
neuralgia – in her dissertation.[23] He considered it a psychosomatic, not
to say hysterical, complaint, but the collaboration of psychiatrists and
gynaecologists was still in its infancy during Treub's professorship. Of
the eighteen women on whom he published a paper, no more than
three were referred to a psychiatrist. Alas, even these three underwent
an operation in the end.

The third woman had first received 'mental treatment' from Treub
himself, the therapy 'consisting of daily lectures, good-humoured to a
greater or lesser degree, and slowly accustoming the patient to sitting upright and to taking walks'. Since she was convinced that she
had a tumour, Treub performed a mock ovariotomy. The woman was
anaesthetized and given a large, but superficial, in her abdomen,
which was then provided with long, thick sutures. Postoperative treatment was of the normal kind, but in her special case the stitches
were removed 'with great cries of joy at the excellent recovery'. The
abdominal pains, however, continued to be severe. After electrocau-

terization of the cervix, Treub decided to 'treat' the 'overly sensitive' patient several times with a branding iron. 'The first time, all went fairly well except for some screaming. The second time, however, it took a great deal of effort to allow my "it's essential" to gain the upper hand over the patient's "I don't want it".' There followed a course of sulphur baths, and Treub also had her treated with 'cold showers for some time'. After having struggled for five months with his patient, Treub, at the end of his tether, referred her to the psychiatrist Winkler. After a while Winkler sent Treub a request to consent to operating, hoping this might have some suggestive effect on the patient by the 'mental method', so the end result was still the removal of her uterus.

To this day, every gynaecologist has patients who insist on an operation from which the doctor expects no improvement because he cannot see any connection between the symptoms and the organ the woman is so keen to get rid of. That can still lead to impotent confrontations, sometimes degenerating into patently sadomasochistic interactions. There is a notorious story about the gynaecologist who wrote to the referring general practitioner, 'There is no point in referring this lady to me, because she no longer has organs for a gynaecologist to deal with.'

Castration was exceedingly difficult to fit into the nineteenth-century view of the world. Those who considered castration a new means of curing mental instability had to take into account that, as a result, they robbed the women of an essential function, reproduction. However, heroic ends call for radical means. Robert Battey, the surgeon from Rome in the state of Georgia who gave his name to the operation for the removal of the normal ovaries, proved above all that he knew how to strike the right note in explaining the motives for his psychiatric investigations:

> I have felt it to be my duty to . . . carve out for myself a new pathway through consecrated ground . . . I have invaded the hidden recesses of the female organism and snatched from its appointed set a glandular body, whose mysterious and wonderful functions are of the highest interest to the human race.

Battey was not the first to remove ovaries, but he was the first to do so with normal and healthy organs. He called it 'normal ovariotomy' in contradistinction to the operation performed on cancer patients. In any case it was believed that after the operation women did not feel that they had been 'unsexed', as men would have felt by castration. There were also eugenic arguments: a woman candidate for castration was likely to bear children that were degenerate.

Follow-ups made at the time show that women deliberately subjected themselves to this assault on their femininity. One woman given to masturbation, then considered a sexual perversion, wrote after the operation: 'My condition is all I could desire. I know and I feel that I am well; I never think of self-abuse; it is foreign and distasteful to me.' And so she was back on the pedestal on which men liked to place women, so much so that they assigned their best indoctrination methods to it. Yet some voices were raised in protest. The British surgeon Sir Thomas Spencer Wells, who had built his reputation on his skill as an ovariotomist, was convinced that his own indications had always been realistic, whereas the psychiatric indications filled him with horror. He described a mirror-image of the medical profession, displaying a society in which women had the final say:[24]

> Fancy the reflected picture of a coterie of the Marthas of the profession on conclave, promulgating the doctrine that most of the unmanageable maladies of men were to be traced to some morbid change in their genitals, founding societies for the discussion of them and hospitals for the cure of them, one of them sitting in her consultation chair, with her little stove by her side and her irons all hot, searing every man as he passed before her; another gravely proposing to bring on the millennium by snuffing out the reproductive powers of all fools, lunatics and criminals; a third getting up and declaring that she found at least seven or eight men in her wards with some condition of his appendages which would prove incurable without surgical treatment . . .
>
> Should we not, to our shame, see ourselves as others see us?

Outside the medical establishment there was one constant opponent of the male attitude to feminine failings, and that was the Christian Science movement, which was mainly led by women. They considered the surgical approach too materialistic, and preferred what they called the 'mind cure'. Christian Scientists ran courses in which one could learn to allow the spiritual to triumph over the physical. To women it seemed as if they were being raised onto the same pedestal but by a means that did not impinge violently on their bodies.

The enthusiasm for performing surgery on the female genital organs had lasting after effects. America is the country with the largest percentage of hysterectomies; nowadays one in three American women in her sixties has had her uterus removed, whereas in France the ratio is no more than one in eighteen.[25] Moreover, in the United States, the ovaries are often taken out as well. The figures might tell us something about French appreciation of the female genitals, but perhaps the way gynaecology is organized in France also has something to do with it. France is the only country in the world where there is such a profession as 'medical gynaecologist' – doctors who have had specialist training not involving surgery. This profession is about to die out, but it is conceivable that it is easier to keep your uterus if you can take your symptoms to a doctor of whom you know for certain that he cannot operate on you.

There is almost no one who doubts that a far greater number of uteri is removed than can be rationally justified. Clitoridectomies were stamped out, but in the 1960s and 1970s female circumcision, that is, the baring of the clitoris by removal of the foreskin, regained some popularity.[26] In 1973, *Playgirl* published an enthusiastic report on the subject. Women who had had the operation joyfully confirmed that their erotic sensitivity had increased. There was a great deal of lobbying to have the operation included in the benefits offered by health insurers, but that did not come to pass. The final verdict of the National Blue Shield Association was that the intervention was 'obsolete or ineffective'.

That might equally well turn out to be the final verdict on one of the most common operations in the world, the medical circumcision of boys. In the United States it has been virtually impossible until quite recently to bring a newborn boy home intact from the obstetric clinic. Sims, incidentally, played some part in the introduction of the circumcision of boys for non-religious reasons in America.[27] A former patient called on him with her five-year-old son, who had had a paralysed leg for some time. Sims, who was indebted to this admirer for a constant stream of new patients, realized that the boy's problem was not in his field and asked Lewis A. Sayre, the most famous orthopaedic surgeon of his day, to come to his office. Sayre obliged, and the boy was given a thorough examination. He lay with his legs drawn up, so that Sims at first had thought that contraction of the flexors was the cause, but Sayre found that the extensors of the leg were paralysed. When he prepared, in accordance with the then most modern methods, to test the reflexes with galvanic impulses, the nurse who had the boy in her care warned the doctor against touching the boy's willie, which had been causing him pain for some time. On inspecting that organ the doctors discovered that the glans and prepuce looked highly inflamed, and this was, in fact, the sole pathology they could discover. Sayre thought it too much of a coincidence, and concluded that the inflamed penis might well have produced a reaction in the nervous system, ultimately causing the paralysis. It seemed obvious that the boy should first be rid of his genital problems, so an operation was unavoidable. Sayre had the boy taken to his own hospital, and since he did not want to keep an experiment so important to himself, he had a large number of students witness it. The operation proved at first to be a disappointment; when the narrowest part of the prepuce had been removed, the inner surface was found to have fused with the glans. But when he, using his nails (it used to be customary to operate with bare hands), brought a little more force to bear, it was possible to expose the glans completely. Sayre's high expectations were fulfilled. The boy improved visibly, had more colour in his cheeks, had a better appetite and was soon afterwards able to walk properly.

To explain his success, Sayre used very nearly the same model as Baker Brown: peripheral stimulation (Baker Brown always referred to excitation; Sayre to irritation) was responsible for the malfunctioning of the nervous system. Reflex neurosis was the name the researchers gave the condition. Soon afterwards, Sayre tried his treatment on children suffering from epilepsy, restlessness and insomnia, but also from intestinal complaints. Between the lines, we can read that with boys, too, genital irritation was sometimes used as a euphemism for masturbation, and circumcision, just like clitoridectomy, was considered a good method of combating self-abuse. Mental illnesses, too, are nervous disorders. Thus Sayre examined the genitals of patients in a mental institution and had 67 of them circumcised. It was alleged that some of these boys improved, but none to such an extent that they could leave the institution.

Although not all Sayre's successors could boast the spectacular results of the master, circumcision became standard practice in the treatment of a variety of conditions, and it is not surprising that in these circumstances it should have occurred to many doctors that different diseases could be nipped in the bud by the preventive removal of the prepuce. That was, moreover, fully in keeping with the spirit of the times. The growing ideas of cultural progress called for better hygiene, based on fear of dirt and germs. Circumcision had always been highly approved in the highest social strata. In the US army, uncircumcised soldiers are taunted, for being circumcised is associated with virility and toughness. The upper classes were also most aware of the threat of venereal diseases, and circumcision was said to render men more resistant to infection. Suddenly the health of Jews attracted general attention, and they were extolled as the fathers of preventive medicine. And yes, it was true: Jews attained a greater age and had fewer venereal diseases and miscarriages; cancer was rarer among them, and degenerative diseases (epilepsy, mental handicap and mental illness) less common. The advocates of circumcision held all the trumps when they compared these two population groups.

All these arguments are of course misleading. An uncircumcised penis poses no health risk, though it does call for a little extra hygienic care. That means that parents must instruct their children in doing things that the most inhibited of them consider near shameful for being reminiscent of masturbation. The undercurrent of the lasting popularity of circumcision of boys in the United States has always been revulsion from masturbation. Dr John Harvey Kellogg, the health apostle who lives on in the corn flakes bearing his name, was most outspoken about his real motives. Because boys were circumcised to rob them of a means of masturbation, he advocated that the operation be performed without the use of anaesthetics. He found it only right and proper that the boys should experience the operation as a punishment, regardless of whether they were already guilty of the sin for which they were being held to account. The educational practices of the Victorian era involved all sorts of obvious sadistic motives, and physicians were not immune to them.

The United States has only thrown up a militant anti-circumcision movement in the last few years, and the best-informed Americans will nowadays think twice before they allow their male offspring to be circumcised. This can sometimes cause a difficult situation: what do you do if you are convinced of the pointlessness of the operation but already have a circumcised son? What emotions are at work between a circumcised and a non-circumcised brother? Will the older boy resent his reshaped anatomy? There have always been people who bitterly regret having been circumcised, and in the United States there is, at the moment, a very active self-help movement that instructs men to practice manipulations of the remains of the foreskin in order to recover a sheathed glans. There have also been groups since the 1990s exalting the uncircumcised state and claiming that uncircumcised males can give and enjoy far greater sexual pleasure.

chapter ten

The Physician and the Uterus

From the time of its founding fathers, medicine has always been concerned with the relationship between women, mental stability and the womb. The general assumption has been that there is a link between disorders of the uterus and the complex of symptoms referred to rather vaguely as hysteria. The nature of the link could vary with the spirit of the age. When Baker Brown used clitoridectomy to bring the surgical treatment of hysteria (among other conditions) out of obscurity into the scientific limelight, he took his place next to a much older medical tradition, as we also know from the admirable *The Technology of Orgasm* by the historian Rachel P. Maines.[1]

'Hysteria' is an elusive concept, but it is bound up with a mysterious organ – the uterus. Plato called the uterus an animal that could wander all over the body. In Chapter 44 of the *Timaeus* we are told:

> [Take] the so-called womb or matrix of women; the animal within
> them is desirous of procreating children, and when remaining unfruit-
> ful long beyond its proper time, gets discontented and angry, and wan-
> dering in every direction through the body, closes up the passages of
> the breath, and, by obstructing respiration, drives them to extremity,
> causing all varieties of disease, until at length the desire and love of the
> man and the woman bring[ing] them together.

Plato probably based this passage on older, Egyptian, sources.[2] The Kahun papyrus (2000 BC) attributes all the complaints of women to the wandering uterus.

For many centuries, physicians relied on the collection of medical writings from the fifth century before Christ which have come down to us as the works of Hippocrates and of a long series of successors, of whom Galen (c. AD 130–200) was the most authoritative. If an index of medical quotations had been kept over the centuries, then

Galen would undoubtedly have been the unchallenged frontrunner, since until far into the nineteenth century disputes among the medical profession used to be finally resolved with 'Galenus dixi' (Galen said so). Throughout the history of medical belief systems the progress of the pattern of complaints combined under the title of 'hysteria', as the wandering uterus came to be called, is reflected. The following fragment is taken from Hippocrates' Diseases of Women:[3]

> . . . when a woman is empty and works harder than in her previous experience, her womb, becoming heated from the hard work, turns because it is empty and light. There is, in fact, empty space for it to turn in because the belly is empty. Now when the womb turns, it hits the liver and they go together and strike against the abdomen – for the womb rushes and goes upward toward the moisture, because . . . the liver is moist. When the womb hits the liver, it produces sudden suffocation, as it occupies the breathing passage around the belly.
>
> . . . When the womb is near the liver and the abdomen and when it is suffocating, the woman turns up the whites of her eyes and becomes chilled; some women become livid. She grinds her teeth and saliva flows from her mouth. These women resemble those who suffer from Herakles' disease [epilepsy]. If the womb lingers near the liver and the abdomen, the woman dies of suffocation.

Since the wandering uterus can suffocate the woman, something must be done to stop it. The Ebers papyrus includes the oldest recipes to return the organ to its proper place. The womb is treated like an undisciplined pet: aromatic substances are introduced through the vagina (generally the smoke of fragrant woods, by means of a hollow artificial penis with holes in it which the woman inserts before squatting over a smouldering fire), while less pleasant odours are admitted through the uppermost orifices of the body. A sensible womb follows its instincts and its sense of smell. In a series of late thirteenth-century English illustrations depicting uterine suffocation, the patient is shown lying on a bier with a bowl of water that has been placed on her chest in order to detect the smallest movement. Another illustration shows her assistants tending to both ends of her body, and the last shows her back on her feet again. This last is also a probable illustration of the women who are predisposed to womb suffocation: widows and young girls who have just attained maturity.[4]

The practice of treating women's complaints with aromatic substances continued for a long time. In Jan Steen's genre paintings on a medical theme, in which the doctor is invariably a man and the patient a young woman who is obviously prey to 'love pangs', somewhere in a corner we sometimes see a fire-pan containing a smouldering shoelace. It is thought that the latter was probably on hand ready to be held under the woman's nose if she felt faint. Some interpreters of Steen's work have suggested that the smouldering material was a pregnancy test of the time: if the woman fainted when she smelled it, she was pregnant. However, one of Steen's contemporaries, the physician Johan van Beverwijck, repeats in his *Schat der Ongesondheyt* (Compendium of ill health) the ancient aroma-therapeutic advice in a chapter on the 'ascent of the life-mother', and recommends the following sources of stench: 'Burnt blue apron strings, burnt feathers, especially those of partridges, and burnt shoe rags'. The most plausible explanation of Steen's laces is that they helped subdue hysterical afflictions.

When medical science was usurped by the Church in the Middle Ages, the treatment was obvious and the womb was addressed in much the same terms as the Devil:

> I conjure you, womb, by our lord Jesus Christ, who walked on the waters with dry feet, . . . , by whose bruises we are healed, by him I conjure you not to harm this maidservant of God, [her name is then filled in], nor to hold onto her head, neck, throat, chest, . . . , ankles, feet or toes, but to quietly remain in the place God delegated to you, so that this handmaiden of God, [her name], might be cured.[5]

The displacement of the uterus and 'love pangs' go hand in hand, and it is left open which is the cause and which the effect. But that it is a bad thing is certain. In 1653, William Harvey deployed all his dramatic powers of expression to convey his concern about the fate of women to the male reader:[6]

> No man (who is but never so little versed in such matters) is ignorant, what grievous *symptomes*, the Rising, Bearing down and Perversion, and Convulsion of the *Wombe* do excite; what horrid extravagancies of minde, what Phrensies, Melancholy Distempers, and Outrageousness, the *preternatural Diseases* of the Womb do induce, as if the affected Persons were inchanted: as also how many difficult *Diseases*, the depraved affluxions of the Terms, or the use of *Venus*, much intermitted and long desired, do forment.

Plato having already postulated that sexual frustration, embodied in the damming up of female 'seed', was the cause of wandering wombs, the solution seemed obvious: the surplus fluid had to be dispersed, by which means the straying organ could be tempted to return to the place where it belonged. In men, too, the damming up of seed was considered to be a source of a multitude of ills, and the 'purging' of sperm was recommended as the best therapy. This view fits in well with the so-called 'doctrine of temperaments', of which Celsus was the great protagonist. Health meant a proper balance of the four body fluids: blood, mucus, white gall and black gall.

For married women sexual congress with their husbands was the most obvious cure, and anyone not yet married sought to remedy that omission as quickly as possible. In the sixteenth century, the French surgeon Ambroise Paré still handed out this piece of advice, adding the rider that they 'bee strongly encountered by their husbands'. If the patient did not have a husband, then the situation was dire. Referring to masturbation was unthinkable at the time, although women had more leeway here than men, since female 'seed' was less precious than male. That appears, for instance, from confessional instruction books: masturbation by young children could be confessed to any priest; boys older than fifteen had to go to special confessors, as did young women over the age of twenty-five (for the sake of comparison: adult homosexuals could only be given absolution by a bishop).[7] Albertus Magnus had a particularly tolerant attitude to girls who had recently reached puberty:

> The girl then starts to desire coitus, but in her desire she does not emit, and the more she performs the sexual act or has recourse to manual practices, the more does she desire; so much so that she attracts the humour, but without emitting it. With the humour, heat is attracted and, as the woman's body is cold and her pores closed, she does not emit the seed of coitus rapidly . . . And if they have no partner, they imagine coitus or the male member, or indulge in practices involving the use of their fingers or other instruments until their channels are opened by the heat of the friction and then the spermatic humour comes out, together with the heat that accompanies it. Thus their groins are tempered and they become more chaste.

The end justifies the means is what this pious writer seems to say. But his view was not widely shared, and so a solution had to be found in a professional medical framework. The physician was given the duty of massaging the vulva and the vagina, so that the sickness could be brought to crisis point, the so-called hysterical paroxysm. The learned writers conveniently glossed over the orgasmic purpose of their activities, but there can be little doubt but that from 500 BC until far into the nineteenth century the satisfaction of unmarried women was a recognized medical intervention.

Advice on the technique of vulvar massage can be found first of all in the writings of Hippocrates. Aretaeus of Cappadocia, Celsus and Galen, the most important ancient writers on medicine whose ideas have come down to us, followed him. Galen has given us the classical description of genital massage therapy, one that was to be repeatedly quoted in subsequent centuries:

> Following the warmth of the remedies and arising from the touch of the genital organs required by the treatment, there followed twitchings accompanied at the same time by pain and pleasure after which she emitted turbid and abundant sperm. From that time on she was free of all the evil she felt.

Pain and pleasure – that combination was essential. The most important mediaeval advocates of the technique were Rhazes and Avicenna. Paracelsus, too, the physician marking the transition from the Middle Ages to the Renaissance, employed the old prescriptions. Harvey, rendered immortal by his discovery of the circulation of the blood, is one of Maines's series of great medical figures, as is the Dutchman Pieter van Foreest, who expressly mentioned the midwife as a paramedical specialist in vaginal massage:[8]

> A widow, 44, . . . in May of 1546 was taken for dead and was lying unconscious, I was urgently called to her . . . it was a case of suffocation because of retained seed. The women present . . . were only making her worse. . . . Because of the urgency of the situation, we asked a midwife to come and apply ointment to the patient's genitals, rubbing them inside with her finger. And thus she was against hope brought back to consciousness.

The nineteenth-century writers whom Maines has been able to discover all came from Francophone territories. In France, vaginal massage by gynaecologists continued to be an accepted method of dealing with vaginismus until well after the Second World War.[9] This was undoubtedly connected with the existence of the profession of medical gynaecology, whose practitioners were not trained in surgical methods and hence were inclined to remain faithful to more conservative techniques.

Those of a prurient bent today will assume that the learned doctors recommended and applied this treatment with a degree of lasciviousness, but that cannot be inferred from their writings. Maines's argument is certainly meant as a critique of the persistent centuries-old androcentric model of sexuality, and she would assuredly not have ignored the abuse of women by men, but she encountered no indications of doctors driven by their own lascivious desires. Vaginal massage was generally administered by midwives, the role of the doctor being confined to the prescription of the aromatic oils required, and sometimes of stimulants to be administered vaginally. Abraham Zacuto described the treatment of a 'virginella' whose problems were so life-threatening that a 'pessarium' had to be administered to her. This device was apparently a kind of dildo made using cyclamen, onion, garlic and ox gall, for it was inserted and manipulated in such a way as to generate warmth and the ejaculation of the juices.

Anyone reading about these practices learns about the then prevailing difficulties of explaining and justifying such intimate procedures. The theologian Vincent of Spain was categorically of the view in about 1200 that the patient must not be allowed to suspect that seed congestion was the cause of her symptoms (Vincent, incidentally, had the same if not greater difficulties with monks suffering from spontaneous seed emission, whom he preferred to leave in ignorance as well).[10] Confessors were in any case skating on thin ice: if the faithful were really to be put back on the right path they had to be helped to put their possible sins into words. However the inevitable questioning of a chaste confessant may well have been counterproductive. Caesarius of Heisterbach tells us about a priest in Brabant who confessed a girl so graphically that for the first time in her life she experienced the temptations of the flesh in her own body.[11] Salacious knowledge was present in abundance in the priesthood; priests were perhaps the only people to know the difference between *a tergo* (anal) and *a retro* (doggy-fashion). This knowledge certainly did not leave them untouched: Rome and Avignon were centres of prostitution, and when the Church councils convened there, business boomed and reinforcements were rushed up from near and far.[12]

Some physician-priests were fully aware of the sexual overtones of their hysterotherapy, and concluded that such cures must be confined to people with 'clean hands and a pure heart'. As Albertus Magnus put it:

> The hand which defiles leads to flabbiness or sodomy, but the hand which cures does not, as we say for women who suffer from a fall in the position of the uterus: it is prescribed that this be put back in place by means of the hand and we say that the hand does not defile

nor corrupt these woman but rather cures them.

On the other hand, the strangest euphemisms and rituals were used when it came to the treatment of female problems. An all-time low was undoubtedly reached with Franz Anton Mesmer (1734–1815), the pioneer of 'animal magnetism'. In his Parisian period, Mesmerite group sessions were important events in the high society calender, and women and girls were the most enthusiastic followers. In 1841 Charles Mackay remembered with shudders what he was told about such happenings.[13] A group of women, sitting round a bath of magnetized water, was being treated by assistant magnetizers. These generally young, muscular and well-shaped gentlemen 'embraced the patient between the knees', and massaged their breasts and torsos while looking deep into their eyes. The rapt sighs of the magnetized patients were accompanied by music, and then one after the other they succumbed to:

> . . . convulsive fits. Some of them sobbed and tore their hair, others laughed till the tears ran from their eyes, while others shrieked and screamed and yelled till they became insensible altogether.

At the height of the pandemonium, the master himself made his entrance, stroked faces, breasts and stomachs and behaved in all respects like a saviour, whereupon the patients regained consciousness. Mackay calls Mesmer a charlatan and a dirty old man, and leaves no one in any doubt about that. In the nineteenth century, the water cure became popular. It was frequently directed at the abdomen (see illus. 25)[14] and we may take it that the powerful jets of water aimed at the clitoris and labia minora brought about erotic stimulation, an effect sought deliberately or otherwise: 'The douche is a very necessary part of the treatment; and, played well on the loins, tends powerfully to facilitate the uterine functions.'

In the nineteenth century, ambiguous feelings about female orgasms must have been at their height. On the one hand, many physicians, following in the footsteps of the classics, maintained that a hysterical crisis opened the window to the classical complex of symptoms. On the other hand, there was the constant fear of triggering off female sexual desires prematurely, thus opening the door to masturbation and 'hence' to mental unbalance. For that reason, even young children had to be kept under close observation. The New York paediatrician Abraham Jacobi declared in November 1875 at a meeting of the New York Medical Association:

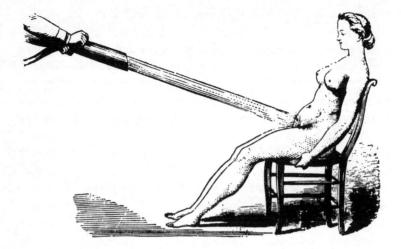

A girl of three years was sent by a medical friend, because of a peculiar form of slight convulsive affections which were reported by the
mother to have lasted a considerable time . . . Redness in the face and
slight twitching about the eyes, with a deep sigh now and then, were
all the symptoms enumerated . . . But for a long time the baby had
lost her former spirits, was not noisy, but rather peevish and listless,
alternately. A few questions and answers sufficed to convince me of
the presence of masturbation in the little girl . . . She always had them
[the slight convulsive affections] when sitting down. She was very apt
to keep her thighs closely joined, or to cross her legs. She moved and
rubbed her limbs violently, got purple in the face, began to perspire,
to twitch about her eyes, which often looked excited, and lean back
exhausted, sighing, or breathing hurriedly . . . Such cases are by no
means rare.[15]

Jacobi appeared to be a good diagnostician; he made the same observations as the girl's mother. However, the conclusions he and many
of his colleagues drew from the observations were less pleasant for
the children. Once the threshold of sin had been crossed, the cutting
medics (the surgeons) were inclined to leave no stone unturned to
eradicate the evil. Surgeons are of course always quicker to intervene
than physicians. They are after all spiritual heirs to the barbers,
whereas physicians are part of a long academic tradition (which
however remained scholastic and authoritarian for a long time;
Molière had good reason to poke fun at them).

Barker-Benfield points out that the doctors who clitoridectomized
or castrated women to rid them of mental disorders quite often tested if

a woman reacted to clitoral stimulation with pleasurable sensations, which, in their eyes, was confirmation of the need to intervene. E. H. Smith published his guidelines for the diagnosis of masturbation in women as late as 1903.[16] If one of the labia was larger than the other, then it was reasonable to suppose that the woman masturbated asymmetrically. It was of course essential to determine whether she indulged in one of the known spurs to masturbation: horse-riding, cycling, using a treadle sewing machine, and, of course, reading French novels. Everything French was greeted with some suspicion. Syphilis was known in English-speaking countries as 'the French disease', and even their sewing machines were more suspect than Anglo-Saxon ones. In a report by the Philadelphia Obstetric Society published in 1873, we find a discussion of the indications for clitoridectomies:

> Dr. Harris said that reference had been made by French physicians to the evil effects of sewing machines. This applied to the French machines only, which were worked by a double treadle, and necessarily with alternate action of the feet. On the other hand, the American machines were worked with a single treadle, on which both feet were placed.

Corsets that were laced too tightly were suspect as well. As a method of direct observation, E. H. Smith advocated watching the patient's response to a weak faradic current through the urethra, as a substitute for the previously prescribed direct clitoral manipulation.

It would seem that, at the time, chance decreed that some women with a certain complex of symptoms finished up with a doctor who got a proficient midwife to relieve them by means of an orgasmic discharge, while other patients fell into the hands of 'radicals' who started off by phrasing their diagnoses in such a way that the entire blame fell squarely onto the woman, after which she was expected to receive gratefully her well-deserved punishment from the doctor's hands.

In his novel *The Road to Wellville*, T. Coraghessan Boyle throws hilarious light on the animosity between these two currents.[17] The story unfolds at the Battle Creek Sanitarium in Michigan, where John Harvey Kellogg is busy administering cures to patients of the American upper class with a firm hand. In his day, Kellogg was an authority in many fields, and in the film of the book his character is played by Anthony Hopkins for all it is worth. The Sanitarium takes an extremely conservative view of sexuality. A young married couple comes to take the cure, but the Spartan diet regime and the sexual abstinence undermine their good intentions. Worse still, unwanted erotic tensions appear between the husband, a nurse and an unmarried TB patient, while the wife (Eleanor) is inveigled by Virginia, a fellow patient, and her friend Lionel into consulting the mysterious German physician Dr Spitzvogel outside the Sanitarium:

> Yes, Eleanor said to herself, but what does he *do*?
> . . .
> 'In German it's called *"Die Handhabung Therapeutik"*.'
> 'Manipulation Therapy,' Virginia breathed.
> 'Well,' Lionel said. 'The doctor manipulates the womb – '
> 'And the breasts,' Virginia put in, lingering over the sibilance of the word as if she couldn't let go of it.
> 'Yes,' Lionel puffed, warming to the subject, 'because this is the seat of the hysterical passions in the female anatomy and the key, many feel, to neurasthenic disorders.'

Naturally, Eleanor has ecstatic moments in Spitzvogel's hands (there is a suggestion that she had never had them before), but when she and her friend delve more deeply into naturism and allow themselves to be massaged together in the open, they are caught by Eleanor's husband. The scene that follows is one of unseemly violence, but after that the married couple leave the Sanitarium, full of vim and set on procreation.

Hysteria has been the subject of even weirder theories. The colleague Freud admired most in the early years of psychoanalysis, the ear, nose and throat specialist Wilhelm Fliess, postulated a neurogenic link between the reproductive organs and the nasal mucosa. For Fliess, the nasal septum was a map of trigger points similar to the sole of the foot or the auricle for today's reflexologists. Spots in the nose corresponding to the sick organs were dabbed with cocaine, and hysteria was one of the ills to be treatd that way. Freud continued to give Fliess the benefit of the doubt for a long time. Now, a century later, it seems obvious that this approach was a compromise between the old-fashioned method of providing direct relief for the uterus and turn-of-the-century prudery: one could be 'penetrated' by a doctor while high on cocaine, yet everything remained above board and a long way above the belt. Incidentally, many of Freud's contemporaries found his ideas about the sexual origin of the neuroses completely unacceptable. There was much backbiting, and in 1910 the psychiatrist Weygandt argued that anyone holding such views ought not to be admitted to a medical congress but sent straight to a police station.[18] To make it clear how perverse he considered psychoanalysts to be, Weygandt argued that Freud's therapy was comparable to the massage of the sexual organs. Perhaps the audience included some old practitioners who said to themselves: so what?

To date, medical practitioners are the only professional group allowed to touch the female genitals. In medical training, serious attention has been paid during the last few decades to the emotional impact of such investigations. Doctor and patient are both aware that their relationship at such moments is very delicate, and that both are expected to remain cool during the process. Most physicians are careful not to touch a patient's clitoris, and that seems a reasonable attitude. Neurologists form the exception, since the bulbocavernosus reflex has to be examined during a complete neurological investigation. This reflex is set off by an unexpected nip of the clitoris, a finger registering the reflex-like tension of the pelvic-floor muscles. Doctors rarely talk about this investigation but it seems to me not unlikely that it is quite often omitted.

In the 1970s, a London sexological clinic looked into the causes of orgasm difficulties in women.[19] The idea was to test the hypothesis that anorgasmic women may have weaker genital reflexes, and because the bulbocavernosus reflex is so difficult to produce and quantify, the response of the pelvic floor to vibrator stimulation of the clitoris was observed instead. If the reaction is positive, the sphincter muscles of the pelvic floor (that is, round the vagina and the anus) can be seen to contract, and the woman is unable to stop that contraction. Women who did not produce this response to vibrator stimulation often proved to be those who had failed to respond to the customary treatment for anorgasmy.

This study was fairly unusual. Nowadays great care is taken to avoid all forms of sexual arousal during clinical examinations. Obstetrics is the exception. We occasionally read advice to doctors to exploit the pain-killing effect of arousal and orgasm during childbirth. Medical professionals who believe that they are serving their patients' best interests by arousing them sexually are few and far between. During preparations for the Tenth World Congress of Sexology in Amsterdam in 1991, the scientific committee was taken aback by an Israeli doctor keen to explain his approach to women with vaginismus. His basic premise was that women with this condition needed above all to be reassured during a physical examination. If the doctor was able to show them during the examination that their vagina was not too tight, and if during the examination they were able to control their fear sufficiently to allow the doctor to probe their vagina with one finger, then their sexual life was bound to improve. This doctor had also noticed that some women were unable to master their fears, and that simultaneous clitoral stimulation increased the chances of success. His outspoken defence of a method his colleagues considered unethical led to a protracted, rather vitriolic correspondence and finally to the acceptance by the Israeli gynaecologist that, if all his colleagues frowned upon his method, he should stop using it. The discussion had something in common with the meeting leading to the expulsion of Baker Brown more than a century earlier. The end did not even in this case justify the means, the Israeli gynaecologist had to concede – with reluctance, because like the castrators and clitoridectomists before him, he was convinced of the validity of his method and he too could boast of many breathlessly grateful patients.

chapter eleven

The Vibrator

What precisely does a vibrator do? It provides oscillations with a frequency beyond the powers of any human finger or tongue. When vibrators first went on the market, their producers emphasized that their product offered an experience beyond compare, and they certainly had a point. Vibrators make use of the vibration sensitivity of the skin, and that is something manual massage does not provide. In this process, it is chiefly touch and pain, together with pressure and sometimes temperature, that determine the cocktail of sensations. Sometimes the skin and mucosa alone are stimulated, though occasionally the underlying muscles, joints and internal organs are included as well. Physiotherapists use vibrators to relax muscles in particular, and that was also the promotional claim issued with the oldest types of vibrator.

There is probably no one who knows as much about vibrators as Rachel Maines, and yet she came upon them by chance. In *The Technology of Orgasm* (1999) she tells us how, as an academic specializing in the history of technology, she collected material on needlework. She was disappointed by the lack of scientific literature on the subject. The explanation she found most plausible was that there is a dearth of writing about activities that are mainly performed by women. She accordingly decided to write a very detailed study of the period from 1880 to 1930, but while collecting the material, for which she drew on countless specialized knitting, crocheting and embroidery magazines, she kept on being distracted by advertisements for massage appliances, and after her dissertation she also came away with a thick folder of advertisements for vibrators. They became her next subject. It had a kick start when she discovered the Bakken Library and Museum of Electricity in Life in Minneapolis. That institution seemed not only to have a complete collection of electrical household goods, but the staff also had a laudable openness of mind. That was anything but the rule in the 1980s. Maines's first publication on vibrators in *Technology and Society* was initially accepted by that journal without demur, but then held back from publication by the editorial board, who were very much afraid the whole article was a satire. Maines had to appear before the annual meeting to convince the members that she was a real person. The way in which the most cautious members of the editorial board had put up a resistance for fear of making fools of themselves had of course a boomerang effect. Maines proudly claims that publicity about the affair had gained the journal quite a few new subscribers.

We know the vibrator as a personal piece of equipment, but that is not how the story began. The first vibrators, dating back to about 1880, were medical instruments for use in the consulting room, and their popularity with doctors quickly grew. What precisely did the doctors do with the device, Maines wondered, and when she started to read the literature she discovered the story of medical genital massage. The success of the vibrator ought to be viewed in the light of this centuries-old medical practice of treating certain feminine complaints by providing them with sexual release. Clearly, quite a few of these patients had need of this treatment with some regularity and, not surprisingly, medical writers occasionally complained about the waste of time and the tedium of this aspect of their professional work. Most of it was delegated to midwives, and unfortunately we do not know what they thought of this form of therapy. A vibrator could do the job more quickly, had to be bought just once, obviated the need for paying midwives, and the medical practitioner could be spared the opprobrium of innuendo.

Remarkably, the introduction of the vibrator into medical practice did not meet many objections. Only twenty years before there had been extremely fierce polemics on the subject of J. Marion Sims's invention of his speculum, an instrument considered to be dangerous because its use could lead to unwanted sexual stimulation.[1] On the other hand, nineteenth-century physicians treated the sick body with all sorts of stimulants, including water cures, electrostatic methods and ozone-producing apparatus. At the Spectacular Bodies exhibition at London's Hayward Gallery at the end of 2000, the American artist Beth B exhibited her installation *Hysteria 2000*, part of which consisted of Charcot's ovarian pressure girdle, a sort of leather corset with two small cushions pushing inwards over the crucial areas, and capable of being pressed into the abdomen with the help of a screw.

Massage (manual, with water or with small hammers and rollers) had traditionally been an integral part of the therapeutic arsenal; what was new was the unashamed concentration on the lower abdomen. The design of the ascending douche, too, made it clear that it was

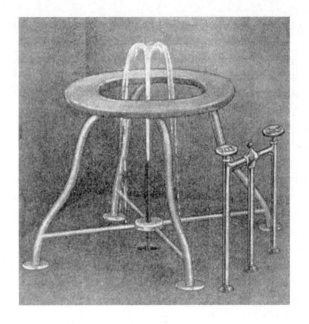

26
The ascending
douche in
Saratoga,
c. 1900.

meant for use on the bottom, and the illustration of Fleury's treatment from 1860 mentioned earlier also speaks volumes. Many clinics were, moreover, equipped with electrically driven vibration chairs and instruments that worked in roughly the same way as modern vibrating weight-loss belts.

The forerunners of modern vibrators were operated by a spiral spring, similar to the type found in many toys. Other sources of vibration were foot pedals (similar to those operating the oldest dentist's drill) and jets of tap water. These sources were specially adapted for domestic use; larger bathing establishments used steam energy.

The use of electro-mechanical movements as a source of energy in vibrator therapy began in 1878 in the famous Parisian psychiatric institution nicknamed La Salpêtrière where Freud was to complete his psychiatric training a few years later. Here the new physiotherapeutic method was tested on hysterical women. Its inventor, Joseph Mortimer Granville, didn't like that at all; he considered hysteria an intangible, if not feigned, condition. The energy source of Granville's apparatus was a powerful accumulator, but it did not take long before town houses were connected to the mains. As a result, the domestic use of vibrators was greatly facilitated, and at the end of the nineteenth century the sale of vibrators considerably increased. Since that time it was stressed in advertisements for the (more expensive) equipment for doctors that the apparatus in question was specifically made for its medical effects, and by its design was a beautiful addition to a doctor's surgery. There was no longer any doubt about the use of vibrations in a broad spectrum of problems; during one of the Balkan wars, vibration equipment was found in British as well as in French field hospitals. A new professional group – electro-masseurs – began to offer their services.

The general public was of course the most interesting target group for the manufacturers. The first advertisement for a home vibrator, the Vibratile, dates back to 1899. In advertisements published at the time, the vibrator shares the honours with the sewing machine, the fan, the electric kettle and the toaster. Housewives would have to wait another ten years or so for the vacuum cleaner and the electric iron. In the advertisement for the first vibrator, neuralgia, headaches and wrinkles were named as ills it was able to treat. Health and beauty were always mentioned in one breath, and the sexual possibilities were no more than hinted at:

> TO WOMEN I address my message of health and beauty.
> Gentle, soothing, invigorating and refreshing. Invented by a woman who knows a woman's needs. All nature pulsates and vibrates with life.
> The most perfect woman is she whose blood pulses with the natural law of being.

The manufacturers balked at specifying the sexual possibilities of their products, understandably so at the time. After all, the medical men who preceded them in treating the sexual frustrations of women had also concealed the orgasmic nature of their massage work for generations. The general public must have picked up the message all the same; in Roger Blake's book *Sex Gadgets* there is an account of a pornographic film, *Widow's Delight*, made in about 1920, in which a lady refuses to embrace her escort at the door but quickly loosens her underwear in her boudoir so that her vibrator can find its way to her most sensitive spot.[2] Maines observes that from 1930 until the sexual revolution in the 1960s, no further advertisements for vibrators or other massage equipment were published, possibly because the true nature of these devices had become generally known. From the 1960s onwards, there was no longer any need to conceal the chief purpose (although photographs in a modern mail order catalogue often still show a smiling woman with a vibrator held against her cheek).

The oldest vibrators were of the hand-mixer type: a handle with a cord, a wider part containing the motor, and a lateral extension to which the various accessories could be attached. The battery-operated shaft vibrator, which from the start of the sexual revolution dominated the entire scene, by its design suggests penetration. That is rather paradoxical, for when it operates deep inside the vagina, most women will feel very little vibration. If the vibrator is used as an aid to orgasms, then the clitoris is the place at which the tip of the vibrator has to be aimed. The principle of the shaft vibrator has been extended in a host of different ways. Towards the end of the 1990s, people could choose between small lateral vibrators (meant for the clitoris), double vibrators (for simultaneous vaginal and anal penetration), and vibrators with a moving shaft which could make their presence felt inside the vagina. The most recent addition is a ring of small beads under the surface, which performs a kind of rolling movement at the entrance to the vagina. Furthermore, vibrators come in various shapes, a curved type enabling the user to stimulate the G-spot. Real connoisseurs frown upon batteries. The corded vibrator is much more powerful, its intensity more controllable, there is less of a hum and no batteries to run out.

Vibrators came out of the cold during the heyday of sex therapy. In the 1970s, women who had never had an orgasm made up a large group, and that was blamed on a simple lack of knowledge. The American psychologist Lonnie Barbach advocated group therapy for women with orgasmic problems, and the group approach became popular all over the world.[3] The mood in those groups was optimistic; the term 'anorgasmy' was replaced with 'preorgasmy', to underline the fact that it was not abnormal for one woman to experience her first orgasm at an earlier age than another. The atmosphere was educational more than therapeutic: homework was set, and the programme designed to achieve a balance between attention to the psychological motives and to proficiency. The vibrator was invariably brought up for discussion and it happened quite often that it was the little extra that had been needed to help a woman to have her first orgasm.

In later years, the New York psychologist Betty Dodson, whom we met earlier, emerged as the guru of orgasm enrichment. She too organized group therapy for women, the aim being an intensification of the erotic experience. The best means to attain that was said to be the communal experience. In her groups joint masturbation was the chosen method for overcoming feelings of shame, and every participant had the use of a vibrator (generally a corded vibrator). Some critics have objected to the exhibitionist element in this approach, but there is undoubtedly something liberating, something anarchistic, about it.

Betty Dodson makes it clear that she thinks little of battery-operated vibrators, but she is one of the few to make known her views on vibrators. Developments in this market sector are rarely driven by good consumer research, and critical observation leads to the conclusion that this line of business does not welcome change. In 1989 the American sexologists Hartman and Fithian told the Sexological World Congress in Caracas about their trials and tribulations in the world of vibrator manufacturers. They had only come into contact with them fairly recently, and that because until about 1970 'sex gadgets' were bought exclusively by men (though often on behalf of their partners even if not always at the partners' express request), and if the purchased device proved not to be up to expectations, it ended up in the bin without further ado. In marketing terms there was thus no call for quality. Only when women themselves looked at what the market had to offer were critical questions about the whys and wherefores of vibrators first raised, and if the product did not fulfil the promises of the vendors, women began asking for their money back. It was at this point that the manufacturers began to consult sexologists.

A special target group, which has been ignored until recently, is made up of those in whom the manual function is impaired. They are physically capable of having sexual pleasure, including orgasm, but cannot achieve it without help. The special circumstances of such people demand special adaptations, and that inspired Joop Steenkamer in the Netherlands to introduce one of the few genuine innovations in the vibrator field.

Steenkamer, a student of industrial design at Delft Technical University, devoted his thesis to this target group.[4] He discovered that the ideal time for people in need of nursing care to masturbate is when taking a bath or sitting under the shower. Ideally, the nurse is only needed to help during the preparations; during the actual masturbation the handicapped persons can proceed on their own (and for men it is important that no one should be required to help in removing the evidence of their activity). Before the bath, he or she has already been helped to undress, and during rehabilitation the possibilities of optimal self-sufficiency in matters of personal hygiene will have been thoroughly explored. One method involving a pulsating jet of water (from the normal shower head) proved to be less than effective, but Steenkamer came up with a device in which the jet of water produced vibrations.

Many years before, the Dutch Council for the Handicapped had already been responsible for an attempt to produce a powerful aid to masturbation, and a prototype, called the Coitron by its maker Robert Trost, was tested.[5] The device did not involve vibration but the direct electrical stimulation by electrodes of the penis (at the level of the frenulum) and the prepuce of the clitoris. 'Electrization' is an old method used in rehabilitation and physiotherapy, and in recent years there has been a keen market in electrical workout aids promising muscle-building without effort. In the genital area, however, it took a long search to discover a form of pulsation that was both painless and erotically stimulating. Trost's experimental subjects did find that they were physically aroused, and a number of women felt that they came close to an orgasm, but the follow-up research for which Trost sought financial support at the time of his publication never materialized.

Direct electrical stimulation fell into desuetude. There was one exception: men with a transverse lesion. If the wish to procreate is blocked by the inability to ejaculate, an attempt is generally made first of all to elicit a reflex ejaculation with a powerful vibrator. If that fails, the mucous membrane of the anus can be stimulated electrically under anaesthesia to produce an ejaculation. Electro-ejaculation has been developed in veterinary surgery; the sperm harvested in this way can then be used for artificial insemination.

Even more futuristic were the experiments conducted by a faculty for nervous diseases in New Orleans during the 1970s.[6] At the time, many medical centres were experimenting with brain surgery for serious psychiatric and neurological disorders. Epileptics had electrodes inserted in the brain that were sometimes left in for years. These electrodes facilitated the observation of spontaneous activity not detectable in an electroencephalogram (EEG) of the skull, but the electrodes could also be used for administering electrical stimuli. In addition, it was possible to administer minute quantities of chemical stimulants through microcannulas. In other centres, such electrodes were also used to administer short, high-dosage current impulses, producing small burns in the nerve centres. This method of adjusting brain functions was a refinement of the much older lobotomy, in which links between parts of the brain were cut, an extremely crude method often used to 'tame' unmanageable patients. Its crudity inspired novelists and filmmakers; the best-known lobotomized troublemaker is played by Jack Nicholson in the film One Flew Over the Cuckoo's Nest.[7]

R. G. Heath has described the emotional reactions of patients to electrical signals registered at various sites. Some areas of the brain invariably produce pleasurable sensations; the septal area in particular is libidinous. That was already known from experiments with rats: if a rat is fitted with an electrode and the means of administering a suitable stimulus to itself (with a pedal) than the rat's life becomes very monotonous. Like a junkie, it spends all day giving itself electrical stimuli.

One of Heath's male patients was fitted with a similar device, and he too liked to stimulate certain cerebral regions every ten seconds. As a result, he felt happy, alert, amiable, and often sexually aroused as well. This externally administered form of arousal was also used in an experiment designed to overcome a male patient's aversion to women. Until his admission, this man had only had homosexual experiences, but he had found these less than satisfying and furthermore marred by his use of prostitutes. First he was given a flavour of heterosexuality in a porno-graphic video; later a female prostitute was hired to provide him with heterosexual experience. After being discharged from hospital, the man functioned better in his social surroundings, and for a time he had an intimate relationship with a woman that was sexually satisfying.[8]

This man and a female epileptic patient were also treated experi-mentally with the administration of drugs to the septal area, the drugs used being acetylcholine and adrenaline. They produced a high state of arousal in both the man and the woman, but only in the woman did that lead to spontaneous orgasms. The investigators ended their article with speculations on possible further developments with the help of new drugs that can be taken orally to produce pleasant sensations. Such developments have already been described in science fiction. In Roger Vadim's film *Barbarella*, made in 1968, Jane Fonda is sent to a distant corner of the universe on a dangerous mission in the year 2300, but on her unfamiliar route she keeps meeting men with whom some sultry sensuality pops up. By this date, we come to learn, sex has been reduced to the taking of a pill, giving rise to a variety of pleasant and meaning-ful inner responses, as suggested by the actors' facial expressions.

Cybersex is the creation of modern science fiction, and Ronald Giphart gives free rein to his imagination in the short story 'The world of things we have left undone', from the 1995 collection *The Love Feast*. He goes home with a girl, Maxime, who does not sleep around, but nevertheless wants to spend a short time making love to him via Teledildonics, something she and her boyfriend have developed. This is an intricate device, a sort of space suit, in which a variety of small motors gives the user the feeling of having a vagina round his penis, a breast in his palm, or a clitoris on his tongue. He can see Maxime on the screen of his fibre-optic helmet, or rather a kind of animated version of her but looking extremely eager and seductive. Only after he and Maxime have had very enjoyable sex and both have come does she tell him that she does not of course have his picture on her screen but that of her boyfriend. With the help of Teledildonics, she can be both faithful and have wild nights while her partner is in a different part of the world.

But back to reality. Industrial design student Ireen Laarakkers graduated in 1995 with a new vibrator design based on consumer research.[9] She questioned a group of female clients of a large sex mail-order concern, and on the basis of their replies formulated a list of requirements. Two brainstorming sessions were then held with some of the respondents, who were encouraged to voice their wishes freely and not to take something as trivial as feasibility into account. The result was a series of visionary designs including large rooms in which warm currents of air continuously caress the body, and telepathic sex smurfs. The conversion of these ideas into concrete products was the work of the designer, who came up with the three prototypes shown in Illus. 21.

> A one-piece battery-operated vibrator, the vibrating section for clitoral stimulation only and constructed so that the noise level is minimized. The handle can be used as a dildo, but does not vibrate.
>
> A mains-voltage device that can be used in conjunction with a Walkman or CD-player, the intensity and frequency of the vibrations varying with the music. The instrument is shaped like a mobile phone. It fits easily in the palm of the hand, can also be sat on, or kept in the panties. It comes with a dildo-shaped end-piece.
>
> A water-filled bag of soft plastic, supplied in various shapes with irregular protrusions, used without a vibrator. It is an aid for women who are used to coming to orgasm by tensing muscles and movements of the hips. Unlike a pillow or a teddy bear this device can be brought to the desired temperature by filling with warm water and the material is soft but also slippery. One type allows penetration.

Laarakkers went back to good old vibration and to frictional and penetrating devices. In this field a great deal of imagination can be used, especially if practical limitations do not have to be taken into account. Everything the participants in the brainstorming session came up with had been thought of before. Tomi Ungerer is best known as an illustrator of children's books, but in his *Fornicon*, published in 1971, he depicted a collection of incredible sexual gratification devices.[10] In his designs sexual satisfaction is often combined with a variety of other activities, such as music, sports, computer games, pinball machines, beauty therapy and bodybuilding exercises. Many of his ideas are technologically feasible. Kienholz has produced comparable suggestions in his installations, and most DIY handymen ought to be able to come up with creative adaptations. A few years ago, a Dutch married couple in an S/M group

Neutral in appearance, an accessible product for women who find it difficult to buy an obvious sex product. Because of its inconspicuous appearance, the magic massager can be obtained at leading stores as a massage device.

Very simple to use. The harder the vibrating head is pressed against the body, the more it vibrates. The vibrating mechanism is set off by even the slightest touch.

Vibration-free handle. Only the head vibrates, so that this product runs more quietly than other vibrators.

Completely enclosed, watertight design. All openings are sealed off with elastic rings. The product is therefore safe, easy to clean and can be used in the shower.

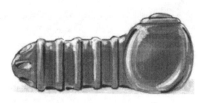

The vibrations of the vibrating head vary with the music that is being played.

Can be used with or without a dildo.

Can also be used in sitting position and needs no hands.

Vibration-free handle. Only the knob vibrates.

Resembles the sensation of water massage since the water inside the product can be set in motion.

The material is odourless, and oil and grease-resistant.

Warm, soft, pleasant to the touch.

No mechanical or electronic parts, user-friendly and natural.

Can be ordered in a variety of shapes and colours.

demonstrated a remote-control vibrator. In this master and slave marriage, their power status was adequately reflected in his ability to arouse her physically whenever he felt like it – not least in congenial company, for instance when she was serving drinks for their guests.

27 The magic massager.

Ireen Laarakkers took her three prototypes to a Berlin sex trade fair, but her experiences there were rather discouraging. There were indeed a few manufacturers who professed to be ready to meet the wishes of the consumers, but in the end she came away empty-handed.

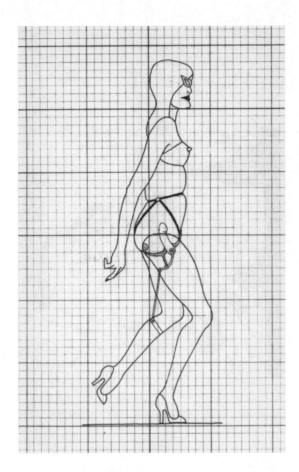

Vibrators have also arrived unbidden on the market: in January 2003 American parents complained to the Mattel company about their toy broomstick, the 'Nimbus 2000', a product sold as part of the Harry Potter marketing boom.[11] The broomstick was designed to fit between children' legs, give off light and could be remote-controlled, but above all, it vibrated. On the manufacturer's website a naïve and enthusiastic uncle reported that his niece played the whole day long with his present to her 'until she is completely worn out'.

It is still possible to make very large profits on the vibrator market with extremely shoddy goods. A woman who, on the advice of her sexologist, bought a vibrator (of the mains type) to deal with her orgasm difficulties, had a partner who worked as a quality-control inspector for a large manufacturer of household appliances. His opinion was scathing. He was truly shocked at the negligence with which the safety aspects of the gadget had been treated, and that at a price and thus a profit margin of which ordinary producers can only dream.

chapter twelve

The Scent of Women

Coyote is in the coffee shop
staring a hole in his scrambled eggs.
He picks up my scent on his fingers
while he's watching the waitresses
Joni Mitchell

A book on female genitals must needs deal with scent and taste, a far
from easy thing to do. Vaginal smells and vaginal secretions are generally disparaged in crude terms. Jokes about vaginal smells are usually evidence of ill-disguised misogyny. In *belles-lettres* there is hardly a mention
of this aspect of erotic life, and so it is left to pornographers to enthuse
about the female perfume of love.

Some nations are more outspoken than others. We know that
Napoleon wrote asking Josephine not to wash herself before His
Majesty's next visit. The French seem to be generally more open and
more exhibitionist about eroticism than, say, the Dutch. The surrealist
playwright and stage director Antonin Artaud ran a radio programme in
the 1950s in which he read a poem with the following lines:

I love cunts because cunts taste of cunt
I love arseholes because arseholes taste of arse.

The French esprit clearly has highly carnal aspects.

The discretion with which we treat sexual odours is at loggerheads
with our biological nature. Now and then we are confronted with this
fact. A woman who had sought therapeutic help for her strong sexual
inhibitions and aversions was putting her five-year-old daughter to bed
one night. The little girl stunned her mother by inviting her 'to smell the
most delicious smell in the whole world'. This was on her finger, with
which she had obviously been touching her genitals – a confusing expe-

rience for a mother so at odds with herself and faced suddenly with the physical directness of her daughter. Maybe the mother had read Philip Roth's *Portnoy's Complaint*.[1] The hero's last great love, to whom he refers scathingly as The Monkey, made shameless use of the magical powers of her smell:

> . . . as in the early days of our courtship, The Monkey retired at one point to the ladies' room at Ranieri's and returned to the table with a finger redolent of pussy, which I held beneath my nose to sniff and kiss at till the main dish arrived . . .

Mother-daughter relationships come in many forms. As against the mother who succeeds in bringing her daughter up with a joyous acceptance of her body, and with everything that goes with it, we have the 'Victorian' matron who checks every night whether her daughter is keeping her hands above the blankets and who completes her investigations by sniffing her daughter's fingers. The reader will not be surprised that this particular mother failed later to offer her daughter any protection when she, by then physically mature, was being sexually abused by her father. On the contrary, the mother justified the father's behaviour, since within her paranoid sexually obsessed vision she had always felt that her daughter deserved to be punished for her wantonness.

In a French coming-of-age film, two elementary-school girls are fascinated by the much older sister of one of them. When the big sister gets undressed (strikingly photographed before a moonlit curtain), she always sniffs at her panties. For the two little girls this becomes a mysterious symbol of adulthood. In the recently published fragments of her diary, Anne Frank describes the solemn feelings with which she observed the products of her vagina:

> I forgot to mention the important news that I'm probably going to have my period soon. I can tell because I keep finding a whitish smear in my panties, and Mother predicted it would start soon. I can hardly wait. It's such a momentous event. Too bad I can't use sanitary towels, but you can't get them any more, and Mummy's tampons can be used only by women who've had a baby.[2]

Exchanging information about vaginal odours is normally the job of medical men; among the many irritations to which genital infections give rise, a strong odour is sometimes the main symptom. Some fifteen years ago, a new diagnosis appeared in gynaecological texts, namely bacterial vaginosis, which can be identified by a pronounced fishy odour. The vaginal secretion is often rather copious but is not unusual in other respects, and there is normally no pain, itching or dryness. Particularly embarrassing for many women is the fact that after sexual intercourse, hence patently as a result of the effect of sperm on the vagina, the smell becomes much stronger. No one will be surprised that some women have quite a struggle with themselves before they are able to visit their doctor with this complaint.

The group of substances responsible for this fishy odour are called amines; they are produced by the breakdown of proteins. The main cause of the complaint is a recently discovered bacterium, *Gardnerella vaginalis*. It is now clear that a group of bacteria, while causing few other untoward effects, accelerates the breakdown of proteins into amines. The treatment of bacterial vaginosis is simple: a single high dose of the antibiotic metronidazole helps to clear up the condition in almost all cases. Very occasionally the treatment has unwanted side effects – some women find after the cure that their vagina has lost its odour almost completely, which was not really what was desired.

How does the sex odour arise and what influences bear on it? Research has shown that the specific aromatic substances involved are short-chain volatile fatty acids.[3] In animal biology they are called copulins, because the presence or absence of these signals determines whether or not the female is sexually attractive to the male. Copulins are produced in the vaginal fluid from proteins, present because the cells of the vaginal wall, like the skin, are constantly being renewed. If you run the tip of your finger over the back of your hand on a hot day, you will pick up a small black roll of dead cells loosened from the substrate. In the vagina, the dead cells break away by themselves and their content becomes available for consumption by bacteria. The wall of the vagina always contains glycogen, the principal carbohydrate reserve. Glycogen is chiefly converted by lactobacilli, the main end products being lactic acid and acetic acid. These lactobacilli, called Döderlein's bacilli after their discoverer, may be considered the most useful commensal inhabitants of the vaginal passage, because their products provide the acid environment of the vagina, and fairly high acidity is an important defence mechanism against all sorts of less desirable bacilli. The lactobacilli themselves flourish at a low pH (that is, a high acidity level).

The vaginal secretion of some women has proved on closer examination to consist almost entirely of lactic and acetic acids, and their odour may be called neutral. In a third of the women, chemical analysis has also revealed the presence of the above-mentioned short-chain volatile fatty acids. In the literature, we speak of 'producers' and 'non-producers'. The fatty acids are the breakdown product of protein components in the dead cells of the wall. Proteins are first broken down into amino acids; this also occurs in the intestine before the proteins from our food can be absorbed. The amino acids are then used as food by another group of bacteria, which effect their conversion into fatty acids. This process also occurs in other parts of the body, for instance in the axillary sweat glands. Sweat only smells sweaty after bacterial conversion. An armpit after a hot bath smells of armpit and not of sweat, much as a fresh seafish does not smell of fish but of the sea. The special aromatic properties of volatile fatty acids are also of culinary importance. The taste of many cheeses is caused in part by roughly the same acids, produced by comparable bacteria. Germaine Greer is therefore right in her attempt to persuade women to take pride in their vaginal odours, on the grounds that many exquisite dishes have a similar taste and smell.

In women who do produce vaginal volatile fatty acids (that is, in the producers), attempts have been made to discover a possible cyclical effect. Such an effect has indeed been found, but only in women who are not on the pill. In a natural cycle, a woman gives off the strongest vaginal smell in the days between menstruation and ovulation, due, it is thought, to the hormonal condition of the vaginal wall. During the days before ovulation, the female cycle is dominated by oestrogenic hormones, and in the vaginal wall this means the storage of a great deal of glycogen. We may take it that during this period there is not only a large supply of food for lactic-acid bacteria, but that in any case there is an extra breakdown of cells, as a result of which the odour producers have more material to convert. With women who are on the pill, the percentage of producers is smaller, and no cycle has been detected (the studies from which this information has been distilled are more than twenty years old, and pill users then were taking higher dosages than women did during the 1990s).

Here we shall digress and take a brief look at the other sex. Among men, too, there are producers and non-producers. In uncircumcised men, the cells discarded from the glans and foreskin remain in a moist environment (the space between the glans and the foreskin) and are open to bacterial attack until the next wash. Circumcised men, by contrast, shed the dead cells into their underwear, and here other conditions prevail. Men who are circumcised later in life will always find that their sexual odours diminish; uncircumcised men who feel unhappy about their smell can do something about it by baring their glans as much and as often as possible.[4]

The research to which we have been referring has been based to a certain extent on chemical analyses, but an important part has always been based on the response of the nasal organ. The nose is highly adapted to telling producers from non-producers, and also to telling the difference before and after ovulation. In that respect man has no need to feel inferior to mammals whose sense of smell has a much better reputation. With a little training, it should be possible to detect the smells we are talking about more reliably. Thus research has shown that most experimental subjects can learn to tell the sex of the producer from the smell of his or her urine. Most people have never learned to do this, first because that ability does not seem to be of particular interest, and second because it is not really done to make a great point of studying the smell of other people's urine. We don't want to be like dogs – wagging our tails as we sniff around lamp-posts.

For human beings do indeed learn about animal responses to smells through living with animals. Many women (and men) have more than once noticed the effect of their smell during an unwelcome confrontation with a dog. The instinctive response with which dogs try to mount human legs is illustrative of the strength of the signals in reproductive behaviour. Biological research in this field is largely based on work with rhesus monkeys, and the substances under investigation were the same volatile fatty acids as are found in human producers. In female rhesus monkeys, the effect of oestrogenic hormones on the production of the attracting smells is quite obvious, as is the reaction of the males. The females get sniffed at and mounted repeatedly, which means that the greatest sexual activity takes place during the period when fertilization can take place. Synthetic short-chain fatty acids can be used to produce the same effects. In human beings, sexual behaviour is less directly governed by such primitive signals, but it would be interesting to discover whether producers arouse greater sexual interest than non-producers, and if this process is cyclical.

Pheromones and behaviour

Some readers will have wondered why the word pheromone has not come up in this book until now. Now and then we read intriguing reports about these biological lures in newspapers and journals. The oldest observation in this field dates back to the beginning of the twentieth century,[5] when the French entomologist Jean Henri Fabre came across a cocoon in a forest, took it back home and watched the cocoon burst into a beautiful female specimen of the emperor moth. He placed it in a cage, and next day he was astonished to find some forty males fluttering round the cage. Fabre tested the attractive power of the female by placing the cage under a glass bell, and discovered that this put an end to the visits.

Later on, research workers demonstrated that a volatile aromatic substance is involved, specific to this butterfly, and that a male can pick up the signal over a distance of three kilometres.

A fascinating new field had thus been opened up to research. The behavioural effect of this first pheromone to be discovered was clear: the enticement of the males had a reproductive motive. In bees, the queen produces a pheromone the moment she leaves the hive on her mating flight, when all the drones follow her and vie with one another for her favours. However, from the same gland the queen also produces a pheromone that suppresses the function of the ovaries of other female bees. This helps to maintain the social system in which just one female in the swarm sees to reproduction (this seems a very primitive form of cohabitation, confined to lower animal species such as insects, but the same social structure is found among marmosets, a genus of small South American monkey).[6] A third pheromone released by the queen bee helps the hive to tell their own tribe from strangers. The creature's behaviour – sexual responses, aggression, the search for food or danger warnings – is automatically controlled by these signals. Pheremones transform their subjects into robots.

Meanwhile all sorts of pheromone applications have found their way into stockbreeding. If a pig-farmer wants to know whether a sow is on heat he uses a spray. Pigs are employed to dig up truffles, and they are particularly good at this job because the smell of truffles strongly resembles their mating pheromone. No wonder then that truffles are sold as aphrodisiacs. There is a Californian spider that has developed into a specialist on imitation insect pheromones. This spider can produce sixteen smells indistinguishable from the real thing to perfume its web with, thus determining what food it gets that day. You may wonder whether this refined power to choose one's menu from Mother Nature's rich store also has repercussions on the character of these spiders. They may well turn out to be insufferably spoilt creatures.

Plants, too, lure insects with imitation pheromones. The bee orchid emits a pheromone for the distributor of its pollen, and externally, too, its flower resembles a willing female, with whom the drone copulates with the same intensity that he would bestow on a female congener. Similarly, artificial insemination centres have no difficulty in getting bulls to mount a wooden railing covered with cowhide.

The pheromone system of behavioural control is part of the most primitive section of the brain, the paleoencephelon, also known as the reptilian brain. A snake is sinister not least because we do not know why it keeps flicking its forked tongue. It was recently shown that these movements of the tongue help to fan the tip of the snout, the seat of the pheromone receptor organ. The latter is completely independent of the olfactory organ and is known as the vomeronasal organ (VNO). We have known for a few years that human beings, too, have such an organ.[7] Two centimetres inside the nasal passage, low against the nasal septum, the ear, nose and throat (ENT) specialist will sometimes see a little red split, the beginning of a funnel-shaped sac about one centimetre in length. This organ is present in all human beings, but many people have variations in the shape of the cartilage sections of the nasal septum, in which case the organ may be camouflaged. Microscopic examination will reveal the presence of a structure similar to that of the olfactory organ (which lies much deeper and higher in the nasal cavity): cells covered with very fine hairs which convert contact with volatile substances into nerve signals, and nerve fibres conducting these signals to the brain.

The vomeronasal organ is still little known, but it will not take long (and will undoubtedly start in the United States) before claims for damages are served on ENT practitioners for destroying the VNO during operations on a deviated nasal septum. These practitioners will have to take the necessary steps to protect themselves. In the information leaflets handed out in preparation for the operation, mention will have to be made of possible damage to the organ and what consequences may be expected.

Recently there has been research involving the inhalation of specific synthetic pheromones while electrical signals (nerve pulses) from the nerve fibre are recorded.[8] It would appear that the VNO is capable of detecting volatile substances which elude the normal olfactory organ, but does not react to some very strong smells. The classical example of such a smell is oil of cloves, which is generally used as a temporary cure for toothache. We must therefore get used to the idea that our behaviour can be influenced by volatile substances that we are unable to detect consciously; by no means all enticing substances are smells. Hence it is best not to refer to the VNO as a sense organ, since sense organs convey signals from the outside world to our consciousness via the senses. The earliest research into synthetic pheromones has yielded another striking result: women react strongly to ER-670, which does not affect men; conversely men react strongly to ER-830, which leaves women unmoved.

This is a remarkable fact, because there are no other organs with this type of selective reaction. If men and women have the same organ, that organ will react identically to say, hormonal stimuli. Men are in theory capable of developing a mammary gland, but throughout their lives that growth potential is never brought into play. To make it happen, high blood levels of female sex hormones are needed, and even girls do not develop these until just after puberty. If men are given high doses of synthetic oestrogen they can quickly catch up to a certain point, as we know from the hormone treatment of male-to-female transsexuals

The pheromone system thus has specific properties. But how are we to fit the function of that system into biology in general? If we look upon an ant colony as a single entity, a single body, then pheromones can be considered as a system of stimulus transmitters from one ant to the next. The first name given to these substances reflected that idea: they were called 'ectohormones' (external hormones). In the body of the individual animal, the transmission of stimuli is effected for the most part through the nervous system and in addition through (endo)hormones – substances formed in some parts of the body and then moved (mostly via the bloodstream) to affect other parts. The various organs keep the organism alive through this collaboration; ectohormones ensure that the individual members of a colony collaborate properly, the better to maintain the social whole and to propagate their kind.

Research into pheromones has naturally been done more intensively on animals than on human beings – their effects on everyday human behaviour is by no means certain. Needless to say, the commercial possibilities of substances that one sex can use to make the other sex more sexually responsive are vast, something that has been known for a long time. Shakespeare's contemporaries spoke of love apples, peeled apples that a woman carried in her armpits for some time before serving them up to the man of her choice.[9] Nowadays men in Greece and the Balkans apparently keep their handkerchief under their armpit during celebrations, then flaunt it invitingly during the dancing so that their pheromones cannot escape the nostrils of their beloved. Folklore is rich in recipes for love potions, and sweat, urine, vaginal secretions and menstrual blood are usually mentioned in these as ingredients.

The main aromatic signals on which this lovers' art relies are, however, drawn from the large arsenal of male sex hormones, which men naturally produce in greater abundance than women. In women, the effects are spectacular, the oldest and best-known example of this transmission of signals being the synchronization of the menstrual cycles of women who have lived together for a long time. This phenomenon, incidentally, is less simple than is generally believed. Among lesbian couples for instance, it seems that 50 per cent menstruate synchronously, but 30 per cent are completely asynchronous. That, too, cannot be an accident.[10] The woman who initiated the research into the pheromonal causes of this phenomenon was called Geneviève; she too was struck by the fact that the women with whom she was in close contact all eventually fell in with her menstrual rhythm. She accordingly designed the following experiment with a colleague: three times a week Geneviève held eight sterile cotton buds in her armpit for a while, and then a cotton bud was brushed across the upper lip of each of eight female volunteers. After four months the dates of the first day of menstruation had drawn significantly closer. An observation that also arises from the same initial period of pheromone research is that, on average, women who have little contact with men have more irregular and slower menstrual cycles than women exposed to the (pheromonal) influence of men. This effect, too, can be transmitted by using cotton buds kept in men's armpits. In men, the lack of female company leads to diminished beard growth.[11]

It is still far from clear what substances have which pheromonal effect on men and women. In any case, they are often the by-products of decomposed male sex hormones. Some of the effective substances (the one most frequently used in experiments is androstenole) have an odour, and that odour is often related to the erotic fragrances commonly used in perfumes of musk and castor oil. It can be said of all sexually stimulating ingredients found in perfumes that the smell is considered repulsive if it is found in high concentrations, but that a small whiff has an erotic effect. Natural musk is obtained from a gland in the abdomen of the musk deer found high in the Himalayas and the Atlas mountains. Some active pheromones smell slightly of urine; of these, androstenone is the one used most frequently for experimental purposes. The kind of experiment carried out using musk and castor oil often has a somewhat domestic air. In a waiting room a chair that has been sprayed with androstenone (urine smell) is avoided by men but preferred by women. In a telephone booth sprayed with androstenole (musk) both men and women tend to have conversations that are longer than usual.

When male experimental subjects are asked to judge the beauty of women on photographs, a whiff of androstenone helps to raise the score. When judging men in the flesh a whiff of androstenole causes women to raise their score and men to lower theirs. This investigation thus bears on a substance that human beings can smell in principle, but which is proffered in doses that do not cross the observation threshold. We cannot tell if the signal is nevertheless transmitted over the normal olfactory system, or via the vomeronasal system. It is a fascinating thought that there may well be human pheromones that cannot be smelled, no matter what the dose, and that can only reach our consciousness through the behaviour they elicit.

We find many examples of inexplicable influences in novels. Thus in Herbjørg Wassmo's *Dina's Book* (1996) the reader is taken to a church on the Norwegian coast on Christmas Day. After the service, the heroine meets her lover in the organ loft and they make passionate love. When they later join the company in the parsonage for the coffee hour, the atmosphere is changed. Everyone is in a special mood, thanks to a 'smell of earth and salty sea winds'.

> But it was present. It affected appetites. Interrupted conversations unexpectedly, as words stopped for a moment and gazes became blissfully distant. Was a stimulating balm that gently dissolved toward the end of the coffee hour. Only to reappear again in memories, long afterward. As people wondered what had created the marvelously good atmosphere at the parsonage on Christmas Day.

The most 'pheromonal' novel is of course Patrick Süskind's *Perfume* (1985). At the end of the book, the brilliant perfumer returns to the surroundings from which he has sprung: the dregs of society sitting round a small fire amidst filth, stench and depravity. When he sprinkles himself with his ultimate perfume, he becomes an angel in everyone's eyes. They all want to be near him, to touch him and possess him, and in a savage orgy he is torn to pieces and devoured. After a few minutes, when nothing is left of him, those present calm down and are filled with great peace of mind. Each of them seems to realize that they have jointly, perhaps for the first time in their lives, done something good, something to which they were driven by love, and love only.

Anyone wanting to use pheromones to attract a sexual partner can obtain them from a sex shop or by mail order, but it is doubtful if the products are subjected to any form of quality control. The serious pharmaceutical industry is of course interested in the commercial exploitation of this new class of drugs, which entails, among other things, a certain amount of trade secrecy. We read that ER-830 works with men and ER-670 with women, but the industry refrains from committing itself on the possible applications of these substances. In a TV documentary about pheromones broadcast in April 1999 it emerged that the Organon company is working on a pheromone that may help to reduce premenstrual tension. The influence of pheromones on the menstrual cycle may well be used to overcome fertility problems in women with an irregular menstrual cycle, and may also be used in a birth-control spray. Volatile substances may even influence the course of a pregnancy. Current research among beauty specialists has shown that women who work a great deal with volatile substances have pregnancies that end more often than usual in miscarriages.[12]

chapter thirteen

Fear and Loathing of Femininity

'Hello, Hans. Do you remember me?' I said, holding out my hand.
He took a step back with a start, as if I had the plague.
'I don't shake hands,' he said. 'Not with women.'
He launched into a long-winded explanation of why he, as an
orthodox Jew, was not allowed to touch me. Triumph shone in his eyes.
I knew that his outrage was feigned. Before me, some twenty other
women had gone up to him with an outstretched hand, and each time he
had enacted the same comedy. He had recoiled from each one and then
inflicted paragraphs from the Talmud and the Torah on each one for
minutes at a time. I had no patience with any of that. While he was still
in full flow, I firmly turned my back on him.[1]

The narrator of the story 'Holy Fire' by Carl Friedman portrays the
development of an inadequate, not very bright Jewish boy into a
religious fanatic who ends up in an Israeli cell after the religiously
inspired murder of a Palestinian youth. His refusal to touch women
fits into the orthodox Jewish tradition, in which the correct handling
of taboos is an important intellectual pursuit. Outsiders are more
familiar with the Jewish dietary laws, the ban on pork and shellfish,
and the strict separation of meat and milk. Less well known is the fact
that Jewish scholars have devoted millions of words over the past two
thousand years to the taboo surrounding a host of aspects of femininity. How is the God-fearing Talmudist to discern a menstruating
woman, and how can he avoid her until she is pure again?

Women themselves have grave responsibilities in this matter, for if
they touch their husbands during their impure days, or hand them
anything, then their husbands, too, become impure.[2] In any case, it
is the women who have the task of ensuring that the religious duties
are scrupulously observed by the entire family. Twelve hours before
menstruation is expected to start, the wife must cease having sexual

intercourse with her husband, and on the presumed last day of menstruation she must perform an internal examination before sunset to make certain that she has stopped bleeding. She must continue to do this twice a day for seven days, using special cloths. There are strict rules concerning what to do about which sorts of spots of blood. In the worst case, the count has to be started all over again. Some women with a short cycle have finished ovulating before they are pure again. Jewish scholars call these women *akarut hilchatit*, infertile according to the *halacha*, the Jewish religious law.[3] Twelve days' abstinence is thus the absolute minimum. And that means not touching each other, and for some not sharing the same bed. Next comes a thorough ablution of the entire body, followed by a ritual immersion accompanied by the appropriate prayers.

The Jewish religion treats female (menstrual) blood differently from male (circumcision) blood.[4] Menstrual blood is deplored; circumcision blood is glorified. The latter is collected in perfumed water, and all the guests wash their hands in the mixture, thus confirming the covenant between God and Abraham. Incidentally, *Al-Qanun fi al-Tibb* (The Canon of Medicine), Avicenna's main work, contains a curious passage in which this Arab scholar attaches different values to male and female urine.[5] The jet of urine from a male is far more sparkling and golden. This is due to the fact that female urine is mixed with vaginal fluids, as well as to the greater width of the female urethra, but Avicenna believed that the differences also reflected an essential qualitative difference, brought about, according to him, by the inquisitiveness of women.

On the Polynesian islands contact between men and women was strictly regulated.[6] There was an isolated menstruation hut to which the women also went to give birth. If a man had contact with a woman while she was menstruating, he could be sentenced to death. Polynesian society used to be so complex that only the richest islanders could afford to observe all the prevailing taboos. In any case, men and women used to cook and eat in separate eating-houses.

Girls had to be taught very early on how to handle their malign powers, something that could prove to be very traumatic. Thus most American Indians tribes had an isolation ritual.[7] Mountain Wolf Woman of the Winnebago was told by her mother that at the first sign of blood she had to hide in the forest. She was not to look at anyone under any circumstances, for the glance of a menstruating woman tainted the blood of the other. When her time came, she did as her mother had told her, but was of course frightened about being left alone in the snow at that moment. Luckily her sister followed her trail, and together they lit a fire and built a wigwam. There she sat for another four days all by herself, cold and hungry, for she had been ordered to fast as well. And she was disgusted with herself, without knowing why. The Old Testament states clearly what this is all about:

> And if a man shall lie with a woman having her sickness, and shall uncover her nakedness; he hath discovered her fountain, and she hath uncovered the fountain of her blood: and both of them shall be cut off from among their people.[8]

Likewise, if a woman continues to lose blood after being confined, sexual congress with her is not allowed, and as mentioned earlier, Pope Gregory extended this prohibition to the breastfeeding period. It was believed that the eye of a menstruating woman emitted evil vapours. In his *De secretis mulierum*, Albertus Magnus describes the eye as a passive organ in which the menstrual fluid can be concentrated, and from which contamination can be spread.[9] If a menstruating woman looks in a mirror, she may well feel pain in her eye, and sometimes a stain will be left on the mirror. It is essential that the female poison be given the monthly opportunity of being drained off. After the menopause, when the evil juices can no longer be dissipated, women are far more poisonous than they were during their fertile years. Because of this belief, older women were the victims of choice in witch-hunts. References to the Fall of Man and the dubious role Eve played in it were common; thus, if a pubic hair from a menstruating woman is placed inside a dung heap, then the heat of the sun will help to turn that hair into a snake.

In the twentieth and twenty-first centuries, there were and still are countless taboos that interfere with women performing various household chores.[10] In Provence, menstruating women are excluded from wine cellars while the wine is fermenting. Milk is said to turn sour and mayonnaise to curdle in the presence of menstruating women; even salt meat can spoil, as can everything that is preserved, bottled or pickled. At the end of the 1960s, many French women gave affirmative answers to questions about menstruation taboos put to them by the ethnographer Yvonne Verdier. In North America, camping out in grizzly bear territory is popular, but menstruating women are warned to be on their guard because grizzlies have a keen nose for menstrual blood.[11] In 1999, a hairdresser made the newspapers with his decision to employ male stylists only in his salon, because women invariably produce inferior work during 'those days'. Recently a friend told me about a café conversation he had overheard in which a greengrocer who still preserved beans every year in the traditional way complained about the failure of his entire crop the previous year. Nothing like that had ever happened to him before, and after long reflection he had hit upon the only possible explanation: he had taken on a woman to help him and she must have been menstruating at the time.

> I can't sleep with you. Why are you so insistent?
>
> I want to sleep with you when you menstruate. It is as if part of me then passes into you and your blood is my own, pouring from a vein that belongs to us both. What do you feel?
>
> I feel the blood defiling both our bodies as if your hardness had made me bleed, as if you had stripped off my skin, had devoured me, leaving me all dried up.[12]

Jerzy Kosinski cites the ultimate taboo: sex with a menstruating woman. There are still many men and women who avoid sex during menstruation, sometimes giving hygienic and practical reasons. Some women certainly consider this taboo frustrating, because the period just before and during menstruation is often when their spontaneous desire is at its height. Kinsey was able as early as 1953 to allude to fourteen published works demonstrating that women are sexually most active in the days round their menstruation.[13] Among the women Kinsey interviewed himself were several who masturbated just once a month, and that was often during menstruation.

The narrator in Kosinski's novel shares a desire with the current Prince of Wales, who, in a much-quoted tapped telephone conversation with Camilla Parker Bowles, confessed that he would love to be her tampon. Anne Vegter, best known as a writer of children's books, also wrote a collection of erotic stories, *Unexpurgated Versions*, in 1995, in which she firmly shed one taboo after another. Her narrator in the story 'Judas's Whispers' builds up erotic tension with her lover Judas to an unbearable pitch by describing to him what has happened at the office that day. These events have been indeed shockingly perverse: the entire female staff dealt out severe punishment to the only male present, Mr Van Niks, whose behaviour in the ladies' room has outraged them. It was his habit to visit the women's cloakroom to 'score' used sanitary towels and tampons, which he then hoarded in a drawer of his desk. Judas and the narrator jointly ensure that this story and their lovemaking are subtly intertwined, and menstruation constitutes an important element of their erotic arousal:

> You put an index finger in your cunt, dig about and feel around, pull your finger back out and then hold the result under your nose. You sniff deeply. You push the finger back in again, repeat the process and give a satisfied nod.

'My period.'

Judas nods, but guardedly. He kneels down in front of you and places his hands on the inside of your thighs. He parts your legs, A sluggish syrup of blood oozes from your cunt and seeps down the perineum towards your back

'My God,' Judas swears reverently.

He creeps closer to you. He follows the red track running between your legs with his eyes, follows with his hands, follows with his tongue.

Judas finds it easy to identify with the abject office colleague:

> He wanted you; of course he did. Who wouldn't, what man wouldn't? God damn it, it's intolerable that you discard that blood, that power, like some sort of disgrace, chuck away that living power . . . Van Niks, my son, I'm with you! I'd like to wallow in that blood too, become as one with the excrement of that fertile body. To be smeared with that smell, the colour of the creative force, oh, Van Niks, I'm with you all the way!

Sex during menstruation is certainly charged with excitement, but oral sex at that time puts many people off completely. Lesbian slang (which, as mentioned earlier, is not averse to calling a spade a spade) includes the terms 'strawberry sex', and 'eating red cabbage' for the oral variety.[14] A book by the criminologist Henk Hagen about (among other things) the meaning of the symbols on Hell's Angels' leather jackets explains that anyone with a black 'wing' has had oral sex with a black woman in the presence of witnesses. If the wing is red and black then the woman was menstruating.

It is quite possible to tell a far more positive story about menstruation. Racing cyclist Leontien van Moorsel waited until she was menstruating to make her second attempt on the world one-hour record because her tolerance of pain and her self-confidence were extremely high at that time. She did indeed break the old record. Penelope Shuttle and Peter Redgrove have listed positive aspects of menstruation in their 1978 study *The Wise Wound*. Their approach leans heavily on Jung's writings, that is, on a cultural heritage handed down in myths, legends and proverbs, and in these the menses are readily interpreted as the time when a woman is closest to her divine core. The Mother Goddess, too, has her menses. Esther Harding has compiled a list of feminine mysteries, and has reported how, in India, the statues of the Mother Goddess were regularly separated from the other images, bloodstained clothes being displayed later as signs of her menstrual period.[15] The clothes, moreover, were highly prized for their curative properties. In Babylon, the moon goddess Ishtar used to menstruate at the full moon. The full moon was Ishtar's day of rest: she neither waxed nor waned; she had her *sabbatu*, the etymological meaning of which is 'heart's rest'. On the other hand, the Sabbath was considered to be an evil and dangerous day. Misfortune lay in wait, so no work or travelling was advisable, and there was also a strong taboo on eating cooked food ('touched by fire'). 'The king shall not ride in his chariot. He shall not sit in judgment. The priest shall not dispense oracles. The healer shall not lay his hands on the sick.' Originally, there used to be one *sabbatu* a month, but later every quarter of the month became a Sabbath. The Jews adopted that custom, and the Christian Sunday can also be traced back to Ishtar's menstruation.

Why do women feel depressed when they menstruate, even though there is so much that is positive about the experience? It seems obvious that such feelings should be seen as a reaction, the reverse of the rage that arises from the frustration they suffer at being forced to suppress their feelings at their most libidinous moments under pressure from men. Shuttle and Redgrove give numerous examples of men begrudging women their special, and above all their spiritual, role in the world. Vegter's Judas was at least aware of his aversion.

Even if one does not accept the Jungian interpretations, one cannot deny that quite a few men feel uncomfortable about this aspect of femininity. Alexandre Dumas tells us about his *Dame aux camélias* that she wore a white rose in her hair for twenty-five days of the month, and a red rose for five. 'No one ever knew the reason for this change of colour, which I simply mention here without being able to explain it.' As for Alex Portnoy:

> It was years later that she called from the bathroom, Run to the drug-store! bring a box of Kotex! immediately! . . . Though her menstrual troubles eventually had to be resolved by surgery, it is difficult never-theless to forgive her for having sent me on that mission of mercy. Better she should have bled herself out on our cold bathroom floor, better *that*, than to have sent an eleven-year-old boy in hot pursuit of sanitary napkins! Where was my sister, for Christ's sake? Where was her own emergency supply?[16]

What is so terrible about confronting a boy with one of the female functions? Why are boys and men not allowed to know that women bleed once a month? The psychoanalytical explanation has many advocates. Little boys can only make sense of their observations of the difference between the sexes by believing that little girls have been stripped of their willies. Such an event must have been horrifying, with a huge loss of blood, and menstruation is the monthly reminder of this mythical drama. The more often men are confronted with menstruation, the greater is their fear of losing their manhood. That leads to all sorts of denigrating, fear-averting names for menstruation, and many jokes are made on the subject. Shuttle and Redgrove give this example:

> A shopkeeper has just engaged a new super-salesman, and is watching his technique. He is amazed to see his new employee sell an entire fishing-kit, waders, hunting-clothes, an outdoor barbecue, a new car, a small aeroplane and a country house to a customer who had simply asked about a fishing-rod on display. 'How do you do it?' asked the amazed shopkeeper. 'Oh, I knew he was a pushover. He didn't even want the fishing-rod. He had just come in to buy a box of sanitary towels for his wife'.

Male ambivalence towards the vagina is reflected in a whole range of emotionally charged ways. Bawdiness is one of them. In 23 letters to Frits van Egters, written in 1997, Thom Hoffman describes his emotions during and after the filming of *The Evenings*, based on the book by Gerard Reve. Hoffman was cast for the 'society scene', a drunken and licentious affair on the day after Christmas. The actors having been rehearsed at length by the director Rudolf van den Berg, and knowing exactly what they needed to do to get the idle chatter about ill health and baldness on film, nevertheless found that the spark was missing because of too much idle time on the set. A private joke was needed to bring out the underlying bawdiness, and the female genitals were naturally the choice to inspire the fit of adolescent giggles. If you should see the film, you will know how the actors managed to be helpless with laughter throughout the scene:

> As Gijs I declaimed on the question of galloping consumption I concentrated on the cunts of first one woman, then another, and as Gijs II discoursed on whooping cough, I pictured this or that bovine vagina. My fellow actors, I realized, were certainly visualizing other tremulous cunts as it was my turn to hold forth on the mystery of baldness and they looked at me with the question in their eyes: 'Whose quivering labia is Hoffmann fantasizing about?' Broad grins were quick to break out and we couldn't help bursting into laughter.

Humour and bawdiness are relatively innocent forms of misogyny, but fear and loathing can assume far more disturbing forms. The dangers the female organ symbolizes are not negligible. The White Knife clan of the Shoshone American Indian tribe believed that a glimpse of the female genitals would result in blindness and disease.[17] For that reason, women's skirts were made of strips; if they should unthinkingly sit down with their legs too wide apart (which they were not meant to do) then a strip would fall over their crotch. If a woman was slovenly about the way she sat down, then it was her brother's duty to reprimand her. He could admonish her, for instance, by throwing a burning piece of wood between her legs.

In some cultures, women can make use of the prevailing repugnance and display their vaginas provocatively to frighten an attacker or to show him their contempt. The vagina has something in common with the head of Medusa – all those who looked at her were turned to stone. It does not take much imagination to think of pubic hair when looking at the snakes that served Medusa as a headdress. And conversely, as we know, the pubic hair of a menstruating woman can turn into a snake.

Monique Wittig's female guerrilla fighters, too, behave like Medusa:

> They say that they bare their genitals so that the sun may be reflected in them as by a mirror. They say that they preserve their brilliance. They say that their pubic hair resembles a spider's web catching the rays. You can see them running by taking big leaps. They are in their centre, beginning at the mons veneris, the encased clitoris, the twice-folded lips, all illuminated. The brilliance that radiates from them when they stop and bend forward causes the eye to be averted, for it cannot bear the sight.[18]

With Polynesians it was generally true to say that everything that was good was male, and everything that was bad was female.[19] The vagina was the seat of the greatest danger. Its negative force was called 'mana'. Polynesian women of the old school would never sit on a chair, for fear a small boy might crawl under it. Women's houses were never built on piles for the same reason, but always on solid platforms. The negative force could sometimes be used for positive ends: if a man had a stomach ache, a woman could try to expel the evil force by sitting on his abdomen.

Christianity has a long anti-sexual tradition. St Odo of Cluny coined the immortal dictum *inter faeces et urinam nascitur* – we are born between faeces and urine. The vagina is seen as the devil's stigma. Thus an itinerant preacher in Idaho is said to have begun a sermon in 1920 with a request to all women to cross their legs. After some shuffling of feet, he continued, 'All right folks, now that the gates of Hell are closed, I can begin my sermon.' The satanic associations attaching to the vagina can also be found in the legend of Pandora's box, from which all the ills in the world have sprung.

Anyone tempted to enter a vagina should be aware that great dangers lie in wait for him. Kubin has given us splendid illustrations of the fear of being swallowed up or being caught in a spider's web. A great deal of misogynist humour hinges round the inexhaustible span of the vagina:

A farmer took his daughter to the cattle market, where he did good business. Satisfied, the two of them were riding back home but – oh, horror! – two heavily armed highwaymen fell upon them. They were looted of everything they had and after a few frightening minutes the dismayed farmer and his daughter watched the robbers make off with their horse and cart. When the highwaymen were at a safe distance, the daughter blushingly confessed that, while she had been unobserved for a moment, she had stowed away all the money they had earned selling the cattle inside her vagina. The blow was thus not as great as the farmer had first feared. 'Pity your mother wasn't with us,' he sighed. 'We'd have been able to keep the horse and cart then as well.'

Women do, of course, sometimes use their vaginas as a hiding place, and prison and customs officers are fully aware of this. How much heroin and cocaine has not been smuggled inside a woman's vagina? *The Illustrated Book of Sexual Records* quotes from *My Secret Life*, the famous picaresque Victorian novel by 'Walter', who describes an exuberant night in a brothel where two women are exhorted to hide as many shillings as possible in their vaginas. The winner comes away with 84 shillings, and when she stands up not a single shilling falls out.[20]

The biggest vagina was created by a woman sculptor. Niki de Saint Phalle called her work *Hon* (the Swedish pronoun 'she'), and *Hon*'s vagina is large enough to accommodate at least ten spectators.

Penis captivus: like dogs

Some male fears have to do with being swallowed up, with man's inability to make any impression on so voluminous an organ. On the other hand, there is also the fear of penis captivus, of a vagina clamped so tightly round the swollen male organ that man and woman cannot separate after coitus. That situation has been the subject of many horror stories told in bars the world over, no doubt in part because our best loved pet, the dog, is quite often found in this compromising situation. In 1992, Midas Dekker, the author of *Dearest Pet*, explained that this locking together is attributed to the joint action of an erectile body at the base of the dog's penis and the reflex contraction of the bitch's sphincter muscles. After ejaculation, the dog remains inside the bitch for a while to add extra prostatic fluid, which increases the likelihood of fertilization. Dekker's book is about sex between humans and animals, and he believes that the human vagina is unlikely to contract to the point of refusing to let go. This comic drama between dogs does, however, make a scene of the same kind between a man and a woman conceivable. In cases where both male and female partners are of the human race, this problem has naturally been examined in the medical literature, but reports are few and far between and generally second-hand. A notorious case history published in 1884 includes this account:

> I was sent for, about 11 p.m., by a gentleman whom, on my arriving at his house, I found in a state of great perturbation, and the story he told me was briefly as follows:
>
> At bedtime, when going to the back kitchen to see if the house was shut up, a noise in the coachman's room attracted his attention, and, going in, he discovered to his horror that the man was in bed with one of the maids. She screamed, he struggled, and they rolled out of the bed together and made frantic efforts to get apart, but

without success. He was a big, burly man, over six feet, and she was a small woman, weighing no more than ninety pounds. She was moaning and screaming, and seemed in great agony, so that, after several fruitless attempts to get them apart, he sent for me. When I arrived I found the man standing up and supporting the woman in his arms, and it was quite evident that his penis was tightly locked in her vagina, and any attempt to dislodge it was accompanied by much pain on the part of both. It was indeed a case of 'de cohesione in coitu'. I applied water, and then ice, but ineffectually, and at last sent for chloroform, a few whiffs of which sent the woman to sleep, relaxed the spasm, and relieved the captive penis which was swollen, livid, and in a state of semi-erection, which did not go down for several hours, and for days the organ was extremely sore.

The author signed his report as Egerton Y. Davis; in the 1880s quite a few readers no doubt recognized this name as the pseudonym of Sir William Osler, a Canadian with a widespread reputation for practical jokes.[21] Those in the know also realized that the Y in the name stood for Yorick, the jester with whose skull Hamlet is so often depicted. This case history has often been quoted as a serious happening in later texts. The dramatic tone is encountered again in the rare subsequent examples. Thus we are told that, in Warsaw, a student couple was caught locked together in the university gardens and exposed in the press, which drove them to commit suicide; in Bremen, a dockworker was found locked inside a woman in a remote corner of the shipyard and surrounded by a crowd of fellow dockers, before the couple were carried off to a hospital.[22] Chloroform was invariably the miracle cure bringing relief. The very few reports that make a slightly more reliable impression are less dramatic, involve domestic sex, and end after a relatively short period of time without medical intervention. In about 1980, there was a keen discussion of the subject in the medical literature, but after 1982 the matter was no longer seriously broached. The last case mentioned dates back to 1947, took place in the Isle of Wight, and concerned a newly married couple.[23]

But however rare such cases may have been, fear of their recurrence is centuries old. In the second half of the thirteenth century warnings on the subject were rife, all stressing that unchecked sexuality could lead to public disgrace, for man and woman alike, and also for a society not strict enough in watching over sexual mores. In the Chevalier de la Tour Landry's book of instructions for his daughters [24] this type of hilarious scene was even repeated twice, no doubt because of the great importance the Chevalier attached to it. In this anecdote,[25] God's anger was aroused by a sergeant who had the effrontery to seduce his sweetheart in church. According to the Middle English translation by Caxton in 1484:

> And thei might never parte, but were fast like a dogge and a biche togedre, that night and the morw all day until the tyme that the pepill yode a procession for them to pray to God and that orrible sight might be ended and hidde and atte the last . . . And they that dede the dede were ioyned to penaince to go naked afore the procession thre sundayes beting them self and recording their synne tofore the pepill.

And the Chevalier's young daughters took note and became very pious.

There is a literary passage in which being stuck together is treated as highly desirable and healing, namely no. 14 in Robert Biggs's book ŠÀ.ZI.GA, a series of incantations circulating in Mesopotamia from the 14th century BC onwards. These incantations are sometimes combined with recipes for magical cures, and are obviously recited by women anxious to help men to an erection:

> INCANTATION.
> Let the wind blow! Let the mountains quake! . . .
> At the head of my bed is tied a buck!
> At the foot of my bed is tied a ram!
> The one at the head of my bed, get an erection, make love
>   to me!
> The one at the foot of my bed, get an erection, make love
>   to me!
> My vagina is the vagina of a bitch! His penis is the penis
>   of a dog!
> As the vagina of a bitch holds fast the penis of a dog
>   (so may my vagina hold fast his penis)!

The recipe to be administered after this incantation consisted of ground magnetic iron ore and *puru* oil.

Vagina dentata

In the Middle Ages powerful men were obsessed with the fear of being poisoned, and it was known quite early on that immunity from all sorts of poisons could be acquired by swallowing ever stronger doses of them every day.[26] As for women, it was believed that every month they built up their tolerance of the poison their menstruation released, so much so that after the menopause their immunity no less than their toxicity was at its most powerful. It was on the basis of this belief that the legend of the poisonous maiden first arose. When Alexander the Great extended his power over large territories at an early age, one king felt particularly threatened by him and decided to take what protective measures he could. He fed poison to a young girl and when she was saturated with it, sent her to Alexander as a present. She was graceful, played the harp beautifully, and Alexander was sorely tempted to embrace her:

> But Aristotle, a servant at court, and his master Socrates, discovered the poison in the girl, and prevented Alexander from touching her. And when they explained things to him, he refused to believe them, but he was afraid of Socrates, his teacher, and did not dare to contradict him. Then Socrates had two slaves brought in and bid one of them to embrace the girl; he dropped dead on the spot; he bid the second slave to do likewise and he too died in the same manner, so that Alexander realized that his teacher had told him the whole truth. But Socrates did not leave it there; he had her touch animals, dogs and horses, and they all dropped dead.

This version comes from the *Dialogues of Placidus and Timaeus*, a popularization of the thoughts of the great churchmen and philosophers of the day. The author obviously knew that Alexander had been taught by Aristotle, but he failed to realize that Socrates was no longer alive when Aristotle was born (Socrates was Plato's teacher, and Plato was Aristotle's).

In the 'vagina dentata' myth, fear of female sexuality is linked directly to a woman's genital organs. This myth exists in many cultures and is therefore frequently used by anthropologists wishing to illustrate the common cultural roots – the collective unconscious – of mankind.[27] An example from the legends of the Wichita Indians, reported by H. R. Hays, tells how the folk hero Son of a Dog was able to avert the danger.[28] On his travels he met the witches Little Spider Woman and Buzzard Woman. Little Spider Woman invited him home, and offered him both her daughters as wives. Buzzard Woman, who was a good witch, privately warned him about the two daughters. They had teeth in their vaginas, and their virginity would cost him his manhood: 'When you lie with them you must not have intercourse even though they try to persuade you. You will hear the gnashing of the teeth in their vaginas.' Son of a Dog was also warned not to fall asleep, and he resolved to follow Buzzard Woman's advice. Lying between the two charming daughters he pretended to be fast asleep and even though Little Spider Woman made a final attempt to smash his skull, he found a way to elude her. Next day Son of a Dog had a secret meeting with Buzzard Woman, who gave him two long whetstones. He was advised to pick the girl he found most attractive and to render her harmless by grinding off her vaginal teeth with one of the whetstones. He should kill the other girl by thrusting the second whetstone up her vagina instead of his penis. Buzzard Woman also gave him a charm to put the evil witch to sleep.

No sooner said than done. One sister did not survive the stony penetration, and the other was indeed fit for sexual intercourse after having been treated with the whetstone. They fled, hotly pursued by Little Spider Woman. Buzzard Woman completed her good work by carrying Spider Woman high up in the sky and then dropping her to her death. So Son of a Dog kept his penis and could use it to exercise his male prerogatives.

A Japanese version starts like the apocryphal story of Tobias and Sarah: a princess has spent a number of wedding nights with bridegroom after bridegroom, consummation being invariably followed by the intrusion of a devil into the bedroom and by his devouring of the bridegroom's genitals. After her father's desperate appeal, a smith sues for her hand. He forges an iron penis on which the devil breaks his teeth.

In life-threatening situations such as wars, disguised castration fears often revolve round enemy women. Thus American soldiers in Germany told stories about German prostitutes with razors in their vaginas, bent on destroying them. The same story was told during the Vietnam War. A psychiatrist, Benjamin Beit-Hallahmi, heard a similar story from a man who had throttled a woman and then mutilated her vagina with a knife before possessing her corpse.[29] During his military service he had twice been picked up by local women in the country to which he had been posted, and where he felt in mortal danger. The personal translation of that danger, namely that female genitals posed a threat to his male organ, can be interpreted as doubt in his own virility.

In 1977, Kate Millett wrote an autobiographical book about her love of Sita. The first time the two of them made love, Sita warned Kate to be careful: once when her car had broken down in the middle of a desert, she had been raped by six men and then cut with a knife. Her clitoris still showed how she had been mutilated.

The vagina arouses far more destructive fear than the penis, when in fact many more women have been injured by penises than men have been hurt by vaginas. In real life, very few penises are cut off, and when it happens it becomes world news. Lorena Bobbitt made the front pages all over the world when she emasculated her husband, who had raped her on many occasions in a drunken stupor.[30] He got away with it fairly well: his penis was successfully reattached to his body and less than a year later the blue film *John Wayne Bobbit Uncut* was screened. His ex-wife did not receive a custodial sentence, the efforts of a feminist support group perhaps playing a part in this. They had threatened that if Lorena were sent to jail hundreds of American men would be castrated.

A Czech woman veterinary surgeon who was raped by two men was able to fool them into thinking that she liked what they had done to her, got them drunk and then castrated both of them. This story too circulated all over the world, and gave rise to a poster with the legend 'Don't rape a woman, she could be a vet'.

Mady Sacks was doubtless inspired by this story when she wrote the scenario for the film *Iris* in 1987. Monique van de Ven plays the eponymous heroine, a capable and devoted veterinary surgeon who has to fight for her right to work in what hostile villagers believe is a male preserve. There follows a series of mind-numbing ordeals, the last of which is a savage rape. When she is sure who is responsible (he turns out to be her extremely unpleasant fiancé, who wants her to return to the big city), she prepares to knock him out with chloroform and to do to him what we have seen her do earlier to male piglets. She has already picked up the scalpel when her conscience gets the better of her, and the last scene of the film is the life-affirming assisted delivery of a calf.

There have certainly been a number of other cases of women damaging a penis, but these are disproportionately few when compared with the number of aggressive acts against the vagina. To put it even more strongly: it is absolutely certain that most mutilations of male genitals have been performed by men, by which we mean war crimes. Psychiatric literature, moreover, regularly reports accounts of men who, generally during a psychotic spell, amputate their own penis. But in women, too, we find examples of genital self-hatred. Thus gynaecologists are regularly confronted with women who have slashed their vaginas, or who have inserted sharp objects or broken glass into them. In some cases this is a recurrent pattern. Women who mutilate themselves are not generally psychotic; genital self-mutilation can be likened to other forms of self-damage, such as slashing one's wrist with a razor, or scarring one's face. In Ingmar Bergman's film *Cries and Whispers* (1972), one of the three daughters of a mother who has just died breaks a wineglass during a quiet but fraught supper with her husband. Later we see her cutting her vagina with the splinters and laughing while smearing her own blood over her face and mouth. The suggestion is that this is an act of retaliation aimed at her husband's sexual prerogatives.

In 1989, the Austrian novelist Elfriede Jelinek published her novel *Lust*, which shocked the world. Not many readers could stomach so much repulsive sex. But as early as *The Piano Teacher* (1983), she had depicted the life of Erika, a lonely piano teacher who lives with her mother and is consumed with unsatisfied, masochistic longings. A relationship with a younger pupil leads to a shocking conclusion. In the film version *The Pianist* by Michael Haneke, Annie Girardot and Isabelle Huppert play the mother and daughter respectively. The fact that Erika mutilates herself fits seamlessly into the story:

> When SHE's home alone, she cuts herself, slicing off her nose to spite other people's faces. She always waits and waits for the moment when she can cut herself unobserved. No sooner does the sound of the closing door die down than she takes out her little talisman, the paternal all-purpose razor . . . This blade is destined for HER flesh. This thin, elegant, foil of bluish steel, pliable, elastic. SHE sits down in front of the magnifying side of the shaving mirror; spreading her legs, she makes a cut, magnifying the aperture that is the doorway into her body. She knows from experience that such a razor doesn't hurt, for her arms, hands and legs have often served as guinea pigs. Her hobby is cutting her own body.
>
> . . . As usual, there is no pain. SHE, however, cuts the wrong place, separating what the Good Lord and Mother Nature have brought together in unusual unity . . . For an instant, the two flesh halves, sliced apart, stare at each other, taken aback at this sudden gap, which wasn't there before . . . Then the blood shoots out resolutely. The drops ooze, run, blend with their comrades, turning into a red trickle, then a soothingly steady red stream when the individual trickles unite . . . Her nether region and her fear are two allies of hers, they usually appear together. If one of these two friends drops into her head without knocking, then she can rest assured: the other cannot be far behind. Mother can check whether or not SHE keeps her hands outside the covers at night; but if Mother wanted to gain control of HER fear, she would have to pry her child's skull open and personally scrape out the fear.
>
> In order to stem the flow of blood, SHE pulls out the popular package whose merits are known to and appreciated by every woman, especially in sports and for any kind of movement. The package quickly replaces the golden cardboard crown worn by the little girl when she is sent as a princess to the children's costume party. SHE, however, never went to a children's party, she never got to know the crown. The queen's

crown suddenly slips into her panties, and the woman knows her place in life. The thing that once shone forth on the head in childlike pride has now landed where the female wood has to wait for an ax.

Reading Jelinek is an ambivalent pleasure, perhaps not entirely unlike cutting your own flesh.

Personal hygiene

By banning advertisements for panty liners and discouraging the use of this product, both physical and mental irritation could be reduced.[31]

Manufacturers of sanitary towels and panty liners keenly exploit revulsion from the female genitals. We can scarcely conceive that less than a century ago women menstruated straight into their clothes, because they thought that otherwise the vital purifying effect of the menstrual flow might be impeded.[32]

Coping with the female genitals has in any case changed markedly over the ages. In the nineteenth century it was unthinkable that a middle-class grown-up woman should wear drawers with a closed crotch, while this type of garment was thought essential for young girls.[33] The emotional experience of overt sexual maturity that their first bra means for modern girls was had by Victorian girls when they put on their first 'open' drawers. An adult woman wearing 'closed' drawers caused as much tut-tutting as a woman with open-crotch panties would cause in the twenty-first century, because that woman was patently flouting the dictates of fashion. Perhaps she also wore long trousers, those recognized symbols of masculinity!

Ask any man to name his standard grumbles, and one will surely be advertisements for feminine hygiene. Sanitary towels and tampons are of course indispensable, and during the fertile phase of their lives women naturally welcome the fact that manufacturers are trying their best to help prevent embarrassing leaks. Everyone responds positively to appealing advertisements in which a sporty mother in white shorts tumbles about gleefully with her child. The panty liner is, however, designed to ward off the dangers of a non-menstruating vagina, and that is a recent invention.

In July 1971 Germaine Greer wrote a savage attack in the *Sunday Times* on the commercialization of vaginal hygiene, in this case vaginal deodorants.[34] Nowadays it is unfashionable to accuse capitalism of bad faith, but Germaine Greer compared the manufacturers to drug dealers who exploit the insecurity of adolescents in order to enslave them to feel-good remedies. Greer was a good observer and recorded a rising trend, the start of which she pinpointed to the middle of 1966; just a few years later she counted fifteen to twenty pages of advertisements for vaginal hygiene preparations in various women's magazines. Indeed, it quickly became clear that chemicals from the spray could damage the mucous membranes. At about the same time many women learned that soap, too, could be an irritant.

By about 1980, most women were firmly convinced that their vagina was too sensitive for deodorants, but the fear fostered by manufacturers that vaginal odours posed a daily threat to feminine self-confidence had meanwhile become firmly rooted in the female collective consciousness. The panty liner has thrived in this environment; in 1999 plans were afoot to market a special type for use with a thong, and in February 2000 this product was advertised for sale. During a period when the colour black was highly fashionable, a black panty liner was marketed. Most women are aware that many doctors are not very enthusiastic about panty liners, but the social pressure, the urge to keep the genitals under control, is greater. For the rest, it cannot be denied that some healthy women inconveniently produce copious vaginal secretions. 'Copious secretion' is not, however, synonymous with 'unhealthy secretion'.

Do panty liners in fact irritate the mucous membranes? If they do, then the manufacturers could be accused of doing something similar to the nineteenth-century brewers who would sometimes add atropine to the beer, which gave drinkers a dry mouth, thus stimulating consumption and increasing the brewers' profits. That practice has since been outlawed.

Germaine Greer mentions a deodorant manufacturer's leaflet claiming that vaginal odours arise because the crotch, an area that is indeed somewhat burdened with sweat and with vaginal secretion, is always covered with clothes and underwear. 'Overheating' is not conducive to vaginal health, which is something most women acknowledge. Germaine Greer stated, wholly in the spirit of her time, that it would therefore be sensible to advise women not to wear panties unless it was absolutely essential. She had her followers, but not very many.

Let us take it that panty liners can indeed lead to vaginal irritation. How can this be explained? The acid vaginal contents (which are a defence mechanism against the 'wrong' bacteria in the vagina) have an irritating effect on the mucous membrane of the labia. The mucous membrane round the hymen is able to cope with this degree of acidity, but outside that region the acid causes irritation. In general the labia are pressed together, and the crotch of a pair of panties, with or without a

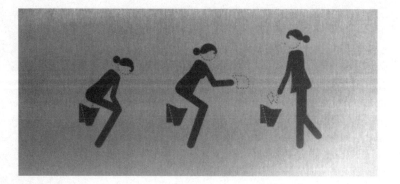

30 Ladies'
urinal *Lady P.*,
by Sphinx.

panty liner, exerts a further degree of pressure, as a result of which the
area between the labia is closed more tightly than normal. The universal belief that women must keep their legs together also plays a part in
this process. Panty liners absorb the vaginal secretion only when it has
seeped further down. If attempts are to be made to stem the harmful
action of the vaginal secretion on the mucous membranes, then the
secretion will have to be caught while it is still inside the hymenal ring.
A simple method, which quite a few women have tried very successfully, is to roll up half a sheet of toilet paper and to place it between the
labia after every urination. Generally such a roll will stay in place until
the next visit to the lavatory. The inner side of the labia remains reasonably dry, encouraging extra keratinization of the mucous membrane.
That renders the labia more resistant to both chemical and bacterial
influences and also to physical injury during sexual intercourse.

All in all, women feel more vulnerable then men when it comes
to genital health. Women become exasperated at the slovenly toilet
behaviour of men and hence are strongly in favour of separate facilities.
Mixed toilets, as shown in the American legal series *Ally McBeal*, are
almost unimaginable in many other countries. Many women consider it unsafe to make physical contact with a lavatory seat on which
other users have sat. Large quantities of toilet paper are used to cover
the seat, and there are several inventions to meet the hygienic demands
of users. One is a lavatory with a button that can be pressed to cover
the seat with a kind of latex sheath. A more recent addition is an automatically revolving seat whose centre rear section is continuously
cleaned. The latest invention encourages women to squat above the
bowl. Sphinx have recently introduced a ladies' urinal in which women
can quickly and efficiently urinate in the 'ski posture'. The pictogram
shows how the device works. It will usher in a kind of revolution in
toilet behaviour, or so the proud inventor of the device hopes.

chapter fourteen

Idealization and Worship of the Female Genitals

They say that books on female parts amuse small girls. For instance, they mention three types of labia minora. The smallest is triangular. It has two narrow jointed folds. It can hardly be seen because it is hidden from sight by the outermost labia. The middle type looks like a lily leaf. It is half-moon-shaped or triangular. You can see it foaming smoothly over its entire length. The large unfolded innermost labia resemble butterfly wings. They are triangular or rectangular, and clearly visible.[1]

Monique Wittig's descriptions are reminiscent of the work of Georgia O'Keeffe, whose paintings of orchids in particular can hardly be viewed without arousing associations with the female genitals. Her landscapes too are sometimes filled with suggestive folds. The visual arts have focused attention on the female genitals over the centuries. Some of this work is highly stylized and has ritual significance. The earliest rock drawings contain phallic as well as vaginal symbols, and are undoubtedly linked to fertility rites. If matriarchal societies ever existed, it goes without saying that they worshipped feminine idols.

Before the invention of photography, illustrations often had fewer artistic pretensions. Prints of the time had a practical use, and what we nowadays admire as seventeenth and eighteenth-century erotic art was simply the saucy literature of the period. Such art was above all descriptive; the illustrations to Pietro Aretino's sonnets are strangely lacking in emotion. The engraver could count on the fact that the viewer would discover the sexual trigger himself while paging through the book (with or without titillating company). It was not until the nineteenth and twentieth centuries that art came to be generally considered a means of conveying the artist's feelings to the spectator, and that was an entirely different form of eroticism. The most famous example is the frontispiece for this book, Gustave Courbet's *L'Origine du monde* (1866) now in the Musée d'Orsay, Paris. In it, the viewer can detect a wide range of emotions, all positive. It is obvious that Courbet wanted to come up with an icon.

The history of this painting is remarkable. For a long time it was owned by the French psychoanalyst Jacques Lacan, but it had been painted for the Egyptian ambassador in Paris, and it used to hang behind a small curtain in his salon. Some discretion was called for; it was similarly said of Goya's *Maja* that the original owner hid the naked version behind a clothed one and that none but intimate friends were allowed to see both. Discretion with regard to explicit sexual themes in art must have been rooted in our Christian past, for there are cultures in which beauty and sexual arousal go hand in hand. Japanese and Chinese erotic art, which has become so popular in Europe, often takes the form of instruction manuals, and used to be traditional wedding presents for the bride. A Chinese pillow book dating back to about AD 100 starts with a poem by the bride to her husband:

> I shed my robes and remove my paint and powder,
> And roll out the picture scroll by the pillow's side.
> The plain girl I shall take as my instructress,
> So that we can practise all the various postures,
> Those that an ordinary husband has but rarely seen,
> Such as taught by Tíen-lao to the Yellow Emperor.
> No joy shall equal the delights of the first night,
> These shall never be forgotten, however old we may grow.[2]

A remarkable feature of Japanese erotic art is that the sexual organs are often drawn with exceptional attention to detail and slightly larger than life size. The close-ups of the vagina are either super-realistic or else extremely stylized, but they invariably reflect great respect for the organ depicted. Even today, Japanese strip shows afford unusually close and extensive views of the vagina, and magnifying glasses are placed beside the catwalk.[3] Japanese drawings allow great expressive freedom, while Chinese art is more precise, using fewer expressive means. What is often reproduced in the greatest detail is the little bound foot. This drastic mutilation of the Chinese woman served as a great erotic symbol and art reflects that fact.

Arthur Golden's *Memoirs of a Geisha* (1997), as we saw earlier, tells us a great deal about Sayuri's training. Among other things she learns about the geisha's special hairdo, the 'pin cushion'. After the hair has been oiled and set in wax, it is piled up high in a knot on top of the head. At the back a small slit is deliberately left open, which is why the official

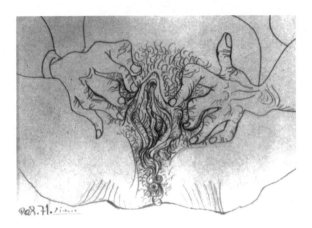

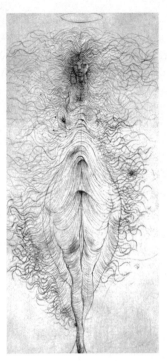

31 Pablo
Picasso,
Untitled, 1971.

32 Hans
Bellmer,
*Madame
Edwarda*, 1965.

name of this hairstyle is the 'split peach'. The pincushion is formed by wrapping the hair around a piece of fabric, and for apprentice geishas the colour of this fabric is red. Sayuri is still fairly ignorant about sexual matters, but some time later a client tells her suggestively what this red slit in her dark shiny hair signifies for men.

Desmond Morris is an ethologist and hence interested in the signals the body sends out to ensure the survival of the species.[4] His explanation of the development of the female breast is well known: because we walk upright and because the human female (unlike the chimpanzee female) does not signal that she is in season, other sexual signals had to be developed. The breast is reminiscent of the buttocks, and the latter are a substitute for the enormous red cushions the female ape displays during her fertile period. Civilization keeps making new rules for subduing forms of behaviour that are too provocative, but nature keeps breaking through with erotic signals in new places. Morris argues (it has to be said on the basis of rather fleeting observations) that the navel became increasingly vaginal during the second half of the twentieth century. On older paintings and photographs, the navel is usually round, but the vertical slit seems to be increasingly prevalent just at a time when the navel is being displayed more and more widely.

In twentieth-century Western art, portraits of sexually accessible women invariably serve to convey sexual feelings, but these can be of various kinds. Picasso cheerfully used a number of pornographic clichés, for instance of the woman who hospitably holds her labia apart. The effect is carefree eroticism. On the other hand, we find male artists who have characterized themselves chiefly as eroto-maniacs can produce very impressive work using their model's gaze, her pose or their synecdochical aesthetic approach. Belmer's rapacious, dripping vaginas may have an exciting effect but the excitement is always mixed with fear and revulsion. Not all erotomaniacs are lovers of women. Ambivalence is part of it all, and sexual enslavement can be a way of warding off fear. Here is Philip Roth:

> Yes, shame, shame, on Alex P. . . . While everybody else has been marrying nice Jewish girls, and having children, . . . what he has been doing is – chasing cunt. And *shikse* cunt, to boot! Chasing it, sniffing it, lapping it, *shtupping* it, but above all, *thinking about it* . . . Every girl he sees turns out (hold your hats) to be carrying around between her legs – a real cunt. Amazing! Astonishing! Still can't get over the fantastic idea that when you are looking at a girl, you are looking at somebody who is guaranteed to have on her – a cunt! *They all have cunts!* Right under their dresses![5]

This is a typical approach to human sexual anatomy. For all the subjects treated here under the heading of idealization and aestheticization also impinge on the fear and revulsion discussed in the last chapter. That is true of cohabiting couples, regardless of whether they are depicted for artistic or for erotic reasons. No matter how much desire and excitement are communicated by the vagina of the beloved, there are many aspects of it that repel. That tension has provided artists with a permanent source of inspiration. Herman de Coninck, the Flemish poet, has used this very ambiguity in his 'Memory's hetaera':

> When with merciless slowness, yawning, peekaboo,
> She sheds her high-priced panties on the floor
> (Sex like luxury has a mysterious x)
> And then proffers her brimming two
> Breasts to his hands, he looks down at her pale
> Legs up to what, three feet above, is his highest goal:
> Lips that are only lips but cannot speak,
> And someone who over his supplications does not show that she smiles.

For women have a mighty sex, a high-up wound,
Venusian mounts, caverns, folds
In which lost nights can never be refound
And play with them down there
Like the Mona Lisa with tourists or the moon with the sea,
Breathtaking, and tinged with slight disdain.

That applies equally to their owner. Even among women overflowing with self-confidence there are not many who are truly proud of their vaginas. During her performance 'Krukje' (The crotch), the photographer Yael Davids transformed her cunt into her face and that made her a very rare exception.

Aesthetic ideals in various cultures

In the early years of one Dutch children's radio programme, letters about labia predominated for a few months. Countless girls seemed to be revolted by the shape, size, colour and other aspects of their labia minora, hoping and longing to be told how they could make their ugly little cunts look a bit more presentable. By 1998 little seemed to have changed, for the editors of a magazine that receives 1,500 letters a month from girls (who were sixteen years old on average) told a reporter that oversized labia continued to be a regular subject of correspondence. Some girls had learnt to camouflage the size of their labia by pushing them inwards. Gynaecologists and plastic surgeons now and then perform cosmetic surgery on the labia. An American journalist interviewed the urologist and plastic surgeon Gary Alter (the name is apt) who describes himself as a 'Female Genital Cosmetic Surgeon', and prides himself on being able to adjust all asymmetrical shapes. The journalist was shown a large number of photographs, and found it amazing to what great extent individual variations could in fact be ironed out, leaving the patients with a kind of standard vulva.[6] Similar adjustments can be made in porn photography by retouching methods, so that the models that young girls aspire to emulate look increasingly less realistic.

What is too large and what is acceptable? Illus. 33 is taken from Dickinson, and serves as a demonstration of the variability of the labia minora.[7] In a French clinic specializing in operations on the external genitals, 163 French women received surgical treatment over a period of 9 years, and here 4 centimetres was considered the boundary between normality and hypertrophy.[8] Apart from cosmetic reasons, some women were also persuaded to have the operation because of complaints during coitus (difficulty in admitting the partner) or while taking part in sports. A good 64 per cent complained of problems with clothing. Tights in particular caused women with large labia some discomfort.

Big is ugly when it comes to female genitals. Yet that is far from self-evident. The Zuni Indians have a special ceremony to confirm the sex of a newborn baby. If it is a girl, a gourd is held over the vagina as an expression of the hope that her sexual organs may grow large. With little boys, the penis is sprinkled with water reflecting the hope that it might remain small. Such were the ideals of the Zuni.[9] Far better known is the case of Hottentot women, who were all believed to have very large labia, combined with a potential to develop excessively fat buttocks (steatopygia). The latter may well be genetically determined, but the large size of the labia is due to stretching and other manipulations. Natalie Angier has described the exploitation of the 'Hottentot Venus', a woman who was brought to Europe in the nineteenth century and was known as Sarah Baartman.[10] She was used as a kind of fairground attraction and after her death her body was dissected. A plaster cast of her impressive body stood in the Musée de l'Homme in Paris until 1981, when protests by a feminist action group lead to the removal from view of this vestige of colonialism. Nelson Mandela asked both the French presidents Mitterand and Chirac for the return of the mortal remains of the Hottentot Venus so that she could be given a decent burial in her own country, and France finally acceded to this request in January 2002. Her remains were buried in August that year in the area of her birth in the Eastern Cape Province.[11] Angier points out that Hottentot women have strong similarities to certain apes, who by trailing their labia over the ground are able to spread their pheromones easily over a large territory. Angier suspects the scientists who were so interested in the Hottentot female genitals of unconsciously rejoicing in a characteristic that seemed to show so clearly that the black race is closer to apes than to human beings.

We have even more anthropological information about Micronesian tribes in the Truk and Ponape islands.[12] Here, too, there is intensive manipulation of the labia and clitoris of young girls (according to the earliest anthropologists, by impotent old men), on the principle of the more the better – better for the pleasure of the woman herself and for that of her partner. She has a 'vagina full of things' (a big clitoris and big labia) and can rightly be proud of them. She can have her labia pierced and suspend all sorts of jingling ornaments from them, and when she gets used to walking with her legs apart, she is also a delight for the ears. If she quarrels with another woman, then

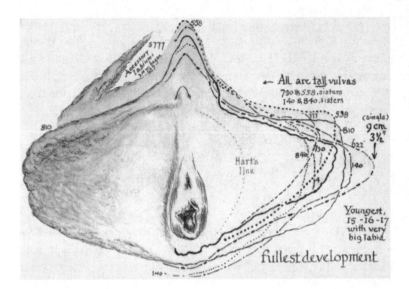

33 Variable size of labia.

the fight is settled by comparing their 'vaginas full of things'. The one who has the most beautiful genitals is in the right. Pubic hair, too, is greatly esteemed, and the effect is further enhanced by tattoos on the inside of the thigh.

Devereux is strongly influenced by psychoanalytical ideas and points out that many of these interventions help to make the female crotch look like the male on superficial examination. This holds true for the Ponape more than for the Truk islanders. Ponape men undergo one-sided ritual castration, as a result of which their genitals are given more median contours. This is said to help overcome general male castration fears. Among the Truk, contact between the sexes may almost be called phallic. It is in any case most important for the man to 'conquer' his woman, that is, bring her to orgasm. Micronesians and Hottentots developed a great love for the clitoris long before Europeans did. During her stay in Africa, Marie Bonaparte, escaping from Europe before the Second World War, was astonished to find that it was possible to meet in a single continent both the most fanatical enemies and the greatest admirers of the clitoris.[13]

Our age is marked in part by an obsession with the body, and the vagina has been dragged into this obsession. First of all there are ways of changing what we find ugly or abnormal. It is possible to reduce the size of the labia, to even out asymmetries, and so on. Hormonal changes during the menopause lead to a reduction in the subcutaneous fat in the labia majora, and there are women who try to offset that by having a cosmetic surgeon inject them with silicon, in much the same way as the mouth can be reshaped in accordance with the latest fashion. A new device, a kind of suction cup, applied to the vagina results in a greatly swollen sex organ, something between a baby's and that of a female chimpanzee on heat. The inventor of this device, Wilhelm Kannengieser, advertised this method among others as a way of preventing post-menopausal atrophy of the mucous membranes and the subcutaneous fatty tissue.[14]

Pubic hair

What are we to make of pubic hair? The attitude to this secondary sexual characteristic varies, in societies as well as in individuals. Anyone studying classical sculpture will notice that many works show men with a fine bush of stylized pubic hair, while there is not even a hint of this in statues of women.[15] In painting, which happened to reflect classical assumptions, the same taboo applied until the nineteenth century; axillary (armpit) and chest hair was also rarely depicted. Goya's *La Maja Desnuda* is considered a milestone, but even in this pioneering painting the pubic hair is adumbrated rather than actually portrayed. Paintings in which the female body was not subordinated to the dominant academic conceptions of art had to be reserved for private use until 1899. Klimt was the first artist to paint an allegorical nude with a flaming bush of red pubic hair, and the title – *Nuda Veritas* – is significant.

Axillary hair was subject to a similar taboo, anyone depicting it drawing a great deal of attention to themselves. The *Maja Desnuda* has none, and the same holds for almost all female nudes. Delvaux is an exception. All his nudes are young and their sexual characteristics are strongly emphasized, not least their pubic and axillary hair. In Japan a porn star emerged from anonymity thanks to her absolute refusal to shave her armpits. Kuroki has ever since been a media phenomenon with a tremendous impact, something between La Cicciolina in Italy and Dr Ruth in the United States.[16]

Does the absence of pubic and axillary hair from most paintings imply that depilation was common in antiquity? In his *Ars Amatoria* (Arts of Love), Ovid advises women to remove the hair from their legs and armpits, but he does not mention pubic hair explicitly. 'De ornatu mulierum' (On the adornment of women), one of the texts in the *Trotula*, the eleventh-century compendium of women's medicine from Salerno, contains a list of depilatories. A steam bath should precede the application of the remedy.

Take juice of the leaves of squirting cucumber and almond milk; with these placed in a vessel, gently mix in quicklime and orpiment. Then add pounded galbanum mixed with a small amount of wine for a day and a night, and cook with this. Once this has well cooked, you should remove the substance of the galbanum and put in a little oil or wine and quicksilver. Having made this concoction, you should remove it from the fire and add a powder of the following herbs. Take an equal amount each of mastic, frankincense, cinnamon, nutmeg, clove. This ointment smells sweetly and is gentle for softening. Salernatan women are accustomed to use this depilatory.

Back in the steam bath, attempts are then made to pluck out the pubic hair and if that proves a problem, the *Trotula* suggests a few alternatives with instructions about what to do if the skin becomes irritated. Henna and egg white play a role in the cure.

Henna and steam baths are also part of the *hamam* (ritual bathing) of Muslim women.[17] For them, depilation is a religious duty. The reason for visiting a *hamam* may be the prospect of a sexual encounter with one's husband (for instance, after a temporary separation), but even after sexual intercourse a Muslim woman is expected to purify herself, and that is best done in a *hamam*. Although Islam has a positive attitude to marital pleasures, quite a few Muslim women seem to feel ashamed of making frequent visits to the bath.

Muslim women shave their pubic hair throughout their lives, and gynaecologists will tell you that in the case of women with thick pubic hair this cannot always be done without irritating the skin and the mucous membranes.

In India, there is an additional rule: widows are not allowed to continue shaving their pubic hair, something most women do while their husbands are alive. Among Western women, the custom of removing all or some of the pubic hair is becoming more widespread. It seems to have turned into a lifestyle issue, sometimes with sexual overtones. Some men and women find a smooth mons veneris more attractive and exciting than the natural 'origin of the world'. In personal ads and on web sites it has become increasingly common for this preference to be stated explicitly, and porn addicts who happen to like 'hairy bushes' were recognized as a separate target group in 2003.

In the past, this preference was anything but widely shared. It is reported that John Ruskin was so shocked by the detail in which his bride differed from the classical nudes he had studied so diligently that he was quite unable to make love to her. The marriage was dissolved. There was a great deal of gossip, and when he planned to get married again, he had to use all sorts of discreet circumlocutions to reassure the bride's family. He did not find that easy to do, since his confidence in his ability to rise to the occasion was naturally based on masturbation, which was something he could not mention except in a thickly veiled manner.[18]

If the husband has a marked predilection for a shaven mons veneris, then that may give rise to arguments in our emancipated age, just like his desire to possess his wife in sexy lingerie or leather. In Paris, there is always a great crush round the customer service counters of the big department stores after Christmas, mainly because women want to exchange the expensive pieces of flimsy lingerie they have been given by their husbands for a decent set of pots and pans. Pubic hair seems a small sacrifice to the male libido, but if after shaving it off you no longer dare to go to the sauna or are ashamed in front of your children, then this male predilection certainly does have undesirable consequences.

In intimate relations, pubic hair can also be of a symbolic importance. Much as parents preserve baby locks, so small tufts of pubic hair can be exchanged as tokens of exclusive ties. In John Irving's *The Cider House Rules* (1985), Homer Wells, the leading character, works in St Cloud's, an orphanage and abortion clinic run by the old and charismatic director Wilbur Larch. His life changes the day when a young couple turns up for an abortion; he falls in love with the girl at first sight. As he tidies the theatre after the operation he discovers a tuft of pubic hair, which then becomes his prize possession. Homer and the girl become very friendly but he keeps his love secret. When a gust of the wind blows the tuft of hair out of his wallet many years later at a cinema ticket counter, the girl helps him to keep his money from being blown away and suddenly realizes that he is not some sort of pathological collector, but that it is all to do with *her* pubic hair. The precious souvenir is carried off by the wind, but love is at last given a chance.

This is a worthy example, but erotic booty is of course also hunted for macho reasons. Naomi Wolf tells us that some American student digs had a special place for exhibiting trophies, for instance on the tiled wall above the toilet.[19] Part of the fun was to watch the reaction of the women. In these digs, there were of course no separate lavatories, and any woman betraying surprise on leaving the bathroom became a ready butt of 'innocent boyish humour'.

Sexual boorishness is part of student life. A notable example is the story told by Willem W. Waterman about his time on the editorial boards of several sex magazines.[20] One day when two pages were still to be filled, the author decided that a bit of a joke would not come amiss. An advertisement was concocted inviting ladies to turn their pubic hair into cash:

It is not generally known that wealthy Arab oil sheiks pay large sums of money today for tablemats braided from pubic hair that has been grown on the slopes of Mount Venus in Europe.

In America, too, this is the latest craze. THE SPECIAL GIFT FOR THE MAN WHO HAS EVERYTHING! Recently the multimillionaire Paul Getty spent $35,000 on a breakfast-table mat made of, among other things, several strands of pubic hair from a natural blonde princess belonging to one of our European royal families.

Do you think that these rich Arabs are mad?

Do you think that Paul Getty is an American social climber?

Don't you understand why these men are mad?

WHAT DO YOU CARE???? IT PAYS WELL.

Women keen to turn their pubic hair into money in this way were invited to send a sample to Public Hair Place Mats, Inc. in Rotterdam. 'Public' was of course a typing error, corrected to 'Pubic' by hand. You also had to give the colour, the type of hair (straight or curly) and rate of growth. Potential vendors were warned that because of the extremely confidential nature of the material, the firm might have to insist on having the pubic hair collected by 'our own representatives from source'. After all, 'the pubic hair of European princesses, for instance, cannot be supplied with an affidavit of origin. Someone at Court has to be paid to collect it.'

Pubic hair was actually sent in, but in fairly small amounts. I have been shown the mural decoration in which this practical joke has been preserved for posterity – large bunches and small tufts in all colours and thicknesses.

O tempora, o mores! On 1 May 2000, a newspaper carried a report about a themed evening in Rotterdam held to glorify pubic hair. Female dancers high above the crowd scattered pubic hair over the dancers below. The pubic hair was synthetic; panties were on sale filled with a thick bundle.

In the New York Museum of Modern Art an ivory-coloured object, elongated and beautifully rounded with perfect spirals expanding concentrically outwards from the centre, used to hang on one wall. Not spectacular but handsome. A card announced that the artist's name was Tom Friedman, and that the materials of his untitled work were 'soap and pubic hair'. It must have been quite a creation, and I like to imagine that it took the artist fifteen years to perfect it. Here the profane was given a particularly effective aesthetic form. When sex is about, double meaning is never far away.

Contemporary embellishments

Trimmed and shaved pubic hair goes with a certain lifestyle, and that applies even more strongly to tattoos and piercings. What used to be associated with primitive cultures and rough sailors can nowadays be part of our erotic imagery. This subject often gives rise to a conflict of generations. Mothers who are happy to accompany their daughters to the jeweller and to hold their hands while they are having their ears pierced, get most upset when their daughters prefer to have their navel pierced. Piercings and tattoos invariably remind the older generation of prostitution and criminality, dissolution and sadomasochism. An acquaintance told me that she agreed with her daughter that she could go ahead with some piercing if she still wanted it on her sixteenth birthday, and that she was then delighted by her daughter's evident satisfaction with her new body ornamentation. Clearly a tattoo or a piercing can be of great value at a time when growing girls and boys are developing a personality of their own.

Piercings of the labia majora and minora and the clitoris have different meanings for different people. Besides the simple 'I think it's beautiful', we sometimes hear that piercing affords both men and women extra excitement during lovemaking. Piercing is then in the same category as the French tickler and the ribbed condom. The most striking emotional impetus is of course masochistic. In Pauline Réage's book *The Story of O* (1954), O's total subjection is completed with a brand-mark and a metal ring through her labia. The latter is a clear indication of a certain status, much as a wedding ring functions as a signal. Sexual bondage can be rendered visible, inside and outside of a particular relationship. In addition to all sorts of highly exhibitionistic sadomasochistic designs, chastity belts as part of the S/M aesthetic are obtainable again nowadays, as witness the photograph by Eric Kroll (illus. 21).

Elasticity

What other characteristics of the vagina lend themselves to idealiza-tion and adoration? In other words, what does a woman have to do in order to conserve an irresistible vagina? Meir Shalev tells us in *The Big Woman* (1998) about a boy who grows up in a family con-sisting of his mother, his sister, his grandmother and two aunts. The feminine influences are overwhelming, and the boy gains a good insight into women's secrets. Looking after their 'pamushka', their genital organs, makes great demands on the ladies. He has to eavesdrop on them, but he manages to gather what is going on when the ladies call out in chorus: 'One, two, three, four. Five, five, five, hold on . . . don't let go . . . ' Four short squeezes and one long one, all to strengthen the pamushka. And behind the bathroom door, he hears his sister being trained: 'There you are, like that, and then another one . . . It's no laughing matter, open up . . . Anyone who's in the know can tell from a woman's face if her pamushka is sweet or sour.'

The tightness and irresistible attraction of the vagina are examined in *F/32* by Eurudice Kamvisseli (1993). The leading character, Ela, has a remarkable love-hate relationship with her genitals, and that is equally true of the hordes of men with whom she shares her organ. The first page reads:

> Ela has the tightest cunt in the world. Every blessing is a curse, Ela reminds herself . . .
>
> Men come to Ela's raving. 'I love your cunt! A real cunt! There's a taste! I love how it is shaved. It's so light. It expands! Like a balmy dream . . . ' 'Bright too! And it swells so much! It gets a hard-on, it stays soft like a fruit, and so dynamic! It pulsates!' 'It's like slipping into the tentacles of a squid, like you are swimming nude and suddenly the entire ocean is condensed into this little powerful fist, it has a rhythm, a double spasm!' 'It smells so fresh, like moist earth, wet paint, cucumber, thunder.' 'It's a delicacy!' 'It's smart!' 'It never breaks down! It even glows in the dark!' 'It's so beautiful! You should be proud of your cunt!'
>
> What inspires these metaphors? Ela wonders. How can I be proud of something I don't control? Ela responds to men's endless linguistic exertions with equanimity: 'Sorry, I wouldn't know'; or 'It is outside my control'; or 'It is independent of me.' But men crack up at the joke and assess that she, too, is good with metaphor.

There is a solution, albeit a gruesome one. A blind old man collides with Ela on the sidewalk in Fifth Avenue and slashes her with a knife. With Ela's big-hearted collaboration, this ecstatic attack, witnessed by many passers-by, results in the complete excision of her cunt. It does not take the cunt long to escape and to render all New York unsafe. Ela follows in its tracks. Cavorting through the zoo (the apes), and men's and women's prisons, Ela's released cunt becomes more and more famous. It appears on David Letterman's TV show under the stage name of V, and with the help of shrewd marketing becomes an image with the same brand recognition as Coca-Cola. Many celebrities cross its path before it is reunited with the woman it came from. The search for a body part that goes its own way is a deliberate paraphrase of Gogol's *The Nose*, and it is quite possible that Gogol chose the nose deliberately because it has such strong associations with the penis.

Tight is good; that goes without saying. The exercises of Meir Shalev's aunts, known as pelvic-floor or Kegel exercises, were in fact advocated in manuals, and an electrical stimulus device – the vagette – was even marketed for the express purpose of increasing the tension of the vaginal muscles. The small Ben-Wah balls sold in sex-shops were said to make these exercises even more effective. There is no doubt that countless women experimented with Kegel exercises during the years of the sexual revolution. In April 1999, a radio programme was broadcast in which a Surinamese woman told listeners about *ketewiwiri*, a herbal steam bath that helps to keep the vagina taut and in pristine condition. After the broadcast, the radio station received so many telephone calls from interested women who had missed the programme that the broadcast was repeated nine days later. The procedure was as follows: a kind of tea was brewed from the herbs and placed in a chamber pot in the lavatory bowl so that the woman could comfortably sit there for about fifteen minutes while the steam rose up between her legs. It appeared from the broadcast that the effects were not very reliable. A warning was issued: if the steam did not work, that could be because the vendor had been menstruating, so that it was best to get your supply of herbs from older women.

Ketewiwiri is an ancient remedy brought to Paramaribo by Maroon women (the descendents of runaway slaves). It consists of various herbs, each with a particular effect. Some do nothing but provide a pleasant odour; others are alleged to give the vagina a vice-like grip. For women who are too ashamed to be seen buying these products, the suppliers have a variety of delivery methods, including the regular use of taxi drivers. Surinamese herbalists adapt the steaming and irrigation technique to the treatment of all sorts of diseases and complaints of the sexual organs, and they are renowned for their work. Heynes Landvel is one of these traditional healers, and he goes on regular tours of the Caribbean and the United States. Whitney Houston is said to be one of his clients.

In Morocco, women use different household remedies for improving vaginal pleasure (for men and women alike).[21] Pepper is one, as is lavender water. The Moroccan sociologist Soumaya Naamane–Guessous has, however, heard few positive reports about these remedies. The oldest recipe for narrowing the vagina (and to prevent female frigidity) can be found in the *Tung-hsüan-tzû*, Master Tung-Hsüan's *ars amatoria*.[22] It includes a series of texts dating back to the Sui dynasty (*c.* 600), but Van Gulik has pointed out that these texts have been handed down since the days of the Han dynasty, that is, since about the beginning of the Christian era.

RECIPE:
Shih-liu-huang (sulphur)   2 grams
Chíng-mu-hsiang (inula incense)   2 grams
Shan-tsái-huang (seeds of *Evodia rutaecarpa Bth.*)
Shê-chúang-tzû (*Cridum japonicum*)

Grind and sift. Apply a small quantity to the vagina before coitus. Choose the dose carefully, for if too much is applied, the vagina will close up.

In the Middle Ages, women also used a number of recipes from the *Trotula*. The vaginal application of remedial substances is as old as medicine itself.[23] Aromatic vapours were particularly popular. Women squatted above a kind of censer, or to improve accessibility they might, for instance, use a perforated hollow dildo. Among the Siberian Samoyed, fumigation was part of the purification ritual following menstruation, the smoke being obtained by burning reindeer hide.[24] Surinamese herbalists work not only with steam, but also with douches, and Surinamese mothers train their daughters very actively in vaginal hygiene, just like the women around Meir Shalev's Israeli hero. And small girls are encouraged to push in their fingers and washcloths a little more deeply.

Vaginal health in body and in mind

Our own education is decidedly more conservative. There are still mothers who try to dissuade their teenage daughters from using tampons:

> She had to fight for permission to use tampons . . . She asked her mother if she could use tampons. No, said her mother. She had tried them herself, they had caused her terrible pain and were dangerous.[25]

The daughter then uses the tampons surreptitiously, but because she cannot insert the first tampon more than halfway, it does indeed prove

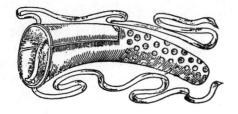
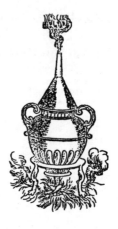

34 Instruments
for vaginal
fumigation
from the
Renaissance.

to be a painful affair. She has to ask her mother's help, and it then emerges that her mother is completely inexperienced. She lied because she did not want to get involved. That makes the girl even more determined. Tampons are an important step on her road to independence.

If women have a vaginal discharge caused by candida (thrush), they can use fungicidal preparations. These used to be administered vaginally, but the pharmaceutical industry has had considerable success with (much more expensive) oral medication, so that women do not have to touch their vagina. Vaginal secretions are far too often considered a pathological symptom, and it would be much better if women were to look upon their discharge more as part of normal personal hygiene. Advertising suggests that women gain considerable self-confidence from regular skin care with moisturizing preparations, and that even signs of a white discharge in panty liners should not shake a woman's poise. The most recent objective findings suggest that women benefit from vaginal douching, particularly if they have frequent intercourse.[26] Perhaps women would more readily resort to this type of personal hygiene if the bidet became more popular.

A healthy vaginal discharge is also to be welcomed, but except for pornography little has been said on this subject. In classical Chinese court life, female sexual fluids were held in high esteem.[27] To the Chinese, sexuality has a religious significance, and in Taoism and Confucianism, lovemaking is part of the quest for immortality. In old Chinese texts, people are constantly encountered who have reached the age of several hundred years, and it appears the meticulous care with which they performed their sexual duties undoubtedly helped their near-immortality.

The male seed is the male life force, which implies that sperm is extremely Yang. Immortality is attained by awakening the sperm time and again, while preventing its escape. The precious Yang essence must be returned with great skill through the spinal cord to the brain. Chinese love manuals contain a wide range of hints on how to prevent loss of seed: the man can open his nostrils wide and hold his breath, or merely breathe in and out vigorously. He can gnash his teeth, roll his eyes, wave his arms about and pinch himself between the anus and the scrotum.[28] During sexual intercourse, the females secretions are awakened. They are extremely Yin, and it is thanks to the combination of the two life juices, pumped up to the brain, that immortality is fostered. A printed text dating back to 1598 (the Ming period), the *Hsiu-chên-yen-i* (The importance of keeping to the truth), mentions three female fluids, each flowing from one of the heights of femininity. Her saliva is the fountain of jade, flowing from the Red Lotus tip, her milk, called the peach of immortality, springs from the Double Lotus tip, and her vaginal fluids are white lead or moon flower, flowing from the Tip of the Purple Mushroom or the Cave of the White Tiger. On the last, Van Gulik who, as we mentioned earlier, was wont to translate sexually explicit passages into Latin rather than English, wrote:

> Emanat ex intima vagina. Ostium eus clausum esse solet; muliere autem in coitu ad voluptatem excita ita ut genae rubescant et haeret vox eus, ostium illut aperitur et humor inde excretus profluit, cum ad summum voluptatis culmen mulier pervenerit. Qui humor ubi in vaginam collectus erit, vir membrum per unius pollicis spatium reducat, deinde promoveat atque retrahat, quo mulieris essentiam hauriat, thereby benefiting his 'original Yang' and nurturing his spirit.

> [The vagina can be seen from the inside. Its entrance is usually closed, but when the woman is aroused during coitus, so that a blush appears on her cheeks and her voice catches, then this mouth opens up and moisture flows from it when the woman has reached the height of her voluptuousness. Once this moisture has collected in the vagina, the man withdraws his member for a few inches, then moves it forward again and pulls it back, thus absorbing the essence of the woman]

Texts such as this were widely read and quoted, in scientific papers no less than in pornographic publications. The sexual pleasure of the woman is as important as is that of the man, who is, moreover, expected to keep a careful check on his ejaculations. Anyone taking his religious responsibilities seriously cannot therefore make do with just one woman. The Tao scholar of the Green Buffalo put it as follows:

If a man keeps changing women during copulation, he will have the greatest advantage. If one is able to copulate with more than ten women in a single night, then everything is for the best. If one keeps copulating with one and the same woman, her life juice will gradually grow weaker until, ultimately, she is no longer in any condition to bestow health upon a man. Worse still, the woman herself will become exhausted.

Ten women a night and that without a single ejaculation! If the women were prostitutes, then the frequency of their sexual contacts yielded so much Yin that the man was compensated for his loss of seed. In about 1500, the texts became more restrained, and Van Gulik assumed that the reason was the rise of syphilis as a new threat to health. Masturbation was considered very unhealthy in all ages, and nocturnal emissions, too, were a cause of concern. In particular, if the man dreamt of a seductive woman, he might well be haunted by female incubi or fox demons. If a man encountered a woman with whom he had had sexual intercourse in his dreams, he had to be on his guard – she might well be an incubus out to rob him of his Yang.

It is hard to tell whether the women who played so important a role in the spiritually guided sexual world really gained a great deal of pleasure from it. The film *Raise the Red Lantern* gives us some idea of domestic life in ancient China.[29] Clearly, men used to bestow great sexual care on their wives and concubines. That was no more than their duty; every woman had the right to sex at least once every five days. But after having done his carnal duty, a man would banish women completely from his mind, and except during nights of lovemaking, they never set eyes upon him. The exalted poem about the wedding night quoted earlier was of course written by a man. Twenty-first-century women have had a hard job to convince their lovers that men are not perfect when it comes to gauging the sexual needs of the opposite sex. Might that also have been the case twenty-five centuries ago in China?

The link between eroticism and spirituality continues to be a topical subject, but can be deceptive. In her short story 'A Man from Singapore',[30] Renate Rubinstein describes her meeting in Hong Kong airport with a man (Mr Jacob), who offers to introduce her to yoga. 'No sex,' he assures her. Renate Rubinstein, who knows herself well enough to realize that yoga is not her kind of thing, nevertheless allows herself to be inveigled into going to the man's apartment, where, accompanied by a hilarious and high-flown commentary, there happens exactly what she might expect to happen in Amsterdam during a one-night stand. She is satisfied with the quality of what is on offer, but nevertheless asks why he made such a point of the fact that this encounter was to be 'no sex'. The man is deeply shocked. How can she possibly compare what she has just experienced with anything so trivial as sex? East is East, and West is West, and never the twain shall meet.

Anxiety about spilled sperm continues to be rife in Asia. Indian physicians have large numbers of male patients with the 'Dhat syndrome', that is, sperm loss combined with all sorts of debilities and anxieties. The Western observer finds it hard to work out whether these patients are common-or-garden hypochondriacs worried about masturbation, or whether there is indeed a sort of physiological condition responsible for 'leaks' of semen. Conversely, as late as 1950, Taoist sects in China offered the public 'Taoist study groups' of a rather orgiastic nature, promising their students immortality and immunity from all sorts of ills.[31]

Not so long ago in Western Europe the spilling of seed was also considered a cause of the loss of mental powers. Thanks to the diaries of the Goncourt brothers, we know that Flaubert, during his regular visits to prostitutes, invariably tried to practise coitus reservatus. 'Hier, j'ai perdu un livre,' (I lost a book yesterday) he told the brothers dejectedly when he wanted to convey that he had once again been caught short by an ejaculation.

Western culture has no songs of praise to the vaginal secretions but anyone reading between the lines will discover a double entendre in Zerlina's aria in Mozart's *Don Giovanni*. During her wedding feast, Zerlina keeps vacillating over Don Giovanni's advances and her fiancé Masetto plots revenge. But Don Giovanni plays him a childish trick and then gives him a good thrashing. Zerlina finds him groaning and bruised, and to console him, tells him that she is able to soothe his pains:

> If you'll be good, my dear,
> you'll see
> the cure I have for you!
> I know, you'll like it;
> It's nature's cure. Though no apothecary
> Can prescribe it.
> It's a certain balm
> I carry within me
> Which I can give you,
> If you want tol try it.
> If you want to know
> Where I keep it,

Then feel it beating
Put your hand here.[32]

And then we read in Lorenzo da Ponte's stage directions that Zerlina places Masetto's hand on her *heart*. Operatic sopranos are physically not very credible in scenes of tender, burgeoning eroticism, but I have heard a great many soubrettes taking the part of Zerlina, and these have included a number of extremely coquettish brides. Masetto is generally played up as a simpleton, and in this aria he has a chance to reach the limits of his expressive powers when it slowly dawns on him what kind of treatment is in store for him. The music of 'Vedrai carino' has a heavenly charm. To use a comparison, the untroubled admiration of the warbling of songbirds has become rather problematic for some readers of the biologist Midas Dekker since he let it slip that these artists are actually purveying smut.

Songs of praise and ritual

If we want to hear all the adoring voices, then vaginal sounds, too, must not be allowed to go uncelebrated. These lines are by the nineteenth-century Arab poet Ibn ar-Róemi:

The sound of a gnarled ramrod
in the crack of a wide-hipped girl,
is like the hand of a baker kneading dough,
or a bricklayer's foot in cement.
A stiff prick in a lush cunt,
in a girl with an abundance to give,
bowed to the ground, not by piety or faith,
beneath a man who is assured of her love,
like a duck bowing before the hawk.[33]

Vaginal sounds are rarely welcomed. Even during erotic encounters, most women will tend to blush when the sucked-in air is released from their vagina. They can easily learn to produce these sounds deliberately, but only in sex clubs in the Far East does this kind of talent come into its own. Anyone approached by a doorman at such a club in Bangkok and addressed with the word 'ping-pong', is actually being invited to witness a number of girls shooting ping-pong balls from their vaginas at the climax of their act. In the film *The Adventures of Priscilla, Queen of the Desert* (1994) such a scene is portrayed with a certain discretion. Smoking a cigarette with the vagina is another displacement of air that is part of the repertoire of most Thai sex performers. The vaginal *pétomane*, who turns passing wind from the vagina into an art form, is a rare bird. In Australia, Elizabeth Bruton does a striptease involving the emission of vaginal sounds in time with the music. Her 'pussy popping', however, seems to be a unique achievement.[34]

The object of an annual festival in Japan is idolization of the vagina. On 15 March, a procession is held in the town of Inuyama, a stylised mussel being the most important object among a host of phallic and vaginal symbols. A small girl is ensconced between the two shells, throwing rice cakes to the assembled multitude. And once every five years, the vagina-idol from the Ogata shrine meets her phallic counterpart from the nearby Tagata shrine.

Idolization of the vagina is not part of Western art, which does, however, contain some extremely suggestive images. Wijdeveld's (never implemented) design for an Amsterdam theatre is an impressive example. We are of course familiar with sex idols, and many people have undoubtedly had quite explicit fantasies about Marlene, Marilyn or Madonna. In the heyday of flower power, groupies were sometimes even more striking and alluring than the rock stars themselves.[35] A well known pair of groupies who called themselves the Plaster Casters were renowned for making plaster casts of erect penises that were exhibited inside domes of Lucite. It was quite an honour for a rock star to be chosen by the Plaster Casters. In Dušan Makavejev's film *WR: Mysteries of the Organism* (1971) this kind of procedure is documented at length as Jim Buckley (1947–1975) is expertly immortalized by Nancy Godfrey. In the twenty-first century things have become simpler: the artists Benno Rehwinkel and Paul Pieck have devised a do-it-yourself kit, which can be ordered from www.w-doubleyou.com.

Casts of vaginas must be more difficult to make. One Berlin silversmith specializes in necklaces with which a woman can adorn herself with a cast of her own clitoris.[36] The manufacturers of sex toys produce, in addition to blow-up dolls, vaginas made of soft plastic, for which quite a few porn stars have allowed their anatomy to be used as models. The contemporary masturbator can, if he so wishes, choose from among a number of extremely accessible idols. He can masturbate using the artificial vagina of the woman of his choice, while having free visual access to her most secret parts with the help of a video. He can also in some cases access her via the Internet. There are thus women today who know that at any given moment of the day

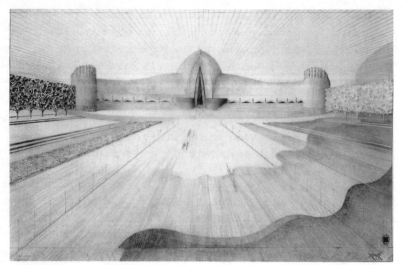

35
Architectural
sketch by
H. T. Wijdeveld.

a few hundred men may be having vicarious sex with them. These women, too, are being immortalized in a way.

Max de Roche's *Cooking for Love* gives an old European recipe that stands out for its charming simplicity: if a girl is interested in a boy, she must take some dough and press it to her vulva before she bakes it. 'Slit bread' is what the recipe is called, and success is said to be guaranteed.

The most intense form of adoration, however, is the personal worship of the beloved's body, although when put into words it often tends to sound cheap. An exception is Kate Millett's novel *Sita*. This love story involving sexual enslavement and constant crises of confidence includes Kate's admission to a 'looney bin'. Sita is ten years older than Kate, obviously much more experienced, with men as well as with women, and, as we heard earlier, she survived a horrifying rape experience during which her vagina was attacked with a knife. Kate's feelings about Sita's cunt are all-embracing:

> Her flesh so warm and delicate, so fragile and aromatic, smooth
> and golden and brown, so utterly dear to me, consumed in it, seen
> as vividly with my eyes closed as open, touched as unerringly with
> my mind as with my hands, putting all the concentration of passion
> in the tips of my fingers, entering her knowing she wants me and
> has made room, made the way smooth and liquid, hungers for my
> tongue as it thirsts to drink her, devour and never finish, that very
> blossom once blasted, damaged, the rapists, the desert – 'they had to
> sew my clitoris back on,' she told me savagely that first time, 'you'll
> find me a little beat up,' warning me gallantly – but how precious

and even dearer to me for its terrible wound, moved with what
particular care and compassion, the most reverential gentleness,
itself the most determined passion, for I would overwhelm it with
tenderness. Make up for, compensate, heal and erase the scars, the
hurts, all the hurts of your life, lady, dearest and loveliest and
most wronged of women, mine now, this moment, entirely mine,
coming as she comes, with the sheer force of adoring her.

Or, to leave the last word to Carlos Drummond de Andrade, I end with
a quotation from his poem 'Chestnut brown anemones, in your unyield-
ing garden':[37]

> Chestnut brown anemones, in your unyielding garden,
> restrain the impassioned hand. Be careful.
> Caress each petal or each sepal leisurely,
> Heavenly; and let the eyes rest,
> like an abstract kiss, even before the ritual kiss,
> on this budding flora, love; all is hallowed.

References

1 ON FEMININITY

1. Wack, 1968.
   Et ex hoc est quod aliqui mulieres quanto
   magis coheunt tanto magis appetunt cohire
   quia habent in collo matricis aliquos vapores
   colericos vel salsos et ideo quanto magis
   coheunt tanto magis habent pruritum.

2 SEARCHING FOR WORDS

1. Anne Frank, 1997.
2. Berriot-Salvadore, 1992.
3. Quoted in Berg, 1995.
4. Blum, 1978.
5. Heer de L∗∗∗, *heelmeester* ('Master de L∗∗∗,
   surgeon'), 1785.
6. Thomasset, 1990.
7. Jacquard and Thomasset, 1988.
8. R. M. Hodes, 1997.
9. Thompson, 1999.
10. In *Sextant*, Autumn 1998.
11. Bornoff, 1991.
12. Jong, 1980.
13. *Livre des blasons du corps féminin*, 1967.
14. . . . non pas . . ., mais petit sardinet,
    . . ., mon plaisir, mon gentil jardinet,
    Où ne fut oncq planté arbre ne souche
    . . ., joly . . . à la vermeille bouche,
    . . . mon petit mignon, ma petite fossette,
    . . . rebondy en forme de bosette;
    . . . revestu d'une riche toyson
    De fin poil d'or en sa vraye saison;
    . . .
    Tout ce qu'on faict, qu'on dict, ou qu'on
    procure,
    Tout ce qu'on veult, qu'on promet, qu'on
    assure
    C'est pour le . . . tant digne decorer,

Chascun te vient à genoux adorer.
Et suis contens de demerurer icy
Près de toy, . . . à te faire service,
Comme celuy qui m'est plus propice.
15. Wittig, 1970.
16. Kunst and Schutte, 1991.
17. Greer, 1971b.
18. Chalker, 2000.
19. Slauerhoff, *Al dwalend*.

**3 THE ANATOMY OF THE FEMALE GENITALS:
THE FACTS**

1. B. Hillen, 'Anatomie' in Heineman et al.,
   1999.
2. Van Voorhis et al., 2000.
3. J. Lowndes Sevely, 1987.
4. Sparks, 1977.
5. Frank and Glickman, 1994.
6. From Sarah Blafer Hrdy, 1999.
7. Steinetz et al., 1997.
8. Frank et al., 1991.
9. Genesis 3:16: 'Unto the woman he said, I will
   greatly multiply thy sorrow and thy conception; in sorrow thou shalt bring forth children
   and thy desire *shall* be to thy husband, and he
   shall rule over thee.'
10. Witz, 2000.
11. De Jong et al., 1999.
12. Van der Putte, 1991.
13. Krantz, 1970.

**4 PHYSIOLOGY: ON THE (SEXUAL) FUNCTION OF
THE GENITAL ORGANS**

1. Masters and Johnson, 1968.
2. Friday, 1973.
3. Kaplan, 1974.

4. Slob et al., 1999.
5. Bancroft et al., 1984.
6. Verhaeghe, 1991.
7. Freud and Andreas-Salomé, 1972.
8. Kinsey et al., 1953.
9. Goozen et al., 1997.
10. Bancroft, 2002.
11. Shafik, 1995.
12. Levin, 2003.
13. Giorgio and Siccardi, 1996.
14. An eighteenth century physician and writer quoted in Barker-Benfield, 1982.
15. 'Geen mop' in Hemmerechts, 1994.
16. Gianotten, 1988.
17. Quoted in Maines, 1977.
18. Ogden, 1944.
19. Chalker, 2000.
20. Ladas, Whipple and Perry, 1974.
21. Hines, 2001.
22. Huffman, 1948.
23. Chalker, 2000.
24. Quoted in Lowndes Sevely, 1987.

5 VIRGINITY

1. C.F.T. Voigt, *De gevaren der jeugd* (The dangers of youth), 1823. Quoted in Van Tilburg, 1998.
2. From Vogels and Van Vliet, 1990.
3. *De Volkskrant*, 2 September 2000.
4. Goosen, 1992.
5. Pinkerton, 2001.
6. Sanders and Reinisch, 1999.
7. Pitts and Rhaman, 2001.
8. Schwartz, 1993.
9. *Nederlands Tijdschrift voor Geneeskunde*, 2001.
10. Naamane-Guessous, 1990.
11. Ranke-Heinemann, 1988.
12. Middleton and Rowley, 1653. The word 'changeling' has two meanings: a) a child believed to have been exchanged by fairies for the parents' true child; and b) a fickle or changeable person.
13. Reyners, 1993.
14. Thiery and Houtzager, 1997.
15. Quoted in Reyners, 1993.
16. Naamane-Guessous, 1990.
17. Tannahill, 1980.
18. *De Telegraaf*, 2 August 2000.
19. Bornoff, 1991.
20. Van Gulik, 1974.
21. Van Gilse, 1942; Goosen, 1992.
22. Jacquard and Thomasset, 1988.

23. Green, 2001.
24. Tannahill, 1980.
25. Huisman, 1998.
26. Naamane-Guessous, 1990.
27. *De Volkskrant*, 22 August 2000; *Vrij Nederland*, 2 December 2000.
28. Cindoglu, 2002.
29. Huisman, 1998.

6 THE POWER OF FREUDIAN IDEAS

1. Van Wissen, 1978.
2. Jacquard and Thomasset, 1988.
3. Fischer, Van Hoorn and Jansz, 1983.
4. Alles am Weibe ist ein Rätsel, und alles am Weibe hat *eine* Lösung: Sie heisst Schwangerschaft.
5. Reprinted in Bonaparte, 1965.
6. Fischer, Van Hoorn and Jansz, 1983.
7. Groenendijk, 1997.
8. *L'Onanisme, Dissertation sur les maladies produites par la masturbation.*
9. Everard, 1994.
10. Ladas, Whipple and Perry, 1974.
11. In Burnes Moore, 1961.
12. Maines, 1999.
13. Chesser, 1941.
14. Roberts et al., 1995.
15. Bezemer, 1990.
16. Bourgeron, 1997.
17. Bourgeron, 1997.
18. Person, 1999.
19. Kapsalis, 1997.

7 ON REPRODUCTION

1. 'Damescomplot' (Ladies' plot), in Ree, 1985.
2. Jacquard and Thomasset, 1988.
3. Niethammer, 1977.
4. Jacquard and Thomasset, 1988.
5. Quoted in Thiery and Houtzager, 1997.
6. Dickinson, 1949.
7. Quoted in Clark and Zarrow, 1971.
8. Settlage et al., 1973, quoted in Levin, 1998.
9. Quoted in Laqueur, 1990.
10. Fox et al., 1970.
11. Baker, 1996.
12. Singh et al., 1998.
13. The account of the physiology of early pregnancy has been taken from Heineman et al., 1999.
14. *De Volkskrant*, 17 June 2000.
15. Seoud et al., 1987.

16. Tilstra, 1997.
17. Wilbers, 2001.
18. Hanson, 1975.
19. Hamerlynck and Mochtar, 1992.
20. Saleh et al., 2000.
21. López, 1967b.
22. Ranke-Heinemann, 1988.
23. Ranke-Heinemann, 1988.
24. Janssens et al., 2000.
25. Fukuda et al., 1996, 1999 and 2000.
26. Fukuda et al., 2001.
27. Fageeh et al., 2002.
28. Renckens, 2000.
29. Saadawi, 1980.
30. Nederlands Tijdschrift voor Geneeskunde, 2000.
31. Tiemessen et al., 1996.
32. Van Roijen et al., 1996.
33. Naamane-Guessous, 1990.
34. The Times of India, 22 April 2001.
35. Askling et al., 1999.
36. Thompson, 1999.
37. Berriot-Salvadore, 1992.
38. Nederlands Tijdschrift voor Geneeskunde, 144 (2000), 1327.
39. Hansen et al., 1999.
40. Mocarelli et al., 2000.
41. Wilcox et al., 1995.
42. Dutroux and Van Gestel, 2003.
43. Quoted in Drenth, 1988.
44. Drenth et al., 1995.
45. Verkuyl, 1988.
46. Reprinted in Nederlands Tijdschrift voor Geneeskunde 143 (1999), 1464.
47. Kaplan and Grotowski, 1996.
48. Beier, 2000.
49. Nederlands Tijdschrift voor Geneeskunde 144 (2000), 1132.
50. Lee and Boot, quoted in Kohl and Francoeur, 1995.
51. Knight Aldrich, 1972.
52. Ranke-Heinemann, 1988.
53. Abram, 1969.
54. Israëls, 1993.
55. Mol and Teer, 1987.
56. Naamane-Guessous, 1990.
57. Reproduction after death has become a real possibility. The male reproductive potential can be preserved in sperm banks for a considerable time, and if an IVF yields more fertilized eggs than can be used there and then, they can be frozen for future use. If the woman who supplied the eggs dies, can another woman help the widower to father his late wife's potential children? A brain-dead man whose organs were removed for transplantation and whose testicles were 'milked' for spermatozoa posed another ethical dilemma. The man had given his consent beforehand, his death (from a cerebral haemorrhage) having been fully expected.
58. Knight, 1960.
59. Van den Akker and Treffers, 1987.
60. De Josselin de Jong, 1922.
61. Cohen, 1949.
62. Van den Akker and Treffers, 1987.
63. Talalaj and Talalaj, 1994.
64. The old man:

> Gelt und gutz genung wil ich dir geben
> Wilstu nach meinem willen leben
> Greift mitter hannde in meiner tasschen
> Des slosz will ich dir auch erlassen.

The woman:

> Es hilft kein slosz für frauen list
> Kein trew mag sein dar lieb nit ist
> Darumb ain slüssel der mir gefelt
> Den wil ich kauffen umb dein gelt.

The young man:

> Ich drag ain slüssel zu solliche slossen
> Wie wol es manchen hat verdrossen
> Der hat der narren kappen fill
> Der rechte liebe kaufen will.

(Quoted in Schultz, 1984)
65. Masters and Johnson, 1968.
66. Hrdy, 1999.
67. Baker, 1996.
68. Penton-Voak et al., 1999.
69. Singh et al., 1998.
70. Van Boxsel, 2001.
71. Heinemann et al., 1999.
72. Black, 1988.
73. Jacquard and Thomasset, 1988.
74. Robinson and Short, 1977.
75. Varendi, Porter and Winberg, 1994.
76. Moors, 2000.
77. Fackelman, 1993.
78. Judson, 2002.
79. Nederlands Tijdschrift voor Geneeskunde 142 (1998), 1110.
80. Nederlands Tijdschrift voor Geneeskunde 143 (1999), 1273.
81. Kitzinger, 1983.
82. Ogden, 1994.
83. Walker, 1992.
84. Nederlands Tijdschrift voor Geneeskunde 141 (1997), 357.
85. Nederlands Tijdschrift voor Geneeskunde 143 (1999), 2369.
86. Nederlandsch Tijdschrift voor Geneeskunde (1901), 618.
87. Ranke-Heinemann, 1988.

88. Naamane-Guessous, 1990.

8 WOMEN'S SEX PROBLEMS

1. Wolfe, 1992.
2. Benard and Schlaffer, 1990.
3. Barbach, 1975.
4. All animals are sad after intercourse.
5. Jacquard and Thomasset, 1988.
6. Graber, 1982.
7. Kitchenham-Pec and Bopp, 1999.
8. Van der Velde, 1999.
9. Drenth, 1990.
10. Van Emde Boas, 1941.
11. Dickinson, 1949.
12. Weijmar Schultz and Van Driel, 1996.
13. Lee, 1996.
14. Quoted in Drenth, 1988a.
15. Scanzoni, 1867.
16. Quoted in Schoon, 1995.
17. Frenken and Van Tol, 1987.
18. Masters and Johnson, 1970.
19. Drenth, 1998a.
20. Thoben and Moors, 1978.
21. Drenth et al., 1995.
22. Drenth, 1998b.

9 CLITORIDECTOMY

1. Lightfoot-Klein, 1989.
2. Reyners, 1993.
3. Lightfoot-Klein, 1989.
4. *Nederlands Tijdschrift voor Geneeskunde* (2002), 801.
5. Lightfoot-Klein, 1989.
6. Kousbroek, 2002.
7. Walker, 1992.
8. Leonard, 2000.
9. Walker, 1992.
10. Barker-Benfield, 1976.
11. Quoted in Barker-Benfield, 1976.
12. Scull and Favreau, 1986.
13. Barker-Benfield, 1976.
14. Bonaparte, 1965.
15. Money and Ehrhardt, 1972.
16. De Jong, 1999.
17. In an undated issue of the Intersex Society of North America.
18. Longo, 1979.
19. Barker-Benfield, 1976.
20. Fistulas continue to pose an enormous health problem in developing countries. The gynae-cologist Kees Waaldijk has been working for nearly twenty years in a special fistula clinic in Nigeria. In the 1990s, the operation became routine: in most cases the condition could be cured in ten minutes under epidural anaesthe-sia, even under the most primitive conditions. Waaldijk intends to open an adequate number of clinics and to train doctors to operate on all women with fistulas. *Nederlands Tijdschrift voor Geneeskunde,* 143 (1999), 1384-5.
21. Rachel Maines, 1999.
22. Quoted in Scull and Favreau (1986).
23. Schoon, 1995.
24. Quoted in Scull and Favreau, 1986.
25. *Nederlands Tijdschrift voor Geneeskunde* 141 (1997), 498-9.
26. Gollaher, 2000.
27. For a detailed account see Gollaher, 2000.

10 THE PHYSICIAN AND THE UTERUS

1. Maines, 1999.
2. Lubsen-Brandsma, 1997.
3. Hanson, 1975.
4. Green, 2001.
5. Bernfeld, 1929.
6. Quoted in Maines, 1999.
7. Jacquard and Thomasset, 1988.
8. Thompson, 1999.
9. Pontanéry-Rougier, 1948.
10. Jacquard and Thomasset, 1988.
11. Laqueur, 2003.
12. Slavenburg, 1996.
13. Quoted in Maines, 1999.
14. Taken from Maines, 1999.
15. Jacobi, 1875.
16. Quoted in Maines, 1999.
17. Boyle, 1994. The film, also produced in 1994, was directed by Alan Parker.
18. Quoted in Steadman, 1979.
19. Brindley and Gillan, 1982.

11 THE VIBRATOR

1. Barker-Benfield, 1976.
2. Quoted in Maines, 1999.
3. Barbach, 1975.
4. Steenkamer, 1992.
5. Trost, 1972.
6. Heath, 1972.
7. Directed by Milos Forman (1975), based on the novel by Ken Kesey.
8. Moan and Heath, 1972.
9. Laarakkers, 1995.

10. Ungerer, 1971.
11. *De Volkskrant*, 18 January 2003.

12 THE SCENT OF WOMEN

1. Roth, 1999.
2. Anne Frank, 1997.
3. Bonsall and Michael, 1978.
4. Drenth, 1998a.
5. Kohl and Francoeur, 1995.
6. Miersch, 1999.
7. Garcia-Velasco and Mondragon, 1991.
8. Monti-Bloch and Grosser, 1991.
9. Kohl and Francoeur, 1995.
10. McClintock, 1998.
11. Kohl and Francoeur, 1995.
12. Kohl and Francoeur, 1995.

13 FEAR AND LOATHING OF FEMININITY

1. From 'Heilig vuur' (Holy fire) in Friedman, 1996.
2. Longman, 2002.
3. Anat Zuria, 2002.
4. Gollaher, 2000.
5. Saadawi, 1980.
6. Hays, 1964.
7. Niethammer, 1977.
8. Leviticus 20:18.
9. Jacquard and Thomasset, 1988.
10. Shorter, 1982
11. Angier, 1999.
12. Kosinski, 1997.
13. Kinsey et al., 1953.
14. Kunst and Schutte, 1991.
15. Quoted in López, 1967a.
16. Roth, 1999.
17. Niethammer, 1977.
18. Wittig, 1970.
19. Hays, 1964.
20. Simons, 1974.
21. Altaffer, 1983.
22. Kräupl-Taylor, 1979.
23. Musgrave, 1980.
24. *Livre du Chevalier de la Tour Landry pour l'enseignement de ses filles.*
25. Jacquard and Thomasset, 1988.
26. Jacquard and Thomasset, 1988.
27. Beit-Hallahmi, 1985.
28. Hays, 1964.
29. Beit-Hallahmi, 1985.
30. Van Driel, 1997.
31. Van de Velde, 1999.

32. Shorter, 1982.
33. Fields, 2000.
34. Greer, 1971a.

14 IDEALIZATION AND WORSHIP OF THE FEMALE GENITALS

1. Wittig, 1970.
2. Quoted in Van Gulik, 1974.
3. Bornoff, 1991.
4. Morris, 1971.
5. Roth, 1999.
6. Gollaher, 2000.
7. Dickinson, 1949.
8. Rouzier et al., 2000.
9. Niethammer, 1977.
10. Angier, 1999.
11. *Volkskrant Magazine*, 2000.
12. Devereux, 1958.
13. Angier, 1999.
14. Schönmayer and Kessel, 1999.
15. Lehmann, 1997.
16. Bornoff, 1991.
17. Naamane-Guessous, 1990.
18. Laqueur, 2000.
19. Wolf, 1997.
20. In the Groningen students' journal *De Nieuwe Clercke.*
21. Naamane-Guessous, 1990.
22. Van Gulik, 1974.
23. Maines, 1999.
24. Hays, 1964.
25. Laurier, 1993.
26. Boon and Van Schie, 1999.
27. Van Gulik, 1974.
28. Bornoff, 1991.
29. Directed by Zhang Yimou, 1991.
30. Rubenstein, 1980.
31. Van Gulik, 1974.
32. *Vedrai carino, se sei buonino*
   che bel remedio ti voglio dar.
   E naturale; non dà disgusto
   e lo speziale non lo sà far.
   E un certo balsamo che porto adesso,
   dare te 'l sposso, se 'l voi provar.
   Saper vorresti dove me stà?
   Senti lo battere, tocca mi quà.
33. Van Gelder (ed.), 2000.
34. Kapsalis, 1997.
35. Wurtzel, 1998.
36. Schönmayer and Kessel, 1999.
37. Carlos Drummond de Andrade, 1992.

Bibliography

Abram, H. S., 'Pseudocyesis followed by true pregnancy in the termination phase of an analysis', *British Journal of Medical Psychology*, 42 (1969), pp. 255–62

Akker, L.P.M. van den and P.D.A. Treffers, 'Een man wordt ouder. Over het begin van het vaderschap', *Nederlands Tijdschrift voor Geneeskunde*, 131 (1987), pp. 2400–405

Altaffer III, L. F., 'Penis Captivus and the Mischievous Sir William Osler', *Southern Medical Journal*, 76 (1983), pp. 637–41

Andehazi, F., *De anatoom*, trans. Fred de Vries (Amsterdam, 1997)

Anon., 'Anonieme bevallingen. Berichten buitenland', *Nederlands Tijdschrift voor Geneeskunde*, 144 (2000), p. 1132

Askling, J., G. Erlandson, M. Kaijser, O. Akre and A. Ekborn, 'Sickness in pregnancy and sex of child', *The Lancet*, 354 (1999), p. 2053

Baker, R., *Sperm Wars* (London, 1996)

Baker Brown, I., 'On the curability of certain forms of insanity, epilepsy, catalepsy, and hysteria in females' (1866), reprinted in R. Barreca, *Desire and Imagination* (London, 1995)

Bancroft, J. 'Sexual effects of androgens in women: some theoretical considerations', *Fertility and Sterility*, 77 (2002), supplement 4S, pp. 55–9

Bancroft, J., R. O'Carroll, A. Mc.Neilly and R. W. Shaw, 'The effect of bromocriptin on the sexual behaviour of hyperprolactinaemic man: a controlled case study', *Clinical Endocrinology*, 21 (1984), pp. 131–8

Barbach, L. G., *For Yourself* (New York, 1975)

Barker-Benfield, G. J., *The Horrors of the Half-known Life* (New York, 1976)

Barker-Benfield, G. J., *The Culture of Sensibility* (Chicago and London, 1982)

Beier, K. M., 'Female analogies to perversion', *Journal of Sex and Marital Therapy*, 26 (2000), pp. 79–93

Beit-Hallahmi, B., 'Dangers of the vagina', *British Journal of Medical Psychology*, 58 (1985), pp. 351–6

Benard, C. and E. Schlaffer, *Laat die mannen toch met rust* (Baarn, 1990)

Bernfeld, W., 'Eine Beschwörung der Gebärmutter aus dem frühen Mittelalter', *Kyklos*, 2 (1929), pp. 272–4

Berg, J. H. van den, *Metabletica van God* (Kampen, 1995)

Berriot-Salvadore, E., 'De vrouw in geneeskunde en natuurwetenschap', in *Geschiedenis van de vrouw*, vol. 3, *Van Renaissance tot de moderne tijd*, ed. G. Duby and M. Perrot (Amsterdam, 1992)

Bezemer, W., 'Vaginisme en dyspareunie en de partnerrelatie. Enkele resultaten van een onderzoek', in *Vaginisme en dyspareunie*, ed. J.P.C. Moors (Houten, 1990)

Biggs, Robert D., *ŠÀ.ZI.GA: Ancient Mesopotamian Potency Incantations* (New York, 1967)

Black, J., *Body Talk* (North Ryde and London, 1988)

Blécourt, W. de, *Het amazonenleger. Irreguliere genezeressen in Nederland 1850–1930* (Amsterdam, 1999)

Blum, L. H., 'Darkness in an enlightened era: women's drawings of their sexual organs', *Psychological Reports*, 42 (1978), pp. 867–73

Bonaparte, M., *Female Sexuality* (New York, 1965)

Bonsall, R. W. and R. P. Michael, 'Volatile odoriferous acids in vaginal fluid', in *The Human Vagina*, ed. E.S.E. Hafez and T. N. Evans (Amsterdam, 1978)

Boon, M. E. and M. A. van Schie, 'Vaginaal

douchen is zo slecht nog niet', *Medisch Contact*, 54 (1999), pp. 546–9

Bornoff, N., *Pink Samurai; an erotic exploration of Japanese society* (London, 1991)

Bourgeron, J. P., *Marie Bonaparte* (Paris, 1997)

Boxsel, M. van, *De Encyclopedie van de Domheid* (Amsterdam, 2001), trans. as *The Encyclopaedia of Stupidity* (London, 2003)

Boyle, T. Coraghessan, *The Road to Welville* (London, 1998)

Breuer, J. and S. Freud, *Studies on Hysteria*, Standard Edition of the Complete Works of Sigmund Freud, vol. 2, trans. James Strachey (London, 1974)

Brindley, G. S. and P. Gillan, 'Men and women who do not have orgasms', *British Journal of Psychiatry*, 140 (1982), pp. 351–6

Bruijn, G. de, 'From masturbation to orgasm with a partner: how some women bridge the gap – and why others don't', *Journal of Sex and Marital Therapy*, 8 (1982), pp. 151–67

Bruijn, G. de, *Vrijen met een man, kan dat dan?* (Baarn, 1985)

Burt, J. C. and A. R. Schramm, 'Plastic surgical postero-lateral redirection extension vulvovaginoplasty', *Annales Chirurgiae et Gynaecologiae*, 72 (1983), pp. 268–73

Chalker, R., *The Clitoral Truth; the Secret World at Your Fingertips* (New York, 2000)

Chesser, E., *Love Without Fear* (London, 1941)

Cindoglu, D., 'Virginity tests and artificial virginity in modern Turkish medicine', *Women and Sexuality in Muslim Societies* (Istanbul, 2001)

Clark, J. H. and M. X. Zarrow, 'Influence of copulation on time of ovulation in women', *American Journal of Obstetrics and Gynecology*, 107 (1971), pp. 1083–5

Cohen, G., 'La couvade (la femme accouche et l'homme se couche)', *Psyche (Paris)*, 4 (1949), pp. 80–93

Coninck, H. de, *De haeteren van het geheugen* (Antwerp, n.d.)

Crenshaw, T. L., *Why We Love and Lust* (London, 1996)

Dekker, M., *Lief dier* (Amsterdam, 1992)

Devereux, G., 'The significance of the external female genitalia and of female orgasm for the male', *Journal of the American Psychoanalytic Association*, 6 (1958), pp. 278–86

Dickinson, R. L., *Human Sex Anatomy*, 2nd edn (London, 1949)

Dirie, W., *Mijn woestijn* (Amsterdam, 1998)

Drenth, J. J., 'Vaginismus and the desire for a

child', *Journal of Psychosomatic Obstetrics and Gynaecology*, 9 (1988a), pp. 125–37

Drenth, J. J., 'What's in a name', *Tijdschrift voor Seksuologie*, 22 (1988b), pp. 145–51

Drenth, J. J., 'A contribution from the past: Coen van Emde Boas's (1904–1981) interpretation of some cases of female dyspareunia', *Sexual and Marital Therapy*, 5 (1990), pp. 175–81

Drenth, J. J., 'The tight foreskin: a psychosomatic phenomenon', *Sexual and Marital Therapy*, 6 (1991), pp. 297–306

Drenth, J. J., S. Andriessen, M. P. Heringa, M.J.E. Mourits, H.B.M. van de Wiel and W.C.M. Weijmar Schultz, 'Connections between primary vaginismus and procreation: some observations from clinical practice', *Journal of Psychosomatic Obstetrics and Gynaecology*, 17 (1996), pp. 195–201

Driel, M. van, *Het geheime deel* (Amsterdam, 1997)

Drummond de Andrade, Carlos, *De liefde, natuurlijk*, trans. August Willemsen (Amsterdam, 1992)

Dutroux, V. and G. van Gestel, *'Mijn zoon Marc Dutroux'* (Antwerp, 2003)

Emde Boas, C. van, 'Coïtusmoeilijkheden (pseudovaginisme) door een variatie der symphysis', *Nederlands Tijdschrift voor Geneeskunde*, 85 (1941), pp. 2178–81

Enoch, M. D and W. H. Trethowan, *Uncommon Psychiatric Syndromes* (Bristol, 1979)

Everard, M., *Ziel en zinnen* (Groningen, 1994)

Fackelman, K. A., 'Hormone of monogamy', *Science News*, 144 (1993), pp. 360–65

Fageeh, W., H. Raffa, H. Jabbad and A. Marzouki, 'Transplantation of the human uterus', *International Journal of Gynecology and Obstetrics*, 76 (2002), pp. 245–51

Fields, J., 'Erotic modesty: (Ad)dressing female sexuality and propriety in open and closed drawers, USA, 1800–1930', *Gender and History*, 14 (2002), pp. 492–515

Fischer, A., W. van Hoorn and J. Jansz, *Psychoanalyse en vrouwelijke seksualiteit* (Meppel, 1983)

Fox, C. A., H. S. Wolff and J. A. Bakker, 'Measurement of intra-vaginal and intra-uterine pressure during human coitus by radiotelemetry', *Journal of Reproduction and Fertility*, 22 (1970), pp. 243–51

Francoeur, R. T., ed., *The International Encyclopedia of Sexuality* (New York, 1997)

Frank, Anne, *The Diary of a Young Girl. The Definitive Edition*, trans. Susan Massotty (London, 1997)

Frank, L. G. and S. E. Glickman, 'Giving birth through a penile clitoris: parturition and dystocia in the spotted hyaena (Crocuta crocuta)', *Journal of Zoology*, 234 (1994), pp. 659–90

Frank, L. G., S. E. Glickman and P. Light, 'Fatal sibling aggression, precocial development, and androgens in neonatal spotted hyenas', *Science*, 252 (1991), pp. 702–4

Frenken, J. and P. van Tol, 'Sexual problems in gynaecological practice', *Journal of Psychosomatic Obstetrics and Gynaecology*, 6 (1987), pp. 143–55

Friday, N., *Diepe gronden* (Utrecht and Antwerp, 1973)

Friedman, C., *De grauwe minnaar* (Amsterdam, 1996)

Fugger, E. F., 'Clinical experience with flow cytometric separation of human X- and Y-chromosome bearing sperm', *Theriogenology*, 52 (1999), pp. 1435–40

Fukuda, M., K. Fukuda, C. Y. Andersen and A. G. Byskov, 'Contralateral selection of dominant follicle favours pre-embryo development', *Human Reproduction*, 11 (1996), pp. 1958–62

Fukuda, M., K. Fukuda, C. Y. Andersen and A. G. Byskov, 'Anovulations in an ovary during two menstrual cycles enhance the pregnancy potential of oocytes matured in that ovary during the following third cycle', *Human Reproduction*, 14 (1999), pp. 96–100

Fukuda, M., K. Fukuda, C. Y. Andersen and A. G. Byskov, 'Does anovulation induced by oral contraceptives favor pregnancy during the following two menstrual cycles?', *Fertility and Sterility*, 73 (2000), pp. 742–7

Fukuda, M., K. Fukuda, C.Y. Andersen and A.G. Byskov, 'Characteristics of human ovulation in natural cycles correlated with age and achievement of pregnancy', *Human Reproduction*, 16 (2001), pp. 2501–7

Garcia-Velasco, J. and M. Mondragon, 'The incidence of the vomeronasal organ in 1000 human subjects and its possible clinical significance', *Journal of Steroid Biochemistry and Molecular Biology*, 39 (1991), pp. 561–3

Gelder, G. J. van, ed., *Een Arabische tuin. Klassieke Arabische poëzie* (Amsterdam and Leuven, 2000)

Gianotten, W. L., 'Zwangerschap en orgasme', *Tijdschrift voor Verloskunde*, 13 (1988), pp. 326–9

Gils, C. van and W. Bezemer, *De gesloten vrouw* (Baarn, 1994)

Gilse, J.B.F. van, 'Beroemde vroedvrouwen', *Nederlands Tijdschrift voor Geneeskunde*, 86 (1942), pp. 573–9

Giorgio, G. and M. Siccardi, 'Ultrasonic observation of a female fetus' sexual behavior in utero', *American Journal of Obstetrics and Gynaecology*, 175 (1996), p. 753

Giphart, R., *Het feest der liefde* (Amsterdam, 1995)

Glastra van Loon, K., *De passievrucht* (Amsterdam and Antwerp, 1999)

Golden, A., *Memoirs of a Geisha* (London, 1998)

Gollaher, D. L., *Circumcision. A History of the World's Most Controversial Surgery* (New York, 2000)

Goosen, L., *Van Andreas tot Zacheus* (Nijmegen, 1992)

Goozen, S.H.M., V. M. Woegant, E. Endert, F. A. Helmond and N. E. van de Poll, 'Psychoendocrinological asessment of the menstrual cycle: the relationship between hormones, sexuality and mood', *Archives of Sexual Behavior*, 26 (1997), pp. 359–82

Graber, B., *Circumvaginal Musculature and Sexual Function* (Basel, 1982)

Green, M.H., *The Trotula* (Philadelphia, 2001)

Greer, G., 'Body odour and the persuaders', *Sunday Times*, 25 July 1971, reprinted in G. Greer, *The Madwoman's Underclothes* (London, 1986) (1971a)

Greer, G., 'Lady love your cunt', *Suck*, 1971, reprinted in G. Greer, *The Madwoman's Underclothes* (London, 1986) (1971b)

Groenendijk, L. F., 'Masturbation and neurasthenia: Freud and Stekel in debate on the harmful effects of autoeroticism', *Journal of Psychology and Human Sexuality*, 9 (1997), pp. 71–93

Gulik, R. H. van, *Sexual Life in Ancient China* (Leiden, 1974)

Halban, J., *Gynäkologische Operationslehre* (Berlin and Vienna, 1932)

Hamerlynck, J.V.T.H. and M. H. Mochtar, 'Het risico van een onbedoelde zwangerschap na een onbeschermde coïtus; beschouwing bij de huidige postcoïtale anticonceptiemethoden', *Nederlands Tijdschrift voor Geneeskunde*, 136 (1992), pp. 2159–61

Hansen, D., H. Moeller and J. Olsen, 'Severe periconceptional life events and the sex ratio in offspring: follow-up study based on five national registers', *British Medical Journal*, 319 (1999), pp. 548–9

Hanson, A. E., 'Hippocrates: Diseases of women 1', *Journal of Women in Culture and Society*, 1

(1975), pp. 567–84

Hays, H. R., *The Dangerous Sex. The Myth of Feminine Evil* (New York, 1964)

Heath, R. G., 'Pleasure and brain activity in man', *Journal of Nervous and Mental Diseases*, 154 (1972), pp. 3–18

Heineman, M. J., O. P. Bleker, J.L.H. Evers and A.P.M. Heinz, eds, *Obstetrie en gynaecologie. De voortplanting van de mens* (Maarssen, 1999)

Hemmerechts, K., *Lang geleden* (n.p., 1994)

Hines, T.M., 'The G-spot: a modern gynecologic myth', *American Journal of Obstetrics and Gynecology*, 185 (2001), pp. 359–62

Hite, S., *The Hite Report* (New York, 1976)

Hodes, R. M., 'Cross-cultural medicine and diverse health beliefs; Ethiopians abroad', *Western Medical Journal*, 166 (1997), pp. 29–36

J. W. Huffman, 'The detailed anatomy of the paraurethral ducts in the adult human female, *American Journal of Obstetrics and Gynecology*, 55 (1948), pp. 86–101.

Hoffman, T., *23 brieven aan Frits van Egters over het maken van De Avonden* (Amsterdam, 1997)

Horney, K., *Feminine Psychology* (New York and London, 1967)

Hrdy, S. B., *Mother's Nature* (New York, 1999)

Huisman, W. M., 'Trans-cultural medicine', *Curare Sonderband* (special issue), 15 (1998), pp. 21–34

Irving, J., *The Cider House Rules* (New York, 1985)

Israëls, H., *Het geval Freud* (Amsterdam, 1993)

Jacobi, A., 'On masturbation and hysteria in young children', *Journal of Medical Association New York* (November 1875)

Jacquard, D., 'De vrouwelijke natuur', in *Geschiedenis van de vrouw*, vol. 2, *De Middeleeuwen*, ed. G. Duby and M. Perrot (Amsterdam, 1990)

Jacquard, D. and C. Thomasset, *Sexuality and Medicine in the Middle Ages* (Cambridge, 1988)

Janssens, R.M.J., C. B. Lambalk, J.P.W. Vermeiden, R. Schats and J. Schoemaker, 'In-vitro fertilization in a spontaneous cycle: easy, cheap and realistic', *Human Reproduction*, 15 (2000), pp. 314–18

Jelinek, E., *The Piano Teacher*, trans.Joachim Neugroschel (New York, 1988)

Jong, E., *Fanny* (New York, 1980)

Jong, J. J. de, R. W. Brouwer, H. F. Veen and J.G.J. Jonkman, 'Vrije lucht onder het diafragma: niet altijd een acuut chirurgisch probleem', *Nederlands Tijdschrift voor Geneeskunde*, 143 (1999), pp. 2033–7

Jong, T. de, *Man of vrouw, min of meer* (Amsterdam, 1999)

Josselin de Jong, J.P.B. de, 'De couvade', *Mededelingen der Koninklijke Akademie van Wetenschappen, Afd. Letterkunde*, vol. 54, series B, 1922

Judson, O., *Dr Tatiana's Sex Advice to All Creation* (New York, 2002)

Kal, J., *1000 sonnetten* (Amsterdam, 1997)

Kamvisseli, Euruduce, *F/3* (Evanston, IL, 1991)

Kaplan, H. S., *The New Sex Therapy* (New York, 1974)

Kaplan, H. S. and T. Owett, 'The female androgen deficiency syndrome', *Journal of Sex and Marital Therapy*, 19 (1993), pp. 3–24

Kaplan, R. and G. Grotowski, 'Denied pregnancy', *Australian and New Zealand Journal of Psychiatry*, 30 (1996), pp. 861–3

Kapsalis, T., *Public Privates* (Durham and London, 1997)

Kinsey, A. C., W. B. Pomeroy, C. E. Martin and P. H. Gebhard, *Sexual Behavior in the Human Female* (Philadelphia and London, 1953)

Kitchenham-Pec, S. and A. Bopp, *Bekkenbodemtraining* (Amsterdam, 1999)

Kitzinger, S., *Het intieme lichaam* (Utrecht and Antwerp, 1983)

Koelman, C.A., A. B. Coumans, H. W. Nijman, I. I. Doxiadis, G. A. Dekker and F. H. Claas, 'Correlation between oral sex and a low incidence of preeclampsia: a role for soluble HLA in seminal fluid?', *Journal of Reproductive Immunology*, 46 (2000), pp. 155–60

Kohl, J. V. and R. T. Francoeur, *The Scent of Eros* (New York, 1995)

Kosinski, J., *Steps* (New York, 1997)

Kousbroek, R., *Scheermesje in opkomst*, NRC, 12 July 2002

Knight, J. A., 'False pregnancy in a male', *Psycho-somatic Medicine*, 22 (1960), pp. 260–66

Knight Aldrich, C., 'A case of recurrent pseudocyesis', *Perspectives in Biology and Medicine*, 16/2 (1972), pp. 11–21

Krantz, K. E., 'The anatomy and physiology of the vulva and vagina and the anatomy of the urethra and bladder', in *Scientific Foundations of Obstetrics and Gynaecology*, ed. E. E. Philipp, J. Barnes and M. Newton (London, 1970)

Kräupl-Taylor, F., 'Penis captivus – did it occur?',

British Medical Journal, 280 (1979),
pp. 977–8

Kunst, H. and X. Schutte, Lesbiaans. Lexicon
van de lesbotaal (Amsterdam, 1991)

L., Natuurkundige beschouwing van de man en
de vrouw in den huwelyken staat
(Amsterdam and Leiden, 1785)

Laarakkers, I., 'Ontwerp van een seksueel
hulpmiddel voor vrouwen', Tijdschrift voor
Seksuologie, 22 (1998), pp. 113–18

Ladas, A. K., B. Whipple and J. D. Perry,
De G-plek (Baarn, 1974)

Laqueur, T. W., Making Sex. Body and Gender
from the Greeks to Freud (Cambridge, MA,
1990)

Laqueur, T .W., Solitary Sex. A Cultural History
of Masturbation (New York, 2003)

Laurier, J., Een hemels meisje (Amsterdam, 1993)

Lawrence, D. H., Lady Chatterley's Lover
(London, 1960)

Lee, P. A., 'Survey report: concept of penis size',
Journal of Sex and Marital Therapy, 22
(1996), pp. 131–5

Lehmann, A.-S., 'Het andere haar', Kunstschrift,
2 (1997), pp. 32–9

Leonard, L., ' "We did it for pleasure only":
hearing alternative tales of female
circumcision', Qualitative Inquiry, 6 (2000),
pp. 212–28

Levin, R .J., 'Sex and the human female
reproductive tract – what really happens
during and after coitus', Internal Journal of
Impotence Research, 10 (1998), pp. 14–21

Levin, R. J., 'Do women gain anything from
coitus apart from pregnancy? Changes in the
human female genital tract activated by
coitus' , Journal of Sex and Marital Therapy,
29 (2003), pp. 59–69

Lightfoot-Klein, H., Prisoners of Ritual (London,
1989)

Livre des blasons du corps féminin, Editions
André Balland, 1967

Longman, C., 'Joodse menstruatieriten: symbool
van vrouwenonderdrukking of vrouwelijke
identiteit?', Tijdschrift voor Seksuologie,
26 (2002), pp. 146–52

Longo, L. D., 'The rise and fall of Battey's
operation', Bulletin of the History of
Medicine, 53 (1979), pp. 224–67

López, E., God als vrouw (Amsterdam, 1967a)

López, E., De prijsstier (Amsterdam, 1967b)

Lowndes Sevely, J., Eve's Secrets (London, 1987)

Lubsen-Brandsma, M.A.C., 'Het veterpotje van
Jan Steen, Zwangerschapstest of gynae-
cologisch therapeuticum in de zeventiende

eeuw?', Nederlands Tijdschrift voor
Geneeskunde, 141 (1997), pp. 2513–16

Maines, R. P., The Technology of Orgasm
(Baltimore, 1999)

Masters, W. H. and V. E. Johnson, Human Sexual
Response (New York,1968)

Masters, W. H. and V. E. Johnson, Human Sexual
Inadequacy (New York, 1970)

McClintock, M. K. 'Whither menstrual
synchrony?', Annual Review of Sex
Research, 9 (1998), pp. 77–95

Middleton, T. and W. Rowley, The Changeling
(London, 1958 [1653])

Millett, K., Sita (London, 1976)

Moan, C. E. and R. G. Heath, 'Septal stimulation
for the initiation of heterosexual behavior in
a homosexual male', Journal of Behaviour
Therapy and Experimental Psychiatry, 3
(1972), pp. 22–30

Mocarelli, P. et.al., 'Paternal concentrations of
dioxin and sex ratio of offspring', The
Lancet, 355 (2000), pp. 1858–63

Mol, E.M.M. and W. Teer, 'Het syndroom van
Münchhausen', Nederlands Tijdschrift voor
Geneeskunde, 131 (1987), pp. 2337–9

Money, J. and A. A. Ehrhardt, Man and Woman,
Boy and Girl (Baltimore, 1972)

Monti-Bloch, L. and B. I. Grosser, 'Effect of
putative pheromones on the electrical activity
of the human vomeronasal organ and
olfactory epithelium', K. Steroid Biochem.
Molec. Biol., 39 (1991) pp. 573–82

Moore, B. E. 'Panel report: frigidity in women',
Journal of the American Psychoanalytic
Association, 9 (1961), pp. 571–84

Moors, J.P.C., 'Seks tijdens zwangerschap en
periode post-partum', Huisarts en Weten-
schap, 43 (2000), pp. 213–18

Morris, D. Intimate Behaviour (London, 1971)

Mouthaan, I., M. de Neef et al., Twee levens.
Dilemma's van islamitische meisjes rondom
maagdelijkheid (Delft, 1997)

Mulisch, H. Het seksuele bolwerk (Amsterdam,
1983)

Musgrave, B., 'Penis captivus has occurred',
British Medical Journal, 280 (1980), p. 51

Naamane-Guessous, S., Achter de schermen van
de schaamte (Amsterdam, 1990)

Narjani, A. E. (pseudonym of M. Bonaparte),
'Considérations sur les causes anatomiques
de la frigidité chez la femme', Bruxelles-
Médical, 42 (1924), pp. 768–78

Niethammer, C., Daughters of the Earth. The
Lives and Legends of American Indian
Women (New York, 1977)

Ogden, N., *Vrouwen en seks* (Utrecht, 1994)

Penton-Voak, I. S., D. I. Perrett, D. L. Castles, T. Kobayashi, D. M. Bnurt, L. K. Murray and R. Minamisawa, 'Menstrual cycle alters face preference', *Nature*, 399 (1999), pp. 741–2

Person, E. S., *The Sexual Century* (New Haven and London, 1999)

Pinkerton, S. D., 'A relative risk-based, disease-specific definition of sexual abstinence failure rates', *Health Education and Behavior*, 28 (2001), pp. 10–20

Pitts, M. and Q. Rahman, 'Which behaviors constitute "having sex" among university students in the UK?', *Archives of Sexual Behavior*, 30 (2001), pp. 169–76

Plasterk, R., *Leven uit het lab* (Amsterdam, 2000)

Pontanéry-Rougier, 'Action de message gynecologique sur le vaginisme', *Comptes rendus de la Société Française de Gynécologie*, 18 (1948), pp. 15–18

Pranzarone, G. F., 'Sexuoerotic stimulation and response in the management of parturition: an immodest proposal', Lecture delivered before the Ninth World Sexology Congress in Caracas

Putte, S.C.J. van der, 'Anogenital "sweat" glands. Histology and pathology of a gland that may mimic mammary glands', *American Journal of Dermatopathology*, 13 (1991), pp. 557–67

Ranke-Heinemann, U., *Eunuchen voor het hemelrijk* (Baarn, 1988)

Réage, P., *The Story of O*, trans. J. P. Hand (London, 1954)

Ree, H., *Een man merkt nooit iets* (Amsterdam, 1985)

Renckens, C., *Kwakzalvers op kaliloog* (Amsterdam, 2000)

Reyners, M.M.J., *Het besnijden van meisjes* (Amsterdam, 1993)

Roberts, C., S. Kippax, C. Waldby and J. Crawford, 'Faking it. The story of "Ohh!"', *Women's Studies International Forum*, 18 (1995), pp. 523–32

Robinson, J. E. and R. V. Short, 'Changes in breast sensitivity at puberty, during the menstrual cycle, and at parturition', *British Medical Journal*, 1 (1977), pp. 1188–91

Rodenko, P., *Vrijmoedige verhalen* (Utrecht, 1980)

Roijen, J. H. van, A. K. Slob, W. L. Gianotten, G. R. Dohle, A.T.M. van der Zon, J.T.M. Vreeburg and R.F.A. Weber, 'Sexual arousal and the quality of semen produced by masturbation', *Human Reproduction*, 11 (1996), pp. 147–51

Roth, P., *Portnoy's Complaint* (London, 1999)

Rouzier, R., C. Louis-Sylvestre, B.-J. Paniel and B. Hassad, 'Hypertrophy of the labia minora: experience with 163 reductions.' *American Journal of Obstetrics and Gynaecology*, 182 (2000), pp. 35–40

Rubenstein, R., 'Een man uit Singapore', in *Over de liefde* (Amsterdam, 1980)

Saadawi, N. el, *De gesluierde Eva* (Leuven, 1980)

Saleh, A., S. L. Tang, M. M. Biljan and T. Tulandi, 'A randomized study of the effect of 10 minutes of bed rest after intrauterine insemination', *Fertility and Sterility*, 74 (2000), pp. 509–11

Sanders, S. A. and J. M. Reinisch, 'Would you say you "had sex" if . . . ?', *Journal of the American Medical Association*, 281 (1999), pp. 275–7

Scanzoni, 'Ueber Vaginismus', *Wiener Medizinische Wochenschrift*, 17 (1867)

Schaik, C. T. van, 'Commentaar', *Tijdschrift voor Psychotherapie*, 1 (1975), pp. 133–5

Schönmayer, S. and M. Kessel, *Lexikon der Lustmittel* (Frankfurt am Main, 1999)

Schoon, L., *De gynaecologie als belichaming van vrouwen* (Zutphen, 1995)

Schreuders-Bais, C. A., M. I. Baas and J.M.J. Dony, 'De waardering voor operatieve behandeling van focale vestibulitis', *Nederlands Tijdschrift voor Obstetrie en Gynaecologie*, 110 (1997), pp. 37–8

Schultz, A., *Das Band der Venus* (Isny, 1984)

Schwartz, I. M., 'Affective reactions of American and Swedish women to their first premarital coitus: a cross-cultural comparison', *Journal of Sex Research*, 30 (1993), pp. 18–26

Scull, A. and D. Favreau, ' "A chance to cut is a chance to cure": sexual surgery for psychosis in three nineteenth century societies', *Research in Law, Deviance and Social Control*, 8 (1986), pp. 3–39

Seoud, M.A.F., H. Khayyat and S. K. Mufarrij, 'Ectopic pregnancy in an undescended fallopian tube: an unusual presentation', *American Journal of Obstetrics and Gynaecology*, 69 (1987), pp. 455–7

Settlage, D. S. F., M. Motoshima and D. R. Tredway, 'Sperm transport from the external cervical os to the fallopian tubes in women: a time and quantitation study', *Fertility and Sterility*, 24 (1973), pp. 655–61

Shafik, A., 'The vagino-levator reflex: description of a reflex and its role in sexual performance', *European Journal of Obstetrics and*

Gynecology, 60 (1995), pp. 161–4

Shalev, M., *De grote vrouw*, trans. Ruben Verhasselt (Amsterdam, 1998)

Shorter, E., *Geschiedenis van het vrouwelijk lichaam* (Baarn, 1982)

Shuttle, P. and P. Redgrove, *The Wise Wound* (London, 1994)

Simons, G. L., *The Illustrated Book of Sexual Records* (London, 1974)

Singh, D., W. Meyer, R. J. Zambarano and D. F. Hurlbert. 'Frequency and timing of orgasm in women desirous of becoming pregnant', *Journal of Sex and Marital Therapy* (1998)

Slavenburg, J., *De mislukte man. Vrouw en seksualiteit in het Christendom* (Zutphen, 1996)

Slob, A. K., C. W. Vink, J.P.C. Moors and W. Everaerd, eds, *Leerboek seksuologie* (Houten and Diegem, 1998)

Sno, H. N., 'Pseudocyesis, een psychogene conceptie', *Tijdschrift voor Psychiatrie*, 27 (1985), pp. 15–25

Sparks, J., *Het hijgend hert en andere hoogstandjes* (Utrecht, 1977)

Steenkamer, J. G., 'Seksueel hulpmiddel voor gehandicapten: het ontwerpen van een masturbatiehulpmiddel voor handge-handicapten', *Tijdschrift voor Seksuologie*, 16 (1992), pp. 237–46

Steinetz, B. G., C. Randolph, M. Weldele, L. G. Frank, P. Licht and S. E. Glickman, 'Pattern and source of secretion of relaxin in the reproductive cycle of the spotted hyena (Crocuta crocuta)', *Biology of Reproduction*, 56 (1997), pp. 1301–6

Strindberg, A., *The Father*, trans. Michael Meyer (London, 1983)

Süskind, P., *Perfume*, trans. John E. Woods (London, 1995)

Talalaj, J. and S. Talalaj, *The Strangest Human Sex Ceremonies and Customs* (Melbourne, 1994)

Tannahill, R., *Sex in History* (London, 1980)

Thiery, M. and H. Houtzager, *Der vrouwen vrouwelijcheit* (Rotterdam, 1997)

Thoben, A. and J.P.C. Moors, *Vaginisme* (Deventer, 1978)

Thomasset, C., 'De vrouwelijke natuur', in *Geschiedenis van de vrouw*, vol. 2, *Middeleeuwen*, ed. G. Duby and M. Perrot (Amsterdam, 1990)

Thompson, L., *The Wandering Womb* (New York, 1999)

Tiemessen, C.H.J., J.H.L. Evers and R.S.G.M. Bots, 'Tight fitting underwear and sperm quality', *The Lancet*, 347 (1996), pp. 1844–5

Tilburg, M. van, *Hoe hoorde het. Seksualiteit en partnerkeuze in de Nederlandse adviesliteratuur 1780–1890* (Amsterdam, 1998)

Tilstra, J., 'Gevorderde abdominale zwangerschap', *Memisa Medisch*, 2 (1997), pp. 30–34

Trost, R.L.A., 'De ontwikkeling van de coïtron, een electronische coïtus-simulator voor de lichamelijk gehandicapte man of vrouw', *Metamedica*, 10 (1972), pp. 263–6

Ungerer, T., *Fornicon* (Utrecht and Antwerp, 1971)

Valins, L., *When a Woman's Body Says No to Sex* (New York, 1992)

Van Voorhis, B. J., A. Dokras and C. H. Syrop, 'Bilateral undescended ovaries: association with infertility and treatment with IVF', *Fertility and Sterility*, 74 (2000), pp. 1041–3

Varendi, H., R. H. Porter and J. Winberg, 'Does the newborn baby find the nipple by smell?', *The Lancet*, 344 (1994), pp. 989–90

Vegter, A., *Ongekuiste versies* (Amsterdam, 1995)

Velde, J. van der, 'The Pelvic Floor. The Mechanism of Vaginismus', thesis, Amsterdam University, 1999

Velde, T. H. van de, *Ideal Marriage*, trans. S. Brown (New York, 1959)

Verhaeghe, P., 'De moderne onbevredigdheid vanuit psychoanalytisch perspectief', *Tijdschrift voor Seksuologie*, 15 (1991), pp. 47–55

Verkuyl, D.A.A., 'Oral conception', *British Journal of Obstetrics and Gynaecology*, 95 (1988), pp. 933–4

Vogels, T. and R. van Vliet, *Jeugd en seks* (The Hague, 1990)

Vroman, L., *Uit slaapwandelen* (Amsterdam, 1957)

Vrouwen en SM (Women and SM, working group of VSSM, the Vereniging Studiegroep Sado Masochisme), *Spelen met macht* (Amsterdam, 1983)

Wack, M. F., 'The measure of pleasure: Peter of Spain on men, women, and lovesickness', *Viator*, 17 (1986), pp. 174–96

Walker, A., *Possessing the Secret of Joy* (London, 1992)

Wassmo, H., *Dina's Book*, trans. Nadia M. Christensen (London, 1996)

Weijmar Schultz, W.C.M. and M. F. van Driel, 'Als het niet past', *Tijdschrift voor Seksuologie*, 19 (1996), pp. 1–7

Wells, J., *The House of Lords* (London, 1997)

Wilbers, D., 'Diagnose in beeld', *Nederlands Tijdschrift voor Geneeskunde*, 145 (2001), pp. 334–5

Wilcox, A. J., C. R. Weinberg and D. D. Baird, 'Timing of sexual intercourse in relation to ovulation', *New England Journal of Medicine*, 333 (1995), pp. 1517–21

Wissen, D. van, *Het mooiste meisje van de klas* (Amsterdam, 1978)

Wittig, M., *Vrouwenguerrilla*, trans. T. Cornips (Amsterdam, 1970)

Witz, C. A., 'Interleukin-6: another piece of the endometriosis-cytokine puzzle', *Fertility and Sterility*, 73 (2000), pp. 212–14

Wolf, N., *Verwarrende tijden. De ontluikende seksualiteit van meisjes in het tijdperk van de pil* (Amsterdam, 1997)

Wolfe, J. L., *Wat te doen als hij hoofdpijn heeft* (Zaltbommel, 1992)

Wurtzel, E., *Bitch. Een lofzang op lastige vrouwen* (Amsterdam, 1998)

Zuria A., 'Purity', videodocumentary, Channel 8, 2002

Acknowledgements

The many people who have assisted me in writing this book and to whom I owe much gratitude include first and foremost my colleagues in the sexological advice team of the Rutgers Foundation: Magda Dijkers, Ank Lammers and Albert Neeleman. All my fellow-workers at the Groningen branch have taken a keen interest in this book, and for that I am extremely grateful to them. Sexologists are a tightly knit family, and hence there were many more colleagues who discussed the various issues with me and may well find their ideas repeated in these pages. In particular, I should like to thank Koos Slob, the editor-in-chief of the *Tijdschrift voor Seksuologie*. Much of what I have written here has previously been published in that journal, and it was Koos who taught me to formulate my ideas and how to deal with criticism. The staff of the library of NISSO (the Netherlands Institute for Socio-Sexological Research) has proved a constant source of expert information, and the same is true of the librarians of the Sophia branch of the Isala Clinics in Zwolle. Mels van Driel introduced me to my Dutch publisher, and has remained an inspiring confidant. Willibrord Weijmar Schultz was a companion on the train with whom I often spent entire journeys exchanging gynaecological ideas, and it was he who introduced me to Dickinson's *Atlas*. Jean Pierre Rawie led me to some obscure poetry and he was always ready to clarify historical subjects and to translate Latin quotations. It is my great pleasure to give him credit for the illustrations in an earlier publication, in which this acknowledgement was omitted. Rosita Steenbeek is probably the only Dutch person who could have introduced me to Tonino Guerra's poem, and she was, moreover, kind enough to translate it for me. Marion Willemsen was a highly critical reader. The members of the Dikkens Society have all, during our animated meetings in Westerwijtwerd, given proof of their various professional knowledge, much of which made me sit up and think. I should like to thank them all, and also the many friends whom I have forgotten to mention and who were never too busy to listen to me. During the revisions made for the third Dutch edition and the present book, the first English-language edition, new advisors came along. Geerd Hayer used his immense library of ancient Middle Eastern texts to find just the right extracts I needed. Matthijs van Boxsel commented on my reproduction of Ms Van de Vorst, and my insecurity concerning the clitoris of monkeys was dealt with by Prof. Van Hooff. Jan Vreeburg gave me insight into the literature on sperm gendering, and Herman Roest on the same literature in the veterinary world.

Finally, of course, my thanks to Lia, who listened to most of the stories and who in exchange for that had to accept my riding roughshod over her own claims to time and attention.

Photographic Acknowledgements

The author and publishers wish to express their thanks to the below sources of illustrative material and/or permission to reproduce it. In some cases locations of artworks are also given below.

©ADAGP, Paris and DACS, London, 2005: 32; from R. L. Dickinson, *Human Sex Anatomy*, (2nd edition, London, 1949): 2, 3, 5, 7, 10, 11, 12, 15, 16, 17, 33; © DACS, 2005: 29; Musée des Beaux-Arts, Dijon: 9; drawing by Chris Drea, from S. B. Hrdy, *Moederschap* (Utrecht, 1999): 4; © erikaroll.com: 21; from Siegfried Giedion, *Mechanization Takes Command* (New York and Oxford, 1948): 25; from Josef Halban, *Gynäkologische Operationslehre* (Berlin and Vienna, 1932): 13, 14; from Guy Hinsdale, *Hydrotherapy* (Philadelphia, 1910): 26; Musée d'Orsay, Paris: 1; drawing © *Nederlands Tijdschrift voor Geneeskunde*: 19; Netherlands Architectural Institute, Rotterdam, Wijdeveld archive: 35 (inv. no. a. 8); from Ambroise Paré, *L'opera ostretico-ginecologica di Ambrogio Paré*, ed. Vittorio Pedore (Bologna, 1966): 34; after A. K. Slob, C. W. Vink, J.P.C. Moors and W. Everaerd, from *Seksuologie voor de arts* (Houten and Diegem, 1998): 6; © Succession Picasso/DACS 2005; from *Tijdschrift voor seksuologie*, vol. 22–23 (1998): 27; from Tomi Ungerer, *Fornicon* (Antwerp and Utrecht, 1971), copyright © 1971, 1980 Diogenes Verlag AG Zurich: 28; after C. van Emde Boas, 1941 in *Nederlands Tijdschrift voor Geneeskunde*, 85, 1941; illustration by J. P. Rawie: 23; after T. Vogels and R. van Vliet, *Jeugd en seks* (The Hague, 1990): 8; x-ray photograph supplied by D. Wilbers, gynaecologist, Medical Centre, Leeuwarden: 18.